HERPES VIRUSES AND VIRUS CHEMOTHERAPY
Pharmacological and Clinical Approaches

HERPES VIRUSES AND VIRUS CHEMOTHERAPY

Pharmacological and Clinical Approaches

Proceedings of the International Symposium on Pharmacological and Clinical Approaches to Herpes Viruses and Virus Chemotherapy, Oiso, Japan, 10-13 September 1984

Editors:

Dr. R. Kono †
Honorary Member of the National Institute of Health of Japan
Professor of Virology Saitama Medical School, Saitama, Japan

Dr. A. Nakajima
Department of Ophthalmology, Juntendo University
School of Medicine, Tokyo, Japan

1985

Excerpta Medica, Amsterdam – New York – Oxford

International Congress Series No. 667
ISBN 0 444 80680 6

Published by:
Elsevier Science Publishers B.V. (Biomedical Division)
P.O. Box 211
1000 AE Amsterdam
The Netherlands

Sole distributors for the USA and Canada:
Elsevier Science Publishing Company Inc.
52 Vanderbilt Avenue
New York, NY 10017
USA

Library of Congress Cataloging in Publication Data

International Symposium on Pharmacological and Clinical
Approaches to Herpes Viruses and Virus Chemotherapy
(1984 : Oiso-machi, Japan)
Herpes viruses and Virus chemotherapy.
(International congress series ; no. 667)
Includes indexes.
1. Herpesvirus diseases--Chemotherapy--Congresses.
2. Herpesviruses--Congresses. 3. Virus diseases--
Chemotherapy--Congresses. 4. Antiviral agents--
Congresses. I. Kono, Reisaku. II. Title. III. Series.
[DNLM: 1. Antiviral Agents--therapeutic use--congresses.
2. Herpesvirus Infections--drug therapy--congresses.
W3 EX89 no.667 / WC 571 I615h 1984]
RC147.H6I59 1984 616.9′25061 85-6800
ISBN 0-444-80680-6 (U.S.)

Printed in The Netherlands

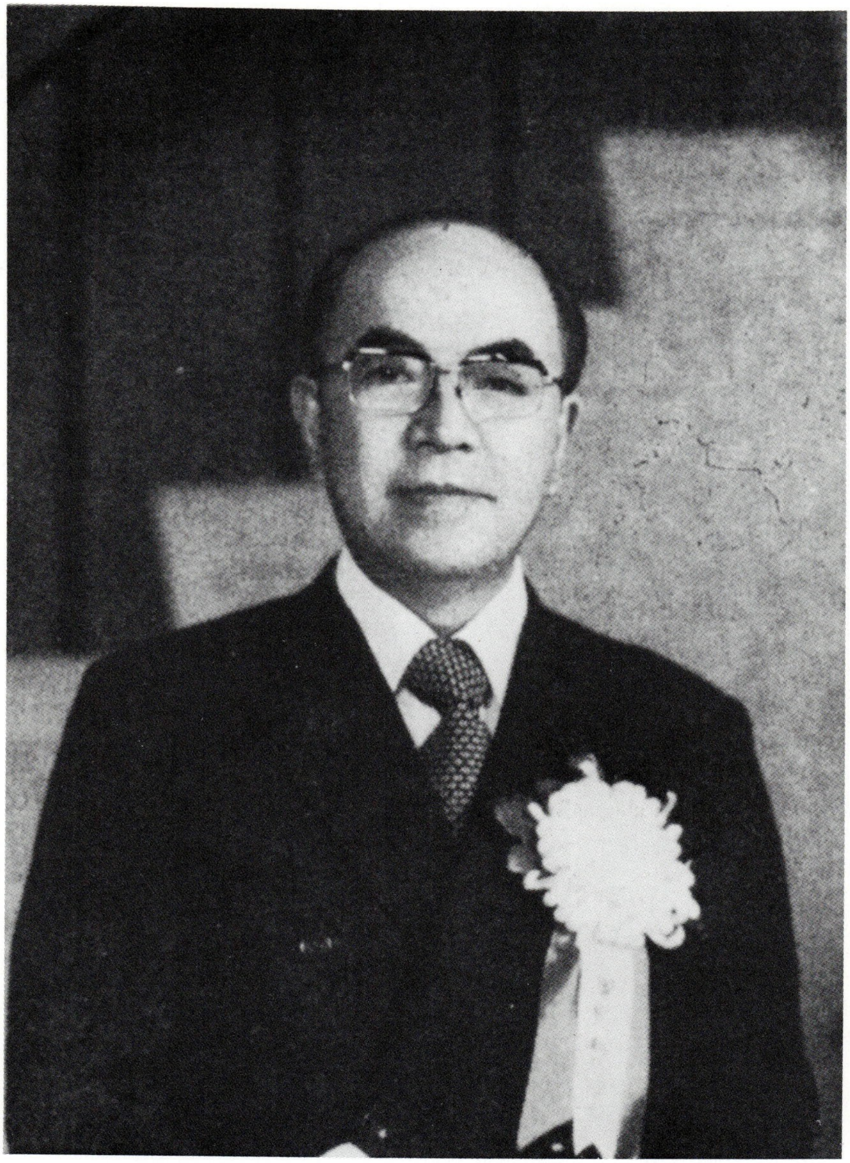

Reisaku Kono †
1915-1985

Obituary

Reisaku Kono, M.D., the president of the Symposium on Pharmacological and Clinical Approaches to Herpes Viruses and Virus Chemotherapy, held on 10-13, September, 1984 at Oiso Prince Hotel, passed away on 23rd January, 1985. We express our deepest sorrow and grievance at his sudden demise, and express our deep sympathy for the bereaved family.

He was born on 4th October, 1915, the eldest son of an ophthalmologist who was the founding president of the Tokyo Ophthalmologists Association. He belonged to the biggest family of scholars in Japan, originating from Gensaku Mitsukuri. He graduated from the University of Tokyo in 1940, and became a virologist. He served as professor at the Virus Institute of Kyoto University, and Chief of Virus Department, National Institute of Health, Japanese Government. He discovered EV70, the causative agent for acute hemorrhagic conjunctivitis. He was the chairman of the committee on SMON (subacute myelo-optico-neuritis) and led the research which established the etiology of the condition to be chinoform and not a virus. He contributed much to the succes of the symposium on Herpes Chemotherapy held in September 1984, in Oiso. He raised funds, visited the USA several times to discuss the programme, set the programme and speakers, and edited various printed matter related to the meeting. He was very good in painting, and the Japanese paintings in the prelims of the programme or the book of abstracts were selected by him. Just before the meeting, his illness was discovered by chance. He underwent surgery a week after the meeting. We were fortunate that he could join us at the meeting. The course of surgery was uneventful, and he was planning to edit a book on acute hemorrhagic conjunctivitis. Malicious cancer cells hidden in his brain killed him suddenly. We sincerely hope that his work will be continued by us and our colleagues for the benefit of mankind.

Akira Nakajima, M.D.
Professor of the Department of Ophthalmology
Juntendo University School of Medicine
Tokyo, Japan

Obituary

We are deeply saddened by the passing of one of the great leaders and teachers-Reisaku Kono. Dr. Kono was honored with the Hideyo Noguchi Memorial Award for Medicine in 1978 for his contribution to the establishment of the causative agent of acute hemorrhagic conjunctivitis. The project of investigating this ocular disease gave me the lucky chance to join his research group. Those who knew Dr. Kono will vividly remember him as a distinguished leader with inspiring ability, sense of organization, and natural kindness to young physicians and investigators. I was able to spend much time with him during our expeditions in West Africa for seroepidemiological study of acute hemorrhagic conjunctivitis, and I can say that he had a profound influence on me because of his outstanding intellect and personal charm. He will be greatly missed not only by his colleagues but also by ophthalmic microbiologists, because he was a virologist who had much interest in ocular infection.

Yukio Uchida, M.D.
Professor of the Department of Ophthalmology
Tokyo Women's Medical College
Tokyo, Japan

Obituary

It was a hot summer afternoon, about a month before this symposium on virus chemotherapy was to be held. Dr. Kono, professor at Saitama Medical College arrived unexpectedly at my office. He looked pale, somewhat uneasy . . . even irritated. It was unusual because he had always been gentle and calm. 'I'm in trouble,' he said quietly, after sitting for a moment's rest on the sofa. 'It seems that I have lung cancer. My luck may finally be running out.' It was so sudden. I was shocked. I could not believe what I had heard, and I could not find anything to say. He briefly explained the results of a physical check-up he had had at the National Cancer Center and told me he would probably have to undergo surgery before or during the symposium to be held in Oiso. 'I think you are rather lucky. From what you say, the lesion must still be fairly small and in the early stage.' These were my words of consolation . . . all I could manage at the moment. 'You know you've always enjoyed good fortune. Didn't you tell me that during World War II, you were luckily saved from a sinking warship when it was bombed?' 'Certainly I have been very lucky, but no more.' He smiled weakly.

In fact, he was not able to have the surgery before the symposium. So, he did his best to carry out his duties, giving the opening address, attending the welcome party, chairing his session and closing the conference. The symposium was successful, as can be seen in this book. To our great regret, however, it will never be read by Dr. Kono, who was one of the most enthusiastic organizers of the symposium. A week after the meeting, he underwent surgery. it seemed successful, but, unfortunately, the cancer had metastasized to other organs including the liver and the brain. About four months later, on January 23rd, 1985, he passed away.

Dr. Kono's sudden death was a great shock to me. He had served as director of the Central Virus Diagnostic Laboratory, National Institute of Health, for nearly ten years, from 1972 to 1981, when I succeeded him. We shared many things, both in our professional and in our private lives. In particular, we worked closely together in virological and epidemiological study of acute hemorrhagic conjunctivitis (AHC) and basic studies for clinical application of interferons. I respected him very much and loved his generous and noble character.

As the discoverer of AHC virus, he naturally had a strong interest in the origin of the virus and epidemiological research. In November, 1977, he organized a scientific research group to carry out an epidemiological investigation of this virus in West Africa, where the first outbreak of AHC occurred in 1969. I participated in the planning for this and spent over 50 days in West Africa on this scientific mission. AHC virus (enterovirus type 70) is naturally temperature-sensitive: it tends to grow at the relatively low temperature of around 33 °C, and it shows a particular tropism to the eyes, where the virus replicates to cause hemorrhagic conjunctivitis. Taking note of these characteristics, which are not shared by other human enteroviruses, Dr. Kono hypothesized that the fly had served as a vector to transmit the virus from eyes to eyes in the first large outbreak of the disease in West Africa. He further speculated that the virus might have been derived either from an animal picornavirus which had mutated to become pathogenic to humans and was transmitted to human eyes by flies, or from an insect picornavirus replicating in flies. Although his hypothesis has not been proved yet – all our attempts to isolate AHC virus from African flies or cattle and to grow the virus in insect cell cultures have so far failed – his adventurous idea stimulated the imaginations of many scientists. One memory of him in Africa remains strongly with me. We were travelling on the Savanna at its hottest. Succumbing to the heat, I sat beneath a baobab tree and dozed off. When I awoke, I saw Dr. Kono out in the harsh sunlight, leisurely sketching women and children drawing water at a well. He was very fond of art, and after he retired from National Institute of Health he most enjoyed painting.

Dr. Kono was an excellent epidemiologist as well as one of the pioneers of clinical virology in Japan. He contributed greatly to the creation and development of a nationwide surveillance system for infectious diseases. He was a hard worker, and, with his profound knowledge and abundant experience, he had a great influence on many young virologists in this country.

During the last several years of his life he devoted himself with great enthusiasm to the progress of clinical study of interferon as General Chairman of the Interferon Scientific Committee (organized by the Ministry of Health and Welfare). In the future, probably within this year, a human natural fibroblast beta interferon is going to be approved as a first new biological drug in Japan. It is my great regret that he cannot see the fruits of his efforts, since I know that he was one of the few who was convinced of the benefits of appropriate use of interferon for the treatment of certain kinds of viral and malignant diseases.

In closing, I would like to say that I think we are all very grateful to Dr. Kono for the idea of bringing us together at the beautiful site of Oiso. I believe the scenic natural surroundings pleased all the participants and made the symposium especially memorable. I also wish to salute Mrs. Kono for her selfless devotion and personal courage in helping her husband to carry out his duties at the conference. I am sure that all participants will readily agree to join me in dedicating this book to the memory of the man who gave so much of himself for the sake of this symposium.

Shudo Yamazaki, M.D.
Director, Central Virus Diagnostic Laboratories
National Institute of Health
Tokyo, Japan

DEDICATION

Dr. Reisaku Kono

1915–1985

Dr. Kono, a giant in the field of virology and a world leader in virological research, has recently died and all of us mourn this great loss. Dr. Kono was born in Tokyo in 1915 and was graduated from Tokyo University in 1940. He worked at the Institute for Infectious Diseases, University of Tokyo and also for the Department of Virology of the National Institutes of Health in Japan, obtaining his Ph.D. in 1950. From 1952 to 1953, he studied in the United States at Johns Hopkins University, Yale University, and Harvard University as a Fellow of the Rockefeller Foundation, obtaining his Master's degree in Public Health from Johns Hopkins University in 1953. In 1958, Dr. Kono became Professor of the Department of Virology at Kyoto University, and Head of its Institute of Virology. He later became Head of the Department of Virology of the National Institutes of Health in Japan, and in 1969, became Chairman of the 18th Annual Meeting of the Society of Virology in Japan, and head of the investigation of subacute myelo-optico-neuropathy, sponsored by the National Institutes of Health. From 1971 to 1981, Dr. Kono was a member of the Japan-United States Cooperative Medical Sciences Program Panel on Viral Disease. In 1980, he was president of the World Symposium on Interferon at Oiso, and in 1984 was president of the International Symposium on Pharmacological and Clinical Approaches to Herpes Viruses and Virus Chemotherapy.

Dr. Kono did landmark research and made major contributions in the area of influenza virus and mumps virus. He developed a polio vaccine used in Japan, and found the causes of acute hemorrhagic conjunctivitis and subacute myelo-optico-neuropathy, as well as doing important work on Coxsackie virus.

Dr. Kono was respected for his brilliance and his creative work in virology. He was loved for his ability to organize, to stimulate students, to be fair and constructive, and to help the world wide advance of man's fight against viral disease. We will all sadly miss him, and we dedicate this work in his honor.

George J. Galasso
Department of Health and Human Services
Public Health Service
National Institute of Health
Bethesda, Maryland
USA

Herbert E. Kaufman
Department of Ophthalmology, LSU Eye Center
Louisiana State University Medical Center
New Orleans, Louisiana
USA

DEDICATION

Dr. Reisaku Kono

It is with great sadness that we learned of the death of Dr. Kono. We did not know him personally prior to our meeting at the International Symposium on Pharmacological and Clinical Approaches to Herpes Viruses and Virus Chemotherapy in Oiso, Japan. However we felt on the basis of our correspondence, which concerned the many problems that evolve normally when such a meeting is being formulated, that he was a very kind, considerate, gentle understanding individual. Thus it was no surprise when we met him that our feelings about him were so correct. He did indeed possess all these wonderful characteristics which we had surmised from his letters to us.

His contributions to science have been of major importance and achieved for him international recognition not only as an outstanding investigator, but also as an exceptional patron of virology. He brought together virologists from all parts of the world and he represented Japanese virology at international meetings with dignity and dedication.

Thus we have lost not only a distinguished scientist, but equally as important a magnificant human being. He will be missed by all who knew him, and we feel very fortunate to have had the opportunity and honor to have known Dr. Kono, even though it was for such a brief period of time. To honor his memory these Proceedings are dedicated to him with great affection and admiration.

William Prusoff
Department of Pharmacology
Yale University School of Medicine
Sterling Hall of Medicine
New Haven, Connecticut, U.S.A.

Yung-Chi Cheng
Department of Pharmacology and Medicine
University of North Carolina
Chapel Hill, North Carolina, U.S.A.

CONTENTS

B. Cutaneous

C. Genital

D. Systemic

IV HERPESVIRUS ASSOCIATED WITH CANCER

VIII ANTIVIRAL AGENTS AGAINST OTHER VIRUS INFECTIONS

IX CURRENT STATUS AND FUTURE PROSPECTS

I BIOLOGY AND RATIONAL DEVELOPMENT OF CHEMOTHERAPEUTIC AGENTS OF HERPESVIRUSES

Herpes Viruses and Virus Chemotherapy, R. Kono, editor

PATHOGENICITY OF RECURRENT AND NON-RECURRENT HERPES SIMPLEX VIRUS STRAINS

YSOLINA M. CENTIFANTO-FITZGERALD

Department of Ophthalmology, LSU Eye Center, Louisiana State University Medical Center School of Medicine, New Orleans, Louisiana 70112, USA

The establishment of latency in the trigeminal ganglia after primary infection with herpes simplex virus (HSV) has been extensively documented.[1-3] Our understanding at the moment is that the virus in residence in the neurons is reactivated from time to time by as yet unknown mechanisms; the virus replicates in the ganglia, travels to the peripheral site, and either causes a lesion or is shed asymptomatically.[4] In humans, virus shedding is seen to occur in the absence of disease, and the frequency of recurrent disease varies.

From the results of controlled animal experiments, it is known that the frequency of shedding and/or recurrent disease varies consistently from one strain to another[5]; furthermore, frequency also varies among animals infected with a common parent stock. These observations suggest that differences in the pattern of recurrences may be regulated by the nature of the virus in residence in the ganglionic tissue, specifically in a particular neuron, as reactivation may be a single event.

In our study of HSV strain differences and ocular disease, we observed different recurrent disease phenotypes: some strains with high frequency of recurrences and shedding, some with low frequency, and some in which neither recurrence nor shedding was apparent. To compare the biological characteristics of the three phenotypes, we selected prototype strains from our library of wild-type HSV strains. We chose the McKrae strain (high frequency of recurrences), the E-43 strain (low frequency of recurrences), and the CGA-3 strain (no recurrences), and examined severity of ocular disease, mortality, recurrence rate, and optimum growth temperature for each strain.

In rabbits, the McKrae strain produces severe epithelial disease that sometimes persists for more than 10 days, but generally clears by day 14. Mortality is about 40-60%. The frequency of recurrent disease is high; in one experiment, 10 of 13 animals had recurrent disease (77%), and in another experiment, 28 of 30 (93%) had recurrences. E-43 strain produces mild dendritic keratitis that usually resolves by day 7, leaving a clear, unscarred cornea. Mortality is low; usually 2 of 25 (12%) animals, in our experience. Clinical recurrences are less frequent, occurring in about 30 to 40% of the animals. CGA-3 strain produces

TABLE: SPONTANEOUS AND INDUCED HSV SHEDDING

Strain	Spontaneous shedding (% eyes)	Iontophoresis (% eyes)	Ganglionic HSV after induction	
			Trigeminal	Superior cervical
McKrae	92	100	100%	100%
E-43	16.7	57.1	100%	78.6%
CGA-3	0	0	25%	0

mild but significant disease. Mortality is nil. Neither recurrence nor virus shedding is seen.

When the same inoculum of each prototype strain was grown at the external temperature of 33°C and at the host core temperature of 39°C, differences were seen. In the McKrae cultures, more plaques developed at 33°C than at 39°C. In the CGA-3 cultures, the virus grew poorly, if at all, at 39°C. E-43 cultures showed results intermediate between those of McKrae and CGA-3.

We looked at virus growth at these two particular temperatures because it seemed that the ability to grow at the external temperature of 33°C might contribute to the development of lesions, but the ability to grow at 39°C would be critical for the reactivation and multiplication process at the ganglionic site; reactivation is essential for the ganglionic virus to migrate to the peripheral site where disease is manifested. It may be that the tendency of CGA-3 to grow poorly at 39°C is related to the non-recurrent phenotype of this strain.

One question is whether these strains grow in the ocular tissue in sufficient amounts to colonize the ganglia, and a second question is whether the strains establish latency. To answer the first question we compared the amounts of infectious virus present in McKrae-infected and CGA-3-infected rabbit corneas. We found that although there were slight differences, the frequently-recurrent McKrae strain and the non-recurrent CGA-3 strain grew equally well in the corneal tissue, with comparable potential to colonize the ganglia.

To determine if the strains establish latency, we quantitated and documented spontaneous shedding and percent colonization of the ganglia in New Zealand white rabbits infected with each of the prototype strains (Table). We found spontaneous shedding in 92% of the McKrae-infected animals; 16.7% of the E-43-infected animals, and, as expected, none of the CGA-3-infected animals. After iontophoretic induction with 6-hydroxydopamine,[6] infectious virus was recovered from 100% of the trigeminal ganglia of E-43- and McKrae-infected animals, but only 25% of the CGA-3-infected animals.

This low rate of recovery for the CGA-3 strain was difficult to reconcile with our findings of sufficient infectious virus in the ocular tissue for successful ganglionic colonization. For this reason, we explored CGA-3 virus recovery from the ganglia in relation to temperature. In the previous study, the percent virus recovery at core body temperature (39°C) was low. However, when six trigeminal ganglia of latently infected animals were explanted and incubated at 33°C for three days, virus was recovered from 100% of the explants.

Our hypothesis is that phenotypic differences, including frequency of recurrence, are attributable to the genetic characteristics of the latent virus; it has already been shown that other characteristics of ocular disease, such as morphology of the lesions, are genetically determined.[7] The ability to grow at the host core temperature of 39°C is important in the reactivation process at the ganglionic site. Assuming that all animals are subject to the same stimuli during latency, the virus will replicate in the neuronal cell, travel to the peripheral site, and cause a lesion or be shed asymptomatically. For virus replication in the ganglia, the ability to grow at 39°C is critical. The CGA-3 strain grows poorly at 39°C and better at 33°C, as evidenced by the fact that 100% of the explanted ganglia incubated at 33°C yielded infectious virus. Hence the inability of the CGA-3 strain to be reactivated in the host animal may be a function of genetically controlled optimum growth temperature. Also, virus shedding in the tear film may be related to the colonization of the superior cervical ganglia. The CGA-3 strain does not colonize the superior cervical ganglia and is not shed in the tear film after iontophoresis with 6-hydroxydopamine.

Recurrent diseases may be caused preferentially in the eye by virus strains that prefer the lower, external temperatures. If the reactivated virus prefers to grow at the higher core temperature, reactivation may take place in a neuronal cell in the ganglion and asymptomatic shedding may occur, but recurrent disease is not established.

That temperature optimum may be important in the mechanisms of recurrent disease is also supported by findings that fresh HSV isolates from patients with confirmed HSV encephalitis and herpes labialis demonstrate preferential growth at 37°C to 39°C. Also, it may be that recurrences triggered by fever or thermal injuries, such as sunburn, or preferential localization on the warmest areas of the body, such as the mucocutaneous junctions (lip), are caused by virus strains that grow better at higher temperatures.

The mechanism of recurrent herpetic disease is a complex one and is governed by many factors, not all of which are understood, including the nature of the reactivation stimuli and their effect on trigeminal or superior cervical ganglia, the genetic make-up of the reactivated virus, and host immune factors that may modify the development of lesions or asymptomatic shedding. In this paper we have demonstrated the existence of different recurrent phenotypes and a possible role for temperature optimum in the recurrence phenomena. Optimum growth temperature is by no means the only factor, but it appears to be at least one determinant in the character of recurrent herpetic keratitis.

ACKNOWLEDGEMENTS

This work was supported in part by PHS grants EY02389 and EY02377 from the National Eye Institute, National Institutes of Health, Bethesda, Maryland.

REFERENCES

1. Kaufman HE, Brown DC, Ellison EM (1967) Science 156:1628.
2. Nesburn AB, Elliott JM, Leibowitz HM (1967) Arch Ophthalmol 78:523-529.
3. Laibson PR, Kibrick S (1969) Invest Ophthalmol 8:346-350.
4. Blyth WA, Hill TJ (1983) In: Rouse BT, Lopez C (eds) Immunology of Herpes Simplex Virus Infection. CRC Press, Boca Raton, Florida, pp. 9-32.
5. Gerdes JC, Smith DS (1983) J Gen Virol 64:2441-2454.
6. Shimomura Y, Gangarosa LP, Kataoka M, Hill JM (1983) HSV-1 shedding by iontophoresis of 6-hydroxydopamine followed by topical epinephrine. Invest Ophthalmol Vis Sci 24:1588-1594.
7. Centifanto-Fitzgerald YM, Yamaguchi T, Kaufman HE, Tognon M, Roizman B (1982) J Exp Med 155:475-489.

BRIEF REVIEW, HERPESVIRUS LATENCY*

JACK G. STEVENS

Department of Microbiology and Immunology and Reed Neurological Research Center
UCLA School of Medicine, Los Angeles, California 90024

INTRODUCTION

The herpesviruses have a complex natural history with the latent state playing a central role. There is a general agreement that in this state viral genetic information is maintained in a "reactivable" form, but infectious virus is not present. While this type of relationship has been definitively proved to exist only in the Epstein-Barr system, all available evidence indicates that it obtains for the other herpesviruses also. The data for Herpes simplex virus have been reviewed elsewhere (1), and rest principally on 1) the appearance of histochemically detectable viral DNA and the virus itself in genome harboring neurons only after explantation and culture of appropriate tissues ("induction") and 2) the capacity of temperature sensitive viral mutants to establish and be maintained in a reactivable state in nervous tissues for extended periods of time.

As is evident from various discussions throughout this meeting, a fundamental, mechanistic description of the latent state is vitally important to have in hand. Aside from obvious intrinsic interest, this description is necessary for practical reasons. More specifically, currently available antiviral substances do not eliminate latent infections, and it is not unlikely that success in this area will come only when a compound can be "tailored" to a biochemical event specifically identified with the latent state.

THE PROBLEMS

The classic problems related to definition of herpetic latency can be outlined as in Table 1. With respect to Herpes simplex virus, in vivo studies are hampered by the fact that only about 1/100 of the cells in the tissue of interest (spinal ganglia for example) harbor latent infections. This limits experimental approaches for study principally to histochemical methods, and information which can be derived from such studies is not extensive. At this time, in vitro studies are hampered because 1) in vitro cultivation of latently infected cells has historically been used as the method to induce virus (a method must therefore be found to reverse this phenomenon), and 2) the general state of the art with

*Because of page limitations, this review will be limited to selected aspects of latency, with Herpes simplex and Epstein-Barr Viruses serving as the models.

respect to culturing nervous tissues is apparently not adequate to preserve the intimate relationships which exist between neurons and supporting cells. With respect to the Epstein-Barr Virus system, an historical problem has been the lack of a lytic system in which significant amounts of virus can be replicated. However, molecular cloning techniques have blunted this problem for studies in which large amounts of viral DNA are needed.

PRESENT KNOWLEDGE OF THE LATENT STATE

For purposes of discussion of the latent state, it is useful to make divisions into events associated with 1) establishment 2) maintenance, and 3) reactivation of the latent virus. With respect to establishment, in herpes simplex virus infections, nearly all available evidence indicate that the latent virus is harbored in neurons (1,4). If it is agreed that this is the case, then two mutually exclusive events follow neuronal infection, and the basis for the "decision" to take one or the other routes is not known. Thus, some neurons undergo lytic infection and produce virus; others do not succumb, but harbor the agent in a latent state. A similar decision seems likely following infection of B lymphocytes with the Epstein-Barr Virus, but this has not been studied.

To establish the latent infection, the viral DNA must first be put into configuration which is compatible with long-term persistence. In mice infected with HSV, Fraser and co-workers (2) have studied this aspect, have ruled out a linear unit length molecule of viral DNA, and have also indicated that there are non-integrated sequences present (3). In an in vitro rat neuronal system modulated by viral inhibitors on the other hand, Wigdahl, et al. (4) found linear non-integrated unit length DNA. A resolution of this basic difference in genomic structure is likely to come when more easily applied technology for in vivo systems is developed. In this regard, it seems important to first establish the physical state in an animal; in vitro systems will always suffer the criticism of relevance if they are used for initial descriptions.

The situation is far more clear in the Epstein-Barr Virus system, since it has been known for over a decade that most EBV genomes exist in B lymphocytes as monomeric plasmids (reviewed in 1). The long standing controversy concerning possible integration of some genetic information has been definitively resolved for at least 2 cell lines. Thus, Kieff and co-workers have found viral-cellular DNA junction fragments (proof for integration) and have also shown that the entire viral genome is present in this integrated state (5). The biologic significance of this finding is not clear and it may well be that these integrated sequences are important for maintenance of the latent state.

With respect to the expression of the viral genome during establishment and maintenance of latency, there is evidence that the immediate early gene ICP 4 and at least one additional gene is involved in establishment and/or maintenance of latency (6), and in situ hybridization experiments indicate that transcripts from the left-hand 30% of the genome are present (7). As is the case with respect to physical state of the genome, there is considerably more known about the Epstein-Barr Virus. Here, there are 9 nuclear transcripts, 3 polyadenylated cytoplasmic messages, and at least 3 translation products in latently infected B lymphocytes (reviewed in 8). The EBNA proteins comprise two of the translation products and a membrane associated protein likely to be LYDMA is the other (9). In addition, the genes encoding all these products have been mapped (8).

With respect to reactivation, there is one study (in the Epstein-Barr Virus system) where a reactivation "gene" has been identified. Here, Miller's group has found a rare HR-1 virus transformed cell in which viral DNA with significant rearrangements and duplication of certain segments has been found. These viruses are defective, induce latently infected cells to produce proteins in addition to the 3 mentioned above, and in certain cell lines, complete virus in replicated (10). How this agent functions is not clear, but a protein product encoded by the defective DNA which serves as an inducer is not an unlikely possibility.

CONCLUSIONS

From this very brief summary, it should be clear that much remains to be learned about herpetic latency, particularly that established by herpes simplex virus. Although exploitable in vitro systems have permitted the interaction to be made more clear with respect to Epstein-Barr Virus, even here more must be accomplished before basic mechanisms associated with the latent state are clearly defined.

TABLE I

CLASSIC DIFFICULTIES, HERPETIC LATENCY STUDIES

1. HSV
    - A. In vivo - approaches limited
    - B. In vitro - "physiologic" conditions for neurons difficult to achieve
2. EBV - No Lytic System

ACKNOWLEDGEMENTS

Research from my own laboratories which is discussed here was supported by grants from the National Institutes of Health (AI-06246), the National Multiple Sclerosis Society (RG 1647-A-1), and the March of Dimes Birth Defects Foundation.

REFERENCES

1. Stevens JG (1977) Adv Cancer Res 26:227
2. Rock DL, Fraser NW (1983) Nature 302:523
3. Fraser NW, Muggeridge MI, Mellerick DM, Rock DL (1984) In: Herpesvirus Rapp F (ed) Allan R. Liss, New York 21:159
4. Wigdahl B, Scheile AC, Zigler RJ, DeClercq E, Rapp F (1984) J Virol 49:205R
5. Matsuo T, Heller M, Petti L, Oshiro E, Kieff E Science In Press
6. Watson K, Stevens JG, Cook ML, Subak-Sharpe JH (1980) J Gen Virol 49:149
7. Galloway DA, Fenoglio CM, McDougall JK (1982) J Virol 41:686
8. Kieff E, Kennessy K, Matsuo P, Dambaagh T, Heller M, Hummel M In: Burkitt's Lymphoma: A Human Cancer Model. Internat'l Agency for Res on Cancer. In Press
9. Hennessy K, Fennewald S, Hummel M, Cole T, Kieff E Proc. Nat'l Acad Sci U S In Press
10. Miller G, Rabson M, Heston C (1984) J Virol 50:174

ANIMAL MODELS OF HERPESVIRUS INFECTIONS

EARL R. KERN, PH.D.
Department of Pediatrics, Division of Infectious Diseases,
University of Utah School of Medicine, Salt Lake City, Utah 84132

The importance of experimental viral infections in the development and testing of antiviral agents is well documented. Our understanding of the pathogenesis of herpesvirus infections and the interaction between the viral infection, the response of the host and a therapeutic agent has been enhanced greatly though the use of animal model systems. When selecting or developing an animal model system for determining the efficacy of an antiviral one should utilize systems that best simulate the corresponding human disease. The properties of an ideal animal model are shown in Table 1.

Table 1. Properties of an Ideal Animal Model

Use natural route of infection and inoculum size, where possible.
Use human virus with minimal alteration by adaptation.
The natural history and pathogenesis of infection are similar to that in humans.
The host's immune response is similar to that seen in humans.
The endpoints used for evaluation of efficacy are similar to human.
The metabolism and toxicity of the drug are similar to humans.

In order to obtain the best information regarding the predictability of an animal model system for efficacy of a potential new compound, a number of guidelines should be considered. These are listed in Table 2.

Table 2. Guidelines for Animal Model Testing

Drug should be evaluated in more than one animal species.
The route, dose and time of drug administration must be varied.
Virus inoculum and route of infection should be varied.
Human infection should be closely simulated.
Sensitivity of virus to drug should be known in same species.
Drug metabolism and toxicity should be known.
Pathogenesis of virus infection and effect of drug should be defined.
Effect of drug on immune system should be determined.
Results from animal models should be compared with data from human trials.

Since the herpesviruses and particularly herpes simplex virus are the etiologic agents of a wide variety of diseases in man, it is important that new antiviral agents be tested in animal models that simulate each of the disease states in humans. A summary of the most often used animal model systems for Herpesvirus infections are shown in Table 3.

Table 3. Animal Models of Herpesvirus Infections

Human Disease	Animal Species	Virus	Inoculation Route
Herpes encephalitis	Mouse	HSV-1	i.c., i.n.
Disseminated neonatal herpes	Mouse	HSV-2	i.n.
Cutaneous infections	Mouse	HSV-1	Orofacial, i.d.
	Guinea pig	HSV-1	dorsal, i.d.
Genital HSV infections			
Primary	Mouse, Guinea Pig	HSV-2, HSV-1	I.vg.
Recurrent	Guinea Pig	HSV-2	I.vg.
Ocular herpes	Rabbit	HSV-1	Intraocular
Cytomegalovirus infections			
Acute, chronic	Mouse	MCMV	i.p.
	Guinea Pig	GPCMV	i.p., s.c.
Primary varicella infection	Guinea Pig	VZV	i.n.
Varicella Zoster	Monkey	Simian Varicella	i.t., i.v.

The following experimental viral infections utilized in our laboratory are used as examples of how animal model infections can be utilized to determine efficacy of antiviral agents. The first experimental system is a model of disseminated neonatal herpes that utilizes intranasal inoculation of mice with HSV-2. After inoculation, virus replication is initially detectable in lung with subsequent dissemination of virus through the blood to visceral organs. Virus is also transmitted by neural routes from the nasopharynx to olfactory lobe, cerebrum, and cerebellum- brain stem. We have reported previously that Acyclovir delivered in drinking water was effective in protecting mice even when therapy did not begin until 96 hours after HSV-2 inoculation. Complete protection was observed in the animals receiving treatment beginning 24 to 48 hours after infection. Similar results were obtained with i.p. treatment. To define the mechanism of successful ACV therapy in this model infection, the titers of HSV-2 in tissues of both untreated and ACV-treated mice were determined. In untreated control mice, virus was first detected in the lung on day 1 with subsequent spread to the spleen and kidney by day 6. During this period of time, virus also spread from the nasopharynx to the pons by day 3 and the olfactory lobe and cerebrum by day 5. In mice that received ACV in their drinking water beginning

1 day after infection, there was complete inhibition of HSV replication in the kidney, spleen, olfactory lobe, and cerebrum and in the lung after day 4. There was a 2-3 log decrease in titers of virus in the pons after day 4. Similar results were obtained in animals treated i.p. with ACV beginning 1 day after viral challenge.

A number of animal species including mice, hamsters, guinea pigs, rabbits, monkeys and non-human primates have been utilized as model infections for genital herpes. Since genital HSV-2 infection in the guinea pig results in the development of primary external lesions similar to those seen in humans and has spontaneous recurrent lesions, the guinea pig is the model that most clearly simulates the disease in humans. After intravaginal inoculation with 5 x 10^4 pfu of HSV-2, initial replication takes place in the vaginal tract with peak virus titers of 10^5 pfu occurring 24 hours after infection. Titers gradually decline until day 10 when most animals have cleared the virus from the vaginal tract. The clinical course of the disease is characterized initially by the appearance of lesions on the external genital skin. These lesions first appear on day 4, peak in severity on days 6-9 and heal completely by days 15-18. After resolution of the primary disease animals begin to exhibit spontaneous recurrent erythematous or vesicular lesions on the external genital skin at the same sites as the primary lesions. The recurrent lesions are small, 1-3 mm, and last only 1-3 days. All infected animals exhibit recurrences and average about one recurrent episode per week.

Since human IFN-αA has about as good activity in guinea pig cells as human cells in tissue culture and is currently being tested in clinical trials of genital herpes, we initiated a series of experiments to determine the activity of this interferon in the guinea pig model. To determine the activity during primary infection, groups of animals were infected and treated i.m. three times daily for seven days with 2 x 10^6 or 1 x 10^7 u/kg of IFN-αA beginning -2, +24, or +72 hours relative to viral inoculation. The external genital lesions were scored daily and the effect of treatment on mean lesion scores was determined. When treatment was begun 2 hours prior to infection, no vesicular lesions developed in any of the animals treated with either concentration. Similar results were obtained when treatment was initiated 24 hours after infection. When therapy was delayed until 72 hours, all animals developed lesions, however, they did not increase in number or severity after day 5 and healed more rapidly than those in the placebo or control groups. Treatment initiated at all three times with either drug concentration also reduced significantly the titers of virus in vaginal secretions and in external lesions.

In a second experiment to determine the effect of IFN-αA treatment on recurrent disease, groups of guinea pigs were infected and left untreated during the primary infection. The animals were then scored daily for three weeks to establish a baseline frequency of recurrent episodes. On day 41, treatment i.m. with placebo, 2×10^6 or 1×10^7 u/kg of IFN-αA was begun and continued three times daily for three weeks. After treatment was stopped the animals were scored for recurrent lesions for three additional weeks. The baseline frequency of recurrent episodes for the groups prior to treatment was 4.0, 4.1 and 3.4. During the three weeks of treatment, the animals receiving IFN-αA had only 1.2 and 1.8 episodes compared to 3.3 in placebo-treated animals. These were both significantly different. After treatment was terminated, however, the frequency of recurrences returned to that of placebo-treated animals.

Due to the strict species specificity of human cytomegalovirus (HCMV), it has not been possible to test potential antiviral agents for activity against HCMV in animals. Inoculation of mice with murine cytomegalovirus (MCMV) provides a model infection that shares many characteristics with the human disease. To determine the effect of treatment on mortality due to MCMV, groups of 15 mice were inoculated i.p. and oral treatment with 50 mg of 9-(1,3-dihydroxy-2-propoxy methyl guanine (DHPG) per kg was begun 6, 24, or 48 h after viral inoculation. There was a significant reduction in mortality when therapy was begun as late as 48h after MCMV infection. Since treatment with DHPG effectively reduced mortality in the lethal infection, we next determined the effect of therapy with DHPG on the pathogenesis of a chronic MCMV infection of mice. Groups of mice were inoculated with a sublethal concentration of MCMV and treated with either placebo or 40 mg of DHPG per kg beginning at 24 h and continuing for 14 days. There was a significant reduction in virus titers of DHPG treated animals in blood, lung, liver, spleen and kidney. In salivary gland, there was a 2 day delay in virus replication, and virus titers were consistently lower for the first 15 days. Both MCMV and HCMV are sensitive to DHPG in vitro and the results from the animal model experiments suggest that this compound may be an excellent candidate for treatment of CMV infections in humans.

The ultimate test of any animal model system is its predictability for human disease. Until recent years there has not been enough experience in testing antivirals both in animal models and human trials to establish the predictability of model systems for HSV infections. The information collected using Ara-A and ACV now allows one to make comparisons of efficacy in animal models of HSV encephalitis and genital herpes with those reported in clinical trials. At the present time, only ara-A, which was effective against encephalitis in mouse models has been shown to be effective in humans. The results with ACV are not yet available. For treatment of genital herpes the comparative data in animal models and human trials for a number of antiviral agents suggest that the mouse and guinea pig models are predictive for treatment of these infections in humans.

PROTECTION AGAINST HERPES SIMPLEX VIRUS INFECTION IN NUDE MICE BY ACYCLOVIR AND ANTIBODY

RYOICHI MORI, YOSHINOBU HAYASHI, MASAHIRO YAMAMOTO AND JIE-LIU TANG
Department of Virology, School of Medicine, Kyushu University, Fukuoka 812, Japan

INTRODUCTION

Acyclovir (ACV; 9-(2-hydroxyethoxymethyl)-guanine, or acycloguanosine) is known to be a potent and selective antiviral agent against herpes simplex virus (HSV) infection [1]. Since HSV can cause severe infections in immunocompromised humans [2], the potential of ACV for therapy of HSV in such patients has been investigated [3-9]. In the present study, we have evaluated protective effects of ACV against HSV infection in nude mice by single use or combined use with antibody. Because of the complete deletion of a mature T cell population, infection with HSV in athymic nude mice provides a useful model of HSV infection in immunocompromised hosts.

MATERIALS AND METHODS

Virus. HSV type 1 (HSV-1), strain Hayashida, was passaged in Vero cells and used for inoculation.

Inoculation of mice. Six-week-old female nude (nu/nu) mice with BALB/c genetic background were used. The mice were inoculated intracutaneously in the midflank with 1 x 10^5 plaque forming units (pfu) of HSV-1 per 0.05 ml [10].

ACV. ACV (kindly provided by Nippon Wellcome Co., Ltd., Osaka, Japan) was dissolved in phosphate buffered saline (PBS) at a concentration of 5 mg/ml and was injected via intraperitoneal route.

Human gamma globulin. Human gamma globulin (kindly provided by The Chemo-Sero-Therapeutic Research Institute, Kumamoto, Japan) is a preparation from pooled human plasma and had a neutralizing titer of 1 : 64 against HSV-1.

Determination of virus titers in mouse tissues. At various times after virus inoculation, mice were sacrificed for the assay of virus titers in their tissues. Tissue samples included the skin, dorsal root ganglia from L (lumbar)-1 to L-5, spinal cord in the lumbosacral area, brain, spleen, liver and kidney. The titers of virus recovered from the various homogenates were expressed as pfu per organ or tissue.

Original form of this paper is as follows: Yamamoto, M., Hayashi, Y., Tang, J.-L. and Mori, R.: Effects of combined use of acyclovir and antibody in athymic nude mice inoculated with herpes simplex virus via intracutaneous route. Antiviral Research (in press).

RESULTS AND DISCUSSION

In the first experiment, protective effects of ACV on the course of HSV infection were studied. In this experiment, treatment with ACV was initiated 3 hours after intracutaneous inoculation with HSV. ACV was administered intraperitoneally, 25 mg/kg of body weight, every 12 hours for a total of 28 injections (700 mg/kg). As shown in Table 1, in the PBS-treated control mice, local skin lesions appeared by day 4 and developed into zosteriform lesions, and all mice died within 20 days after infection. In the ACV-treated mice, the local skin lesions appeared after day 9, and later development of skin lesions was also suppressed as long as the ACV treatment was continued. The lesion remained at the site of inoculation for up to 15 days and developed into zosteriform lesions after day 20. Five of six ACV-treated mice eventually died from day 21 to day 30.

Table 2 shows virus titers of tissue homogenates from control and ACV-treated mice at various intervals after infection. The organs from which the virus could be recovered were the skin, dorsal root ganglia, spinal cord and brain. No virus could be recovered from the liver, spleen and kidney.

TABLE 1.
PROTECTIVE EFFECTS OF ACV ON THE COURSE OF HSV INFECTION

	No. of mice with lesions (zosteriform lesions)/No. of mice alive at day							
	4	7	10	13	16	20	25	30
Control	6(0)/6	6(4)/6	3(2)/3	3(3)/3	1(1)/1	0	0	0
ACV	0/6	0/6	4(0)/6	4(0)/6	5(1)/6	5(3)/6	2(2)/3	0/1

TABLE 2.
EFFECTS OF ACV ON VIRAL GROWTH IN MOUSE TISSUES

		virus titer ($\log_{10}$ pfu / organ ± S.D.) at day				
Tissue	Drug	4	7	13	16	25
Skin	PBS	5.0 ± 0.4	5.1 ± 0.7	6.3 ± 0.9	n.d.	n.d.
	ACV	3.1 ± 0.7	2.7 ± 0.2	2.6 ± 1.0	4.3 ± 1.3	6.2 ± 0.7
Dorsal root ganglia	PBS	1.8 ± 0.8	2.0 ± 0.9	3.6 ± 0.6	n.d.	n.d.
	ACV	<1.0	<1.0	<1.0	1.4 ± 0.6	3.0 ± 0.9
Spinal cord	PBS	<1.7	2.7 ± 0.9	2.9 ± 1.1	n.d.	n.d.
	ACV	n.d.	n.d.	<1.7	<1.7	2.6 ± 0.6
Brain	PBS	<1.7	<1.7	3.7 ± 0.6	n.d.	n.d.
	ACV	n.d.	n.d.	<1.7	<1.7	3.9 ± 0.5

Tissue samples from the ACV-treated mice showed a striking reduction in the viral titers. However, with the cessation of ACV-treatment, titer rose along the development of the skin lesions.

Since cessation of administration of ACV caused multiplication of HSV and finally death of nude mice, effects of combined use of ACV and human gamma globulin were studied in the next experiment. ACV was administered intraperitoneally, 25 mg/kg, beginning 3 hours after the virus inoculation and was given every 12 hours for a total of 22 injections (550 mg/kg). One milliliter of human gamma globulin was injected intraperitoneally only once 3 hours after virus inoculation. Mice which received only ACV, gamma globulin or PBS served as controls.

The development of skin lesions in each group is shown in Table 3. Effects of ACV were almost the same as those shown in the first experiment. In the human gamma globulin-treated mice, the development of zosteriform skin lesions was delayed and survival time was also prolonged as described previously [11,12].

The use of ACV plus human gamma globulin was more effective. The development of skin lesions was suppressed and the mean survival time was significantly prolonged. The most important observation was that 5 out of 17 nude mice that were treated by ACV plus human gamma globulin did not develop diseases. The mice which failed to develop any skin lesions were killed 60 days after challenge and tested for the virus, but no virus was recovered from the dorsal root ganglia even after cocultivation with Vero cells. This is the indication of lack of latent infection of HSV.

TABLE 3.
EFFECTS OF COMBINED USE OF ACV AND HUMAN GAMMA GLOBULIN

	No. of mice with lesions (zosteriform lesions)/No. of mice alive at day						
	5	10	15	20	25	30	35
Control	15(0)/16	13(11)/13	7(7)/7	2(2)/2	0	0	0
ACV	4(0)/10	6(0)/10	9(2)/10	6(6)/7	0/1	0/1	0/1
HGG*	13(0)/17	16(7)/17	16(13)/17	14(14)/15	10(10)/11	2(2)/3	0/1
ACV + HGG	3(0)/17	7(0)/17	11(1)/17	12(7)/17	6(5)/11	4(4)/9	1(1)/5

*HGG: Human gamma globulin

These observations indicate that the use of ACV combined with human gamma globulin would be effective in the prophylaxis of HSV infection in immunocompromised hosts and may even inhibit the latent infection of HSV when they are used at an early stage of infection.

REFERENCES

1. Elion GB, Furman PA, Fyfe JA, de Miranda P, Beauchamp L, Schaeffer HJ (1977) Proc Natl Aca Sci USA 74:5716-5720
2. Nahmias AJ, Roizman B (1973) N Engl J Med 289:781-789
3. Mitchell CD, Bean B, Gentry SR, Groth KE, Boen JR, Balfour Jr HH (1981) Lancet 1:1389-1392
4. Saral R, Burns WH, Laskin OL, Santos GW, Lietman PS (1981) N Engl J Med 305:63-67
5. Meyers JD, Wade JC, Mitchell CD, Saral R, Lietman PS, Durack DT, Levin MJ, Segreti AC, Balfour Jr HH (1982) Am J Med 73(1A):229-235
6. Straus SE, Smith HA, Brickman C, de Miranda P, McLaren C, Keeney RE (1982) Ann Intern Med 96:270-276
7. Wade JC, Newton B, McLaren C, Flournoy N, Keeney RE, Meyers JD (1982) Ann Intern Med 96:265-269
8. Gluckman E, Latsberg J, Devergie A, Zhao XM, Melo R, Gomez-Morales M, Mazerton MC, Perol Y (1983) J Antimicrob Chemother 12(Suppl B):161-167
9. Prentice HG (1983) J Antimicrob Chemother 12(Suppl B):153-159
10. Nagafuchi S, Oda H, Mori R, Taniguchi T (1979) J Gen Virol 44:715-723
11. Hayashida I, Nagafuchi S, Hayashi Y, Kino Y, Mori R, Oda H, Ohtomo N, Tashiro A (1982) Microbiol Immunol 26:497-509
12. Kino Y, Hayashi Y, Hayashida I, Mori R (1982) J Gen Virol 63:475-479

Herpes Viruses and Virus Chemotherapy, R. Kono, editor

EFFECT OF ARA-A AND ACYCLOVIR TREATMENT ON EXPERIMENTAL HERPES SIMPLEX VIRUS ENCEPHALITIS IN RABBITS

TAKESHI KURATA, SUGISHI OHTANI, ATSUKO YAMAMOTO, RYO HONDO, YUZO AOYAMA, KOZABURO HAYASHI AND *HIROMICHI MIZUTANI

Department of Pathology, Institute of Medical Science, University of Tokyo, Shirokanedai 4-6-1, Minatoku, Tokyo 108 and *Department of Virus Research, Kanto Teishin Hospital, Higashigotanda 5-9-22, Shinagawaku, Tokyo 141,(Japan)

INTRODUCTION

Herpes simplex virus (HSV) encephalitis has the highest incidence and serious prognosis as the acute sporadic encephalitis in our country after marked decline of Japanese encephalitis. 9-β-D-arabinofuranosyl-adenine (Ara-A) and 9-(2-hydroxyethoxymethyl)guanine (Acyclovir; ACV) are known to interfere the replication of viral DNA in vitro and to be beneficial for in vivo experiments (1-4). In humans, Ara-A or ACV decreased the mortality and improved the clinical signs in HSV encephalitis (5-7). In any reports of HSV encephalitis, necessity of rapid correct diagnosis and an early application of the drug for therapy have been suggested. In this report, the validity of drugs on the encephalitis induced in rabbits was examined. Histopathological and immunofluorescent studies (IF) were done to confirm the disease. Also practical value of enzyme-linked immunosorbent assay (ELISA) and complement fixation test (CF) for rapid diagnosis of specific antibody rise in cerebrospinal fluid (CSF) and serum were examined.

MATERIALS AND METHODS

Rabbits. New Zealand white rabbits, weighd 2.2-2.4kg, were obtained from Experimental Animal Research Center of our Institute.

Virus inoculation. Two strains of type 1 HSV (CHR-3, $1x10^7$pfu/ml, and Tomioka, $9.2x10^7$pfu/ml) were used. After scratching the bilateral corneas with needles, virus solution ($5x10^5$pfu/0.1ml) was inoculated. With this method, it was possible to produce HSV encepahlitis or neurological sign in all rabbits.

Drugs. Ara-A and ACV were kindly supplied by Mochida Pharmaceutical Co. and Wellcome Foundation Ltd., respectively. Drug solutions were given slowly intravenously twice a day from the 3rd or 6th day after virus infection for 9 or 10 days, respectively. As placebo, the same amount of physiological saline was used.

Antibody in CSF and serum. Sera and CSF were collected every other day from all rabbits after infection with/without drug therapy. Rise of antibody was tested by ELISA of which method was written elsewhere (8). CF was done according to the Kolmer's method using microplate.

Viral antigens. Brains, bilateral corneas and conjunctiva, and trigeminal ganglia were removed from all rabbits. All tissues were divided, and one piece was frozen in n-hexane at -70°C and the other was fixed in 10% buffered-formalin for paraffin embedding. Frozen and paraffin sections were used for direct and indirect IF, respectively (9).

Histopathology. Morphological changes were examined with hematoxylin and eosin stained specimens.

RESULTS

Clinical signs. The first signs were hair errection, congestion and tears in eyes and a large amount of sebum was noted as days went by. A week after infection, rabbits with/without therapy showed crouching, lower appetite, irritability, convulsion and hyperreflexia, and they seemed typical signs of HSV encephalitis. In rabbits with therapy from early course of infection, signs were improved well and at 30th day corneal lesions were completely cured or with slight scars, without any neurological signs(Fig.1-A). Drug from 6th day could not improve so well the ocular lesions (Fig.1-B) nor neurological symptoms such as wryneck, paralysis of under extremities or emaciation which remained as sequelae. No serious signs were observed in rabbits infected with Tomioka strain after therapy.

Effect of the drug on survival rate.(Table I) A dose was determined according to the human application (6-7). As it is clear from Table I, therapy in the early course of infection rescued 90% of rabbits from death, on the contrary 40% of animals could survive with placebo. Drug administration, after typical neurological signs completed, was not so beneficial. With Tomioka strain mortality was 10% in two therapy groups, suggesting the difference of virulence to nervous tissues.

TABLE I

SURVIVAL RATE OF RABBITS WITH HERPES SIMPLEX VIRUS ENCEPHALITIS BY DRUG THERAPY

Experiment	Virus strain	Number of rabbits	Drug mg/day	Survived rabbits at day 30	Clinical sequelae
I	CHR-3	10	Ara-A 20mg(day 3-11)	9	- ~ +
	"	10	placebo (")	4	++
II	CHR-3	10	ACV 30mg(day 3-11)	9	- ~ +
	"	10	placebo (")	3	++
III	CHR-3	20	Ara-A 20mg(day 6-15)	12	+
	"	20	placebo (")	6	++
IV	Tomioka	10	Ara-A 20mg(day 6-15)	9	- ~ +
	"	10	ACV 20mg(")	9	- ~ +
	"	10	placebo (")	6	+

Antibody in CSF and serum. This experiment was done to know the rise of antibody in CSF and serum after HSV infection and to get exact reason for therapy as HSV encephalitis. CSF was obtained via cerebello-medullary cisterna. Kinetics of

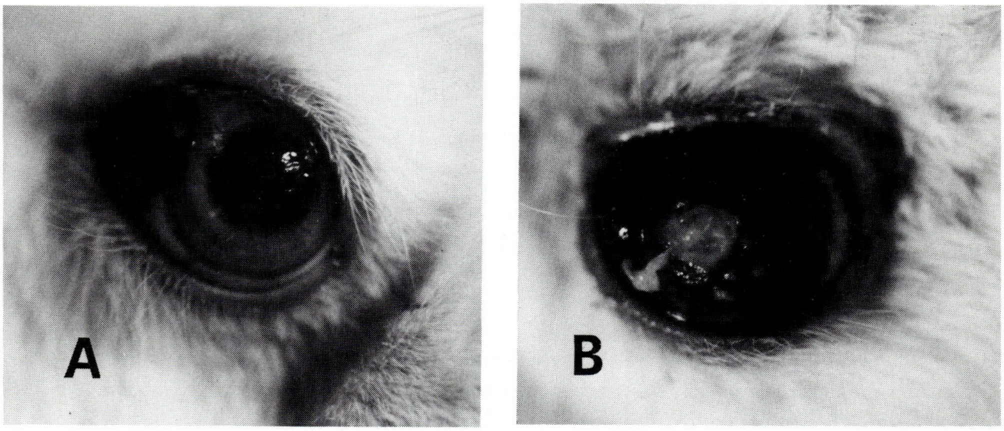

Fig.1. Corneas of rabbits

Fig.1-A shows the cornea with almost complete cure by treatment of Ara-A(day 3-11) and 1-B is the cornea with pus and granulation of survived rabbit treated with Ara-A(day 6-15)

antibody rise were determined by ELISA and CF. Referring to the IgG in CSF, measurable rise of antibody appeared during 4-6 days and increased rapidly until day 10, and in sera antibody started to rise about two days later of CSF, 6-8 dasy after infection. No significant difference in antibody rise between treated and non-treated animals during the course of experiment was observed. ELISA could catch antibody in CSF in earlier stage than CF.

Distribution of viral antigens and histopathological changes. Distribution of viral antigens in paraffin specimens were similar to that in frozen materials. In eyes, specific fluorescence was detected in the corneal epithelia and propria, and in conjunctiva. Neurons, Schwann's cells and satellite cells had viral antigens in trigeminal ganglia. Pons also showed antigens in nuclei nervi trigemini, glial cells and neuronal fibers. In cerebrum, viral antigens were observed widely in neurons and glial cells, especially neurons of hippocampus. No basic difference was noted between drug-treated or non-treated fatal rabbits in the antigen distribution. Distribution of viral antigen suggested the neurogenic spread of HSV. In fatal rabbits, irrespective of therapy, histopathological changes were similar in eyes and nervous tissues. Hypertrophied conjunctiva, corneas with granulation and/or pus, and infiltration of a large amount of plasma cells and leukocytes were noted. Trigeminal ganglia showed wide infiltration of small round cells, hemorrhages, and lobulated intranuclear inclusion bodies in neurons. In cerebrum, hemorrhages, perivascular cuffs, degeneration of neurons, and typical Cowdry A or full type inclusion bodies in neurons and glial cells were observed.

DISCUSSION

In the experimentally-induced HSV encephalitis of rabbits, therapeutic effect of antiviral drugs and propriety of antibody rise for establishment of definitive diagnosis were examined. The earlier application of the drug in the course of infection, the better survival rate and improvement of clinical signs were obtained. Without doubt, for definitive diagnosis of viral diseases, causative virus has to be isolated from the foci. If so, how should be established the early and rapid diagnosis of HSV encephalitis ? Lee (10) has recommended to find viral particles in the biopsied brain tissues by electronmicroscopy. Nahmias (11) began to change opinion to recommend to detect IgG in CSF by passive hemagglutination or by IF instead of brain biopsy. In suspected cases of HSV encephalitis, frequent testing of CSF or serum should be tried to catch significant rise of antibody specific to HSV for early diagnosis. ELISA in our hand is quite sensitive method and seems useful for application for human cases (8). In animal experimental system, false positive with cross reaction of IgG was not recognized. In conclusion, drug therapy in HSV encephalitis at the early course of infection was quite effective for cure and ELISA is a useful tool for detection of early rise of antibody, especially in CSF.

REFERENCES

1. Shannon WH (1975) In: Pavan-Langston D, Buchanan RA, Alford A Jr (eds) Adenin arabinoside: An antiviral agent. Raven Press, New York, pp 1-43
2. Sloan BJ (1975) ditto, pp 43-94
3. Schaeffer HJ, Beauchamp L, de Miranda P, Elion GB, Bauer DJ, Collins P(1978) Nature 272:583-585
4. Collins P, Oliver NM(1982) Am J Med 73:96-99
5. Whitley RJ, Soong SJ, Hirsch MS, Karchmer AW, Dolin R, Glasso GJ, Dunnick JK, Alford CA, NIAID Collaborative antiviral study group (1981) New Engl J Med 304:313-318
6. Ohtani S, HSV encephalitis study group (1982) J Japan Assoc Infect Dis 56:799-823
7. Ohtani S, HSV encephalitis study group (1983) Clin Virol 11:104-117
8. Mizutani H, Mizutani H, Kamei S, Takasu T, Kurata T, Yamamoto A, Aoyama Y, Ohtani S (1984) J Japan Assoc Infect Dis 58:187-196
9. Kurata T. Hondo R, Sato S, Oda A, Aoyama Y (1983) Ann New York Acad Sci 420:192-207
10. Lee FK, Visintine AN, Takei Y, Whitley R, Dannenbager J, Nahmias AJ (1981) Am J Surg Pathol 5:565-572
11. Nahmias AJ, Whitley RJ, Visintine AN, Takei Y, Alford CA Jr, Collaborative antiviral study group (1982) J Infect Dis 145:829-836

© 1985 Elsevier Science Publishers B.V. (Biomedical Division)
Herpes Viruses and Virus Chemotherapy, R. Kono, editor

LABORATORY DIAGNOSIS OF HERPESVIRUS INFECTION

G. D. HSIUNG and M. L. LANDRY

Virology Reference Laboratory, V. A. Medical Center, West Haven, CT. and
Yale University School of Medicine, New Haven, CT. U. S. A.

INTRODUCTION

In order to select an effective chemotherapeutic agent for a herpesvirus infection, an accurate laboratory diagnosis of the specific virus involved is imperative. This will be particularly important as drugs become available with a narrow spectrum of action on the replication of a specific herpesvirus.

Morphologically, all herpesviruses are alike - either in thin section or in negatively stained preparations (Figure 1). Therefore, it is not possible to

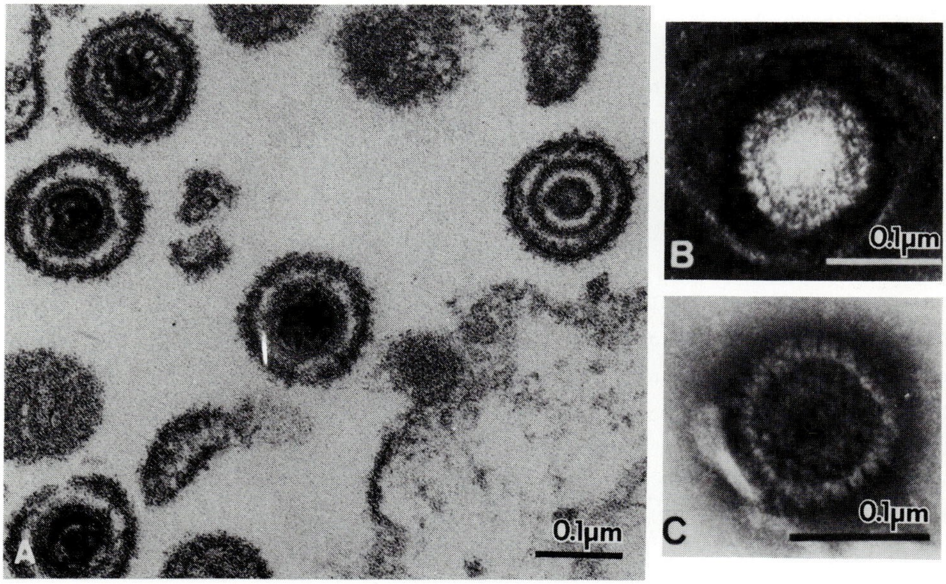

Fig. 1. Enveloped particles in thin section (A), enveloped herpesvirus particle (B) and naked herpesvirus particle (C) in PTA stained preparations.

differentiate members of the herpesvirus group by their morphological structure alone. There are five serologically distinct human herpesvirus types. These are herpes simplex virus (HSV) types 1 and 2, varicella-zoster (VZV), cytomegalovirus (CMV), and Epstein-Barr virus (EBV). Clinically, each of these five herpesviruses produces distinct disease syndromes. A diagnosis can be made based on clinical observations. However, misdiagnoses have been made from time to time and dual or multiple infections can occur (1).

LABORATORY DIAGNOSIS OF FIVE HUMAN HERPESVIRUS TYPES

Biologically, the five human herpesviruses are distinct in their replication properties in cell cultures. Table 1 shows the host range of the five herpesvirus infections in cell cultures and in experimental animals (2). HSV-1 and HSV-2 show a wide range of host cell infections. Rapid cytopathic effects are easily observed in human fibroblasts, Hep-2 passaged cell lines, rabbit kidney/ guinea pig embryo fibroblasts and many others. HSV are pathogenic for infant mice

Table 1. HERPESVIRIDAE

Herpes-Virus	CPE in Cell Culture				Mouse Pathogenicity
	HEF	HEP-2	VERO	RK	
HSV-1	++	+	+	++	+
HSV-2	++	+	+	++	+
VZV	+	-	-	-	-
CMV	+	-	-	-	-
EBV	-	-	-	-	-

and produce lesions on chorioallantoic membrane of embryonic hen eggs. In contrast, VZV and CMV are extremely host-specific replicating only in human fibroblast (HEF) cells. Thus, the latter cell system must be utilized in order to facilitate the isolation of these two viruses. In addition, virus-induced cellular changes by VZV and CMV often require days or even weeks. Detection of EBV infection requires even more specialized and tedious procedures, such as the transformation of cord blood lymphocytes, a technique which is not available in a routine clinical laboratory; thus, serologic diagnosis of EBV infection is commonly applied including detection of antibodies to viral capsid antigen and/or EB nuclear antigen. Thus, methods for detection of CMV or EBV nucleic acid in clinical specimens have been recently developed for rapid diagnosis (3, 4).

Isolation of HSV in Cell Cultures

Obtaining a rapid and accurate diagnosis of herpes simplex virus (HSV) infections is one of the major concerns for the clinical virology laboratory today, especially for genital herpes in pregnant women. The critical first step in making a successful HSV isolation is obtaining a proper specimen and rapidly transporting it to a laboratory. The availability of a highly sensitive cell system has facilitated the detection and diagnosis of HSV infection in less than 24 hours. Although HSV has a wide host range, a most sensitive cell system is necessary in order to detect a minimum amount of infectious virus. For example, the same amount of HSV will induce cytopathic effect in primary rabbit kidney(RK) cells in less than 24 hours, whereas 72 hours of incubation time are necessary if insensitive HEF cells are used. This is illustrated in greater detail in Table 2. When 10 infectious virus particles are present in the clinical specimen, one or two days are necessary for virus induced CPE in primary RK cells, whereas 10-100 infectious virus particles are necessary in order to see changes in HEF cells in two days or even longer in Vero or Hep-2 cells. This delay in obtaining laboratory results causes the delay of reports from the clinical laboratory, thus adversely affecting chemotherapy.

Table 2. COMPARATIVE SENSITIVITY OF CELL CULTURES TO HSV INFECTION

HSV	CPE Induced by HSV in Different Cell Cultures											
	RK			HEF			HEP-2			VERO		
($TCID_{50}$)	1*	2	4	1	2	4	1	2	4	1	2	4
10000	+++**	+++	+++	0	+	++	0	+	++	0	++	++
1000	++	++	+++	0	+	++	0	0	++	0	+	++
100	+	+	+++	0	0	+	0	0	0	0	0	0
10	0	+	++	0	0	0	0	0	0	0	0	0
1	0	0	+	0	0	0	0	0	0	0	0	0

*Days post inoculation; ** degree of CPE

Differentiation of HSV-1 and HSV-2

Because of antigenic similarities between HSV-1 and HSV-2, several nonimmunologic techniques have been developed over the years for distinguishing the two types. These include cell culture selection, bromovinyl deoxyuridine (BVDU) sensitivity tests and restriction endonuclease analysis. In our laboratory, 42 isolates were typed by biological and biochemical properties and by restriction enzyme analysis (Table 3) and 100% agreement between these three methods was obtained. In addition, 33 isolates typed by nucleic acid hybridization at San Diego VA were sent to our laboratory with coded numbers. Again, 32 were in

Table 3. COMPARISON OF METHODS FOR TYPING HSV ISOLATES FROM CLINICAL SPECIMENS

Source of Virus Isolates	Methods for Typing	Cell Culture Selection and/or BVDU Sensitivity HSV-1	HSV-2	Total No. Tested
West Haven VA	Restriction Endonuclease Analysis	20	22	42
San Diego VA	Microneut, Elisa-RIA, Nucleic Acid Hybridization	20	12	33*

*One virus stock was not sufficient for typing.

agreement with the cell culture selection and BVDU sensitivity system. Recently, monocloncal antibodies became available for typing HSV-1 and HSV-2 either by immunofluorescence or by immunoperoxidase methods, thus facilitating identification of HSV-1 and HSV-2 significantly.

Speed of Diagnosis of HSV Infection

How fast can one make a diagnosis of HSV infection? What is the best method for detection of HSV? The method of choice depends upon the number of virus particles present in the clinical specimen. If there are less than 10 infectious virus particles, one or two days may be necessary if the most sensitive cell culture system is used. On the other hand, if there are 10^6-10^7 virus particles present in the specimen, only 30 minutes are necessary for a positive result when electron microscopic examination is used. Detection of viral protein or viral nucleic acid require 10^4-10^6 virus particles in the specimen. However, such high concentrations of virus particles are uncommon in clinical specimens.

ANTIVIRAL SENSITIVITY TESTING

Drug sensitivity testing of clinical isolates is an important function of clinical microbiology laboratories and is essential for the administering of appropriate and effective drugs. Antiviral susceptibility testing will also be necessary and is within the capability of a virology laboratory, but performance standards need to be established. Two methods are commonly used in the laboratory for testing drug sensitivity to a virus; one of the methods is to determine the virus yield in the culture medium. Basically, this is done by adding varying concentrations of drug to the culture medium of virus-infected monolayers and assaying aliquots of the medium for the yield of virus. The resulting reduction of virus yield can be plotted against virus yield without drugs. The second and perhaps the simplest method of antiviral assay which can be performed by a routine laboratory is a plaque reduction assay. Plaque formation in the absence of test drug is compared to plaque formation in the presence of drug at different concentrations. However, different results are obtained when different cell culture systems are used for plaque reduction assay. For example, only 1 uM of acyclovir is necessary to inhibit HSV-1 strain NYU-78 when Vero cells are used for the assay, whereas 16 uM of the drug is needed to inhibit the same amount of virus completely when GPE cells are used. Thus, the importance of selection of cell culture system for drug sensitivity tests is apparent.

SUMMARY

With the current increased interest in studying herpesvirus infections and the availability of anti-herpesviral agents, laboratory diagnosis for herpesvirus infections is even more pressing. In the early 1960s, only a few studies on herpesvirus infections were published (5). Today, as chemotherapy becomes a reality, and more antivirals become available, the interest in studying herpesviruses will undoubtedly increase not only for herpes simplex virus but also for other herpesviruses as well. Thus, the development of accurate and rapid laboratory diagnosis of all herpesvirus infections deserves high priority if chemotherapy for herpes infection is to be used rapidly and successfully.

ACKNOWLEDGEMENTS

This study was supported in part by research contract #AI 12665 from the National Institute of Allergy and Infectious Diseases, NIH, and Veterans Administration Research Funds.

REFERENCES

1. Landry ML, Mayo DR, Hsiung GD (1982) Comparison of guinea pig cells, rabbit kidney cells and human embryonic lung fibroblast cell strains for the isolation of herpes simplex virus. J Clin Micro 15: 842-847.

2. Hsiung GD (1982) Diagnostic Virology, Yale Univ. Press, New Haven, pp.195-217.

3. Chou S, Merigan TC (1983) Rapid detection and quantitation of human cytomegalovirus in urine through DNA hybridization. N Eng J Med 308: 921-925.

4. Andiman W, Gradoville L, Heston L, et al. (1983) Use of cloned probes to detect Epstein-Barr viral DNA in tissues of patients with neoplastic and lymphoproliferative diseases. J Infect Dis 148: 967-977.

5. Hsiung GD, Mayo DR, Lucia HL, Landry ML (1984) Genital herpes: Pathogenesis and chemotherapy in the guinea pig model. Rev Infect Dis 6: 33-50.

Herpes Viruses and Virus Chemotherapy, R. Kono, editor

A LIVE VARICELLA VACCINE (OKA STRAIN)

MICHIAKI TAKAHASHI

Department of Virology Research Institute for Microbial Diseases,
Osaka University Suita, Osaka, 565 Japan

DEVELOPMENT OF A LIVE VARICELLA VACCINE OF THE OKA STRAIN

The Oka strain of varicella-zoster virus(VZV) was isolated in primary human embryonic lung cells from the vesicles of a 3-year-old child with typical chickenpox. It was passaged 11 times in human embryonic lung cells at 34C and 12 times in guinea pig embryo (GPE) cells at 37C. The virus was then passaged in human diploid cells (WI-38 and MRC-5) several times to prepare an experimental vaccine[1)2)3)].

BIOLOGICAL AND BIOPHYSICAL MARKERS OF THE VACCINE VIRUS

1)Temperature sensitivity tests on the vaccine and wild-type strains

The vaccine strain was slightly temperature sensitive at 39C unlike the wild-type strains. The foci of the vaccine strain were also smaller than those of wild-type strains at high temperature but similar in size to the latter at lower temperature.

2)Difference in infectivity on GPEF and HuEF cells of the vaccine and wild-type strains

The vaccine strain showed a higher ratio of infectivity on GPEF to that on HuEF than any of the wild-type strains examined. This test is convenient and the results are reproducible. Therefore, it can be employed as a marker test on clinical isolates from vaccinees[4)].

3)Cleavage profiles on DNAs of vaccine and wild-type strains by restriction endonuclease

In DNA digests with restriction endonucleases, the Hpa I-K fragment of the parental and vaccine Oka strain differed in mobility from that of other wild-type strains[4)].

SUMMARIZED CLINICAL AND IMMUNOLOGICAL RESULTS OF VACCINATION IN JAPAN FROM 1973 TO 1983

The clinical and immunological results of vaccination between 1974 and 1983 in 54 hospitals in Japan have been summarized which are divided into 3 groups, i.e. children with malignancies, children with underlying diseases other than malignancies and normal children. Viral doses used were 100 to 2,500 PFU/dose, mainly 500 PFU.

VACCINATION OF CHILDREN WITH MALIGNANCIES

1)Vaccination of children with acute leukemia

By the end of 1983, a total of 309 acute leukemia children were immunized with the varicella vaccine in 39 hospitals. In general, the following conditions had to be met; 1)the patients should be in remission 2)cell-mediated immunity assessed by phytohemagglutinin or other reagents should be normal and 3)all anticancer therapy except 6MP should be suspended one week prior to and one week after vaccination.

Of the 240 patients that received vaccination under the above condition, 40(16.7%) developed mild clinical reactions, except one T cell leukemic patient who developed numerous vesicles and high fever. Of the 69 patients who received emergency vaccination or received vaccination without suspension of chemotherapy, 30(43.3%) developed mostly mild clinical reactions, but one T cell leukemic patient developed numerous vesicles lasting 40 days. Immune responses were observed in most of the vaccinees by IAHA (Immune adherence hemagglutination)test or FAMA(fluorescent antibody to membrane antigen) test and varicella skin test. Clinical varicella infection in the vaccinees has been reported in 34 cases(11.0%); mild cases 17, moderate cases 11, severe cases 3; one contracted varicella during meningeal leukemia and another contracted it while receiving intensive chemotherapy. Eighteen patients received revaccination to maintain immunity, of whom no clinical varicella infection has been reported.

2)Incidence of zoster in patients with malignancies

A comparison was made in three study groups on the incidence of zoster in the vaccinated luekemia children group and the leukemic children that had experienced natural varicella. Both groups had received the same kind of chemotherapy. Incidence of zoster in the vaccinated group is less and its clinical symptoms is also less severe than those in naturally infected group.

VACCINATION OF CHILDREN WITH UNDERLYING DISEASES OTHER THAN MALIGNANCIES

Approximately 1,500 children with underlying diseases other than malignancies were vaccinated, including those with neurological disorder, heart diseases, allergic disposition, congenital diseases, nephrotic diseases, endocrinal diseases, metabolic diseases. Mild clinical reaction were observed in only about 3% of them, and an antibody response was observed in about 96%. Of the vaccinated, 171 had nephrotic syndrome and 96 of them were on steroid therapy. Eleven cases with nephrotic syndrome developed mild clinical symptoms and an immune response was detected in almost all of them.

VACCINATION OF NORMAL CHILDREN

In a study group, 915 normal children were vaccinated between 1978 and 1982. As clinical reaction after vaccination, fever and slight rash were observed in only 10 children. Serological response was observed in all the susceptible children examined. Of the 854 children who could be followed, 602 children contact with varicella patients, but only 5 of them developed extremely mild varicella. Mild zoster occurred in one child who was admitted to hospital with mycoplasma pneumonia.

A LONG-TERM (7-10 YEARS) FOLLOW-UP STUDY ON THE VACCINE RECIPIENTS

A long-term (7-10 years) follow-up study has also been made in other study group [5]. Questionnaires were sent to the parents of 282 children that had received vaccination during 1973-1976. Answers were obtained from 103 parents, and 100 could be evaluated. Among them, 33 children had underlying diseases, and of them nine had been receiving steroid therapy at the time of vaccination. They had a total of 147 contacts with varicella patients (family 26, school 66, playmate 55) after vaccination. Of the 100 vaccinees, five children developed varicella. Four of them contracted varicella within one year after vaccination, the symptoms being very mild, and one exhibited typical varicella symptoms three years after vaccination. No case of zoster has been reported. For the examination of persistence of immunity to VZV in the vaccinees, blood was collected from 38 of the 100 vaccinees. Twenty nine children who had natural varicella over the last ten years were included as controls. FAMA antibody of >1:4 was detected in 37/38 (97.4%) cases with a geometric mean titer (GMT) of $2^{3.1}$ in the vaccinees while 29/29 (100%) of the natural varicella group were FAMA positive with a GMT of $2^{3.5}$.

By the VZV skin test, 37/38 were positive (97.4%) in the vaccinated group (one negative case had chronic nephrisis and an antibody titer 1:16), while 28/29 (96.6%) were positive in the natural varicella group (one negative case had bronchial asthma). From these results, it is evident that immunization with the live varicella vaccine confered a long lasting (7-10 years) immunities.

ISOLATION OF VZV FROM BLOOD CELLS OF NATURALLY INFECTED CHILDLEN AND VACCINATED CHILDREN

Ozaki et al[6] demonstrated VZV could be recovered from mononuclear cells of children with no underlying diseases just after onset of the diseases (from 4 out 6 patients within day 1 of the diseases and none out of 3 patients day 2 and 3). Later Asano et al [7] showed that the viruses could be isolated from 4 of 4 children one day before onset of the diseases, 4 of 4 two days before, one of 2 four days before, and one of 2 five days before onset of the diseases. No virus was isolated on 6,7 and 11 days before onset of varicella.

No VZV could be recovered from a total of 27 children on day 4 to 14 days after vaccination who received the vaccine with dose of 5,000 PFU. These results suggest that the magnitude of replication of the vaccine virus in the susceptible organs and blood cells in human is far less than that of wild-type VZV, which seems be related to the attenuated nature of the vaccine virus.

REFERENCES

1. Takahashi M, Otsuka T, Okuno Y, Asano Y, Yazaki T, Isomura S.(1974) Lancet ii:1288-1290

2. Takahashi M, Asano Y, Kamiya H, Baba K, Yamanishi K. (1981)"The Human Herpesviruses" edited by Nahmias A.J. Elsevier, New York 414-431

3. Takahashi M, Baba K.(1984)Medical Virology III edited by de la Maza L.H. and Peterson E.M. Elsevier, New York 255-278

4. Hayakawa Y, Torigoe S, Shiraki K, Yamanishi K, Takahashi M. (1984) J.Infect.Dis. 149:956-963

5. Asano Y, Nagai T, Miyata T, Yazaki T, Ito S, Yamanishi K, Takahashi M. (in press) J. Pediatrics

6. Ozaki T, Ichikawa T, Matsui Y, Nagai T, Asano Y, Yamanishi K, Takahashi M. (1984) J.Pediatrics 104:85-87

7. Asano Y, Itakura N, Hiroishi Y, Hirose S, Nagai T, Ozaki T, Yazaki T, Yamanishi K, Takahashi M. (in press) J.Pediatrics

Herpes Viruses and Virus Chemotherapy, R. Kono, editor

PHARMACOLOGICAL CONSIDERATIONS OF ANTIVIRAL COMPOUNDS

W.H. PRUSOFF, T.-S. LIN, S.A. SIEGEL, M. ZUCKER, W.F. BRUBAKER, JR. AND J.J. LEE

Department of Pharmacology, Yale University School of Medicine, New Haven, Connecticut, USA

Some of the questions that may be raised in a discussion of pharmacologic considerations relative to antiviral agents include:

1. How does one design an effective but non-toxic antiviral agent?
2. Can we deliver the drug to the target site and maintain an antiviral concentration for the required period of time? Here we are concerned with adsorption, distribution, metabolism and excretion of the drug.
3. How can we avoid or minimize the emergence of a resistant population of virus?
4. How can we prevent the virus from going into the latent state, but once there how can we control its reactivation?

The first question is concerned with the design of an antiviral drug. To date serendipity has played a major role in the development of the antiviral drugs that are in clinical use, and this approach will continue to make additional contributions.

Ideally we would like to have a drug that exerts its antiviral activity as a consequence of interaction with a target that is unique to the virus, and hence of little or no concern to the uninfected host tissues. Such an example is the preferential or specific activation of a compound in the virus infected cell by a virus encoded enzyme. Compounds such as Acyclovir, BVdU; FIAC; 9-[1,3-dihydroxy-2-propoxymethyl] guanine, 5'-amino analog of IUdR and of thymidine, etc., are indeed preferentially phosphorylated by the herpesvirus encoded thymidine kinase, and compounds such as phosphono formate preferentially inhibit herpesvirus encoded DNA polymerase.

I will discuss in the last session on Thursday other approaches that are, or may be taken, for the future development of antiviral agents.

The second major pharmacologic consideration concerns the efficient or selective transport of the drug to the viral infected tissue. Before a drug can reach the target site it must be absorbed, transferred from the capillary into the extracellular fluid, and transported into the infected cell. Several experimental approaches have been reported with the objective of improving transport or drug delivery to the target area.

For example the use of prodrugs. A prodrug is a compound that is converted either enzymically or chemically to the active or parent drug. Although a prodrug may decrease the rate of excretion or the rate of degradation of the parent drug prior to reaching the target site, this does not imply preferential or specific uptake by the infected cell. If there is no preferential retention by the infected tissue then the therapeutic index is not affected. Improved uptake into both target and normal tissues could result in enhanced toxicity. An example of a prodrug is the 5'-phosphate or 5'-valeric acid ester of ara-A. Both of these have the desirable property of increased solubility.

The poor solubility of ara-A requires its administration in a large fluid volume, and this may exacerbate an edema, already present in patients with herpes encephalitis, or may increase the risk of congestive heart failure.

A prodrug may have a decreased rate of degradation and hence prolong the biological half-life of the parent drug. This would obviate the necessity for frequent administration of the parent drug.

INHIBITION OF DEGRADATIVE ENZYMES

Another way of increasing the concentration of active drug is to prevent its metabolic degradation by inhibition of the responsible catabolic enzyme or modification of structure, such as Cyclaradine or 2-fluoro-ara A.

There have been many attempts to prevent cleavage of pyrimidine nucleosides either by structural modification of the nucleoside analog or by coadministration of inhibitors of the pyrimidine nucleoside phosphorylases. Unfortunately humans possess 2 phosphorylases which degrade pyrimidine nucleosides--uridine phosphorylase and thymidine phosphorylase, but inhibitors of only the uridine phosphorylase have been developed.

Pyrimidine nucleosides such as IUdR, F_3dThd and BVdU are rapidly cleaved by thymidine phosphorylase or by the non-specific uridine phosphorylase, and hence their biological half-life is very brief. Whereas the cleaved free pyrimidines derived from IUdR or F_3dThd are rapidly removed from the blood stream, significant levels of (2-bromovinyl)uracil formed from BVdU remain in the blood stream of the rat for up to 24 hours.

Of interest is the recent observation that after BVdU had been completely converted to BVUra in rats, the administration of thymidine had regenerated BVdU by a transfer of the deoxyribose moiety of thymidine to BVUra. Whether this procedure will have clinical utility is an intriguing pharmacologic consideration.

An interesting approach to overcome the problem of toxicity of an antiviral drug was based on an observation made by Cheng over 10 years ago. 5'-Amino-5'-deoxythymidine inhibited the phosphorylation of IUdR by the cellular thymidine kinase, but both were substrates for the herpesvirus thymidine kinase.

Although IUdR is a clinically useful antiviral agent for topical administration, it cannot be used for treatment of systemic herpesvirus infections, because uninfected cells that are synthesizing DNA will also utilize this compound. A consequence of the incorporation of IUdR into the DNA of such cells is cytotoxicity, and hence systemic administration of IUdR may result in bone marrow toxicity, alopecia and stomatitis. Thus by combining the two analogs, Paul Fischer found phosphorylation of IUdR in normal cells was prevented, but antiviral activity in the virus infected cells was retained and was additive for the 2 compounds.

Another approach to eliminate an undesirable property of a drug is modification of its structure but with retention of antiviral activity. An example of this will be presented by Dr. Vince who synthesized cyclaradine, the carbocyclic analog of ara-A and found it to be resistant to enzymic degradation. This affords a longer antiviral activity *in vivo*.

Another example is the synthesis of the 5'-amino analog of IUdR, which eliminated the toxicities attributed to IUdR because of its being a substrate for the HSV-encoded thymidine kinase, but not for the cellular TK. Unfortunately the decrease in antiviral activity, relative to IUdR, has not encouraged its further development.

Another pharmacological consideration relates to the dichotomy that although a concentration of a drug required to inhibit the virus *in vitro* may be attained in the blood stream, it may have no effect on the viral infection *in vivo*. This may be related to the need to attain the antiviral concentration within the infected cell, because the concentration in the blood stream may not necessarily reflect the intracellular concentration.

Failure of the drug to attain an antiviral concentration for the required period of time at the target site, within the cell, could be a consequence of poor transport, rapid intracellular degradation, or by deviation of the drug from the viral target site by diversion to a non-critical metabolic reaction.

The third pharmacologic consideration concerns the emergence of resistance by viruses when exposed to an antiviral drug. Darby and Field recently published a superb review concerned with the problems of viral resistance and latency. Resistance could be a consequence of a genetic alteration in the viral genome, or it could be an apparent resistance that is related to the cell type that is infected, or it could be related to pharmacokinetic parameters unique to the animal species or to a unique peculiarity of an individual within the same species.

Herpesvirus exposed to antiviral agents that require phosphorylation by the viral encoded thymidine kinase (TK) may express a phenotype that is resistant, because it is either TK^-, or one that produces low levels of TK, or one that produces TK with altered substrate specificity.

Herpesviruses may also become resistant because they induce a DNA polymerase with altered substrate specificities.

Different sensitivities to a drug by a single viral isolate have been found under conditions where different methods of assay or different cell lines were used. However, a lack of clinical response may be because of bona fide genetic resistance of the virus, or may be related to a failure to transport the drug into the infected cell, failure to reach or maintain in the infected cell the required antiviral concentration for an appropriate amount of time, variation of pool sizes of endogenous competing substrates (Harmenburg), variation of rates of excretion, etc. For one or more of these reasons a lack of clinical efficacy may be observed, even though the isolated virus may be sensitive to the drug.

One approach to avoid or minimize emergence of resistance, true or apparent, is the use of combination therapy in which the two drugs are used which have different target sites, use different enzymes for activation, and preferably have different pharmacokinetic properties relative to transport and excretion.

Finally the last pharmacologic concern is how can we avoid the problem of allowing the virus to enter a latent state, but once established what can be done to either destroy the latent genome or to prevent or modify its expression. What pharmacologic considerations should we be concerned with? Darby and Field in their recent review listed a dozen uncertainties relating to latent infections. Once the answers to their concerns are found, we will be in a better position to approach the solution to this problem.

There have been some probes to deliver an antiviral drug into the cell body of a ganglion, the site of latent herpesvirus, by retrograde axonal transport. This was accomplished by the use of a protein that had previously been shown to be taken up, by pinocytosis, and subsequently transported into the nerve cell body by retrograde axonal flow.

Thus, the carbohydrate portion of horseradish peroxidase was partially oxidized with sodium metaperiodate to produce aldehyde moieties which form a Schiff base with the 5'-amino group of 5-iodo-5'-amino-2',5'-dideoxyuridine. The ratio of AIdUrd to protein in the conjugate ranged from 2 to 9. Retrograde transport of the complex was established by autoradiography of the trigeminal ganglion neuron 24 hours after corneal injection of $[^{125}I]$-drug-protein complex. These experiments demonstrated that it is possible to get an antiviral agent to the site of the latent virus. Whether one can attain by this procedure an antiviral concentration of a drug in the ganglion, and what the consequences would be remains to be determined.

Finally, regardless of drug, there is great variation in patient's response and hence the same dose will not be effective in all patients. Those patients who slowly inactivate a drug or excrete it slowly may experience accumulation of the drug with associated toxicity. Hence one would want to decrease the dose or the interval of administration. The reverse picture emerges in those patients who catabolize or excrete a drug rapidly, and hence increased dosage or frequency of administration is indicated. The reasons for variation are numerous and include: age, sex, preganancy, disease, exercise, dietary factors, g.i. functions, renal function, liver function, fever and many more factors. Thus an understanding of the pharmacokinetics of a drug (absorption, distribution, biotransformation and excretion) enables the clinician to choose appropriate dosage schedules for a particular patient.

We have attempted to present some of the problems in the use of antiviral agents and have also indicated various directions that have been pursued in an attempt to circumvent problems associated with these drugs.

ACKNOWLEDGEMENTS

The research performed in this laboratory was supported by United States Public Health Service Grant, CA-05262, from the National Cancer Institute.

II NEW ANTIHERPETIC DRUGS IN ANTIVIRAL CHEMOTHERAPY

DEOXYNUCLEOTIDE METABOLISM OF HERPESVIRUS AND THE IMPLICATION IN CHEMOTHERAPY

YUNG-CHI CHENG, SUSAN P. GRILL, LOUISE M. NUTTER, KENNETH F. BASTOW, KARL B. FRANK, AND JWO-FARN CHIOU

Department of Pharmacology, School of Medicine, University of North Carolina, Chapel Hill, North Carolina, 27514, USA

Herpesviruses are DNA viruses. One of the prerequisites of virus replication is the continuous supply of deoxynucleotides for DNA synthesis. In order to ensure that there are sufficient deoxynucleotides in virus infected cells, severel host cellular enzymes will have to be functional or the virus will induce several enzymes to bypass the requirement of host enzymes. In the case of herpes simplex virus type 1 and type 2 (HSV-1 and HSV-2 respectively), these are thymidine kinase, ribonucleotide reductase, bifunctional DNase, dUTP pyrophosphatase, DNA polymerase, and Uracil DNA glycosylase (1). Their presence in virus infected cells could serve as the basis for devising strategies in designing selective antiviral compounds. The development of antiviral compounds based on virus specified thymidine kinase (2,3) and DNA polymerase (4,5) yielded several interesting antiviral compounds which are at different stages of clinical development. These are: fluoroiodoarabinosylcytosine (FIAC), fluoromethylarabinosyluracil (FMAU), bromovinyldeoxyuridine (BVdU), acyclovir (ACV), 2'-nor-2'-deoxyguanosine (DHPG) and phosphonoformic Acid (PFA). Since virus variants could arise as the natural consequence of virus DNA replication, it is conceivable that the resistant variants could be a common clinical problem, particularly in the future (6,7,8). Combinations of drugs with different sites of action or selection of compounds with multiple independent sites of action should be considered in antiviral chemotherapy in order to overcome the intrinsic heterogeneity of virus populations.

Several new targets are being considered for developing antiviral compounds. One of the proposed targets is viral induced ribonucleotide reductase. Ribonucleotide reductase is known to play a critical role in supplying deoxynucleotides de novo for DNA synthesis in uninfected cells, and it was assumed that it may play a similar role in virus infected cells. Genetic evidence seems to support such a hypothesis (9). Furthermore, the properties of viral induced ribonucleotide reductase are quite different from the host enzyme (10,11,12). Thus, attention was given by several groups in designing a selective inhibitor of this enzyme with the hope of it being a selective antiviral compound. Recently, we examined the functional role of this enzyme in HSV-2 infected cells. Greater than 95% of intracellular activity could be inhibited with a less than one log decrease of virus yield, and less than one fold alteration of deoxynucleotide pools (13). These studies were performed in culture employing proliferating cells as the host for HSV-2 infection. This observation raised the question of whether the development of selective inhibitors of virus ribonucleotide reductase is a viable approach in designing antiviral compounds. It could be argued that virus induced ribonucleotide reductase may play an important role in the viral reactivation process since neuron cells are the host for latent virus. This will require further exploration.

The physiological roles of virus induced DNase, dUTP pyrophosphotase and Uracil DNA-glycosylase are not clear at the present time. Virus induced DNase has both exonuclease and endonuclease activities (14). The product of exonuclease is 5'-dNMP which is the precursor for DNA synthesis (15,16). Thus, virus DNase may play a key role in virus infected cells in supplying deoxynucleotides for viral DNA synthesis by digesting host DNA. Its associated endonuclease activity is specific for supercoiled DNA (14). This unique property suggests its possible involvement in maturation of virus DNA. Uracil DNA-glycosylase, which removes uracil from DNA, is a key enzyme in the DNA repair mechanism. If uracil which resulted from the deamination of cytosine in the DNA, was not removed, point mutations or mistranscription at the point of deamination could occur. dUTP pyrophosphatase could selectively breakdown dUTP to dUMP. An effective pathway of removing dUTP in cells is critical, otherwise the incorporation of dUTP into DNA could lead to the disruption of DNA synthesis due to the presence of an apyrimidinic site resulting from the action of Uracil DNA-glycosylase. HSV-1 and HSV-2 are capable of inducing virus specific Uracil DNA-glycosylase and dUTP pyrophosphatase (17) which have different physical properties from the host enzyme. Furthermore, there was no host enzyme activity remaining in the cells eight hours post infection (17). These two viral induced enzymes may be worth further investigation as targets for developing antiviral compounds.

In summary, deoxynucleotide metabolism in virus infected cells is sufficiently different from that in uninfected cells. Inhibition of virus replication without damaging host DNA synthesis could be achieved by taking advantage of those differences.

REFERENCES

1. Cheng Y-C, Nakayama K, Derse D, Bastow K, Ruth J, Tan RS, Dutschman GE, Caradonna SJ, Grill S (1982) In: Shiota H, Cheng Y-C, Prusoff WH (eds) Herpesvirus, Clinical, Pharmacological and Basic Aspects. Excerpta Medica, Amsterdam-Oxford-Princeton, pp 47-56
2. Cheng Y-C (1977) Ann NY Acad Sci 184:594-598
3. Cheng Y-C (1984) In: Becker Y (ed) Antiviral Drugs and Interferon: The Molecular Basis of Their Activity. Martinus Nijhoff, Boston, pp 59-70

4. Cheng Y-C, Derse D, Frank K, Bastow K (1984) In: Becker Y (ed) Antiviral Drugs and Interferon: The Molecular Basis of Their Activity. Martinus Nijhoff, Boston, pp 117-126

5. Eriksson B, Oberg B (1984) In: Becker Y (ed) Antiviral Drugs and Interferon: The molecular Basis of Their Activity. Martinus Nijhoff, Boston, pp 127-142

6. Derse DD, Bastow KF, Cheng Y-C (1982) J Biol Chem 257:10252-10260

7. Bastow KF, Derse DD, Cheng Y-C (1983) Antimicrob Agents Chemother 23:914-917

8. Crumpacker CS, Schnipper IE, Marlowe SI, Kowalsky PN, Hershey BJ, Levin MJ (1982) N Engl J Med 306:343-346

9. Dutia BM (1983) J Gen Virol 64:513-521

10. Cohen GH (1972) J Virol 9:408-418

11. Ponce de Leon M, Eisenberg RJ, Cohen GH (1977) J Gen Virol 36:163-173

12. Averett DR, Lubberg C, Elion GB, Spector T (1983) J Biol Chem 258:9831-9838

13. Nutter LM, Grill SP, Cheng Y-C (1984) Biochem Pharm, In Press

14. Hoffman PJ, Cheng Y-C (1979) J Virol 32:449-457

15. Keir HM (1968) Mol Biol of Viruses 18:67-99

16. Hoffman PJ, Cheng Y-C (1978) J Biol Chem 253:3557-3562

17. Caradonna SJ, Cheng Y-C (1981) J Biol Chem 256:9834-9837

BIOCHEMISTRY AND PHARMACOLOGY OF ACYCLOVIR

Gertrude B. Elion
Wellcome Research Laboratories, Burroughs Wellcome Co., Research Triangle Park, NC 27709 (USA)

Acyclovir (9-(2-hydroxyethoxymethyl)guanine; ACV) is an analog of deoxyguanosine containing an acyclic side chain in place of the deoxyribose. This compound is highly inhibitory to the replication of herpes simplex viruses types 1 and 2 (HSV-1, HSV-2) with ID_{50} values = 0.1-1 μM, and to varicella zoster virus (VZV) with ID_{50} = 3-4 μM. On the other hand, it is non-toxic to uninfected Vero cells (ID_{50} = 300 μM) and to WI38 cells (ID_{50} > 3000 μM) which act as host cells for HSV and VZV respectively. Human cytomegalovirus (HCMV) is less sensitive than HSV or VZV (ID_{50} = 115 μM for strain, AD169) but more sensitive than the uninfected host WI38 cells (1-4).

The reason for the high selectivity of ACV for the herpesviruses HSV and VZV is the phosphorylation of ACV to a monophosphate (ACV-MP) by a virus-specified thymidine kinase. The large amount of ACV-MP formed in the virus-infected cell is then transformed to the diphosphate (ACV-DP) by cellular guanylate kinase and to the triphosphate (ACV-TP) by other cellular enzymes. It is the ACV-TP which is the true inhibitor of viral DNA synthesis by its action on the viral DNA polymerase. In uninfected cells, very little phosphorylation of ACV takes place even at high concentrations of drug; the enzyme responsible for this activity appears to be a 5'-nucleotidase (J.J. Fyfe, personal communication). The amount of ACV-TP formed in uninfected cells is very much lower than in HSV or VZV-infected cells at all concentrations of ACV.

The extent to which DNA polymerase is inhibited is a function not only of the amount of ACV-TP formed but also of the apparent inhibition constant, K_i, for the particular polymerase. Each virus specifies its own DNA polymerase and each is different from the cellular DNA polymerases. The K_i values used for Fig. 1 were determined in a cell-free system for DNA polymerases purified by passage through DEAE-cellulose and phosphocellulose columns and calculated from initial rates of the inhibited reactions. Since the template used was activated calf thymus DNA, not viral DNA, the K_i values may be considered valid only when compared relative to one another, but not as absolute values. The amounts of ACV-TP formed were determined by the high pressure liquid chromatography of extracts of virally infected and uninfected cells exposed to 100 μM or 1 μM ACV for 7 hours. The ratio of the amount of ACV-TP formed in a virally infected cell to the K_i value for that specific viral DNA polymerase determines the degree of inhibition of viral DNA replication (Fig. 1). In general, the viral DNA polymerases specified by HSV-1, HSV-2, VZV are much more sensitive to inhibition by ACV-TP than are the cellular DNA polymerases. The combination of high ACV-TP concentration and low K_i values for the viral DNA polymerases makes the ratio ACV-TP/K_i much higher than for uninfected cells. For Epstein-Barr virus (EBV) where no viral-specified TK is present, the amounts of ACV-TP is low. However, since the K_i for the EBV DNA polymerase is exceedingly low, inhibition of EBV replication occurs at low levels of ACV.

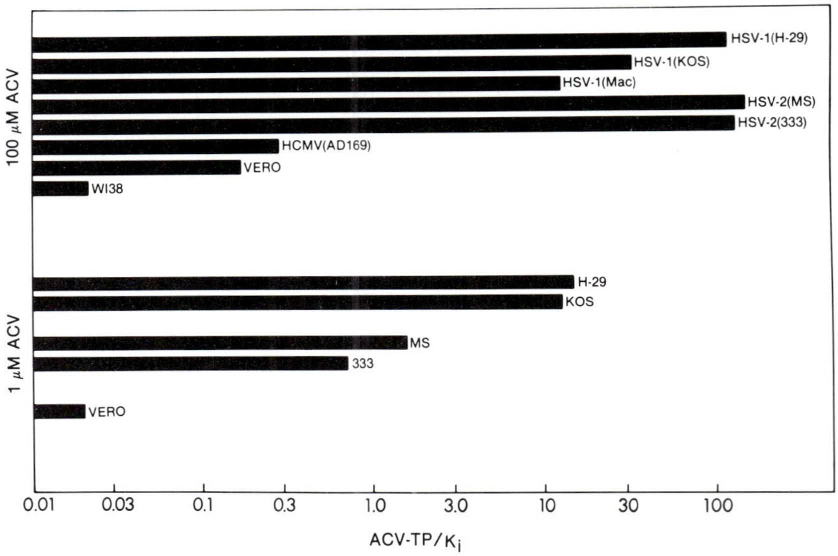

Fig. 1. Ratio of the concentration of ACV-TP to the K_i for the DNA polymerases of various viruses and cells (Reproduced from Ref. 4).

Another aspect of the inhibition of HSV replication by ACV-TP is the chain termination which occurs when HSV DNA polymerase uses ACV-TP as a substrate. If ACV is incorporated into a growing viral DNA chain, the chain is terminated, since there is no group on the side chain corresponding to the 3'-hydroxyl group of deoxyribose. Any viral DNA synthesized therefore consists of small fragments (4). Not only is the chain terminated, but the viral DNA polymerase becomes inactivated during the process. This inactivation of the DNA polymerase is essentially irreversible. If fresh DNA template and dGTP are added after the enzyme reaction has stopped, the reaction does not resume. If fresh enzyme is added, together with a large amount of dGTP to prevent further reaction with ACV-TP, the enzymatic polymerization proceeds again (5). Studies of the enzyme kinetics suggest that the first interaction of ACV-TP and enzyme is reversible and dGTP is competitive at this step. However, the ACV-TP-enzyme complex quickly change to an irreversible form, where dGTP can no longer compete and the enzyme becomes inactive. This inactivation does not occur with the cellular DNA polymerase α.

Many investigations on the absorption, distribution, and metabolic disposition of ACV in various species have been performed. The compound is metabolically stable in mice, rats, dogs and humans (6,7). In man only about 10% of the drug is metabolized to 9-carboxymethoxymethyl guanine, which is excreted in the urine together with unchanged ACV (7). The $t_{\frac{1}{2}}$ of ACV in human plasma is approximately 3 hours. It is best administered to man as one-hour infusions at 8 hour intervals to avoid high urinary concentrations which may produce crystalluria. The drug penetrates all tissues and the steady-state level in cerebrospinal fluid in man given ACV intravenously is about one-half the plasma level. The drug is cleared by renal excretion at 2 to 3 times glomerular filtration rate, indicating some tubular secretion in the kidney. The compound has no effect on the antibody response or on cellular immunity in animals. The extent of oral absorption of ACV varies in different species. The order of oral absorbability is dog $>$ mouse $>$ man $>$ rat $>$ monkey.

Extensive toxicological studies with ACV have been conducted in a variety of species. The compound has been found to be non-carcinogenic, non-teratogenic and to have no effect on reproduction or fertility in laboratory animals. The detailed toxicological studies have been reported in a group of 5 papers published in 1983 (8).

Although ACV administered orally to man can produce peak plasma levels of 8 μM, the limited oral absorption has made it necessary to give the drug at 4 hour intervals at doses ranging from 200-800 mg. It would obviously be desirable to have a more bioavailable form of the drug. Recently it has been found that a suitable pro-drug for ACV is 2-amino-9-(2-hydroxyethoxymethyl)purine (BW 515U). This compound is converted by xanthine oxidase _in vitro_, as well as _in vivo_, to ACV (9). In man BW 515U is extremely well absorbed orally and its conversion to ACV is essentially complete. Thus, plasma levels of ACV can be achieved with oral BW 515U which are the same as those obtained with intravenous ACV at the same dose level. This should greatly facilitate the treatment of out-patients. Clinical trials with pro-drug are currently in progress.

REFERENCES

1. Elion GB, Furman PA, Fyfe JA, de Miranda P, Beauchamp L, Schaeffer HS (1977) Proc Natl Acad Sci 74:5716-5720
2. Schaeffer HJ, Beauchamp L, de Miranda P, Elion GB, Bauer DJ, Collins P (1978) Nature 272:583-585
3. Elion GB (1982) Am J Med 73(1A):7-13
4. Elion GB (1983) J Antimicrob Chemotherapy 12 (Suppl B):9-17
5. Furman PA, St. Clair MH, Spector T (1984) J Biol Chem 259:9575-9579
6. de Miranda P, Krasny HC, Page DA, Elion GB (1982) Am J Med 73(1A):31-35
7. de Miranda P, Blum MB (1983) J Antimicrob Chemotherapy 12 (Suppl B):29-37
8. Tucker WE Jr et al(1983) Fundamental Applied Toxicol 3:559-602
9. Krenitsky TA, Hall WW, de Miranda P, Beauchamp LM, Schaeffer HJ, Whiteman PD (1984) Proc Natl Acad Sci 81:3209-3213

CLINICAL POTENTIALS OF BROMOVINYLDEOXYURIDINE (BVDU) : IN PARTICULAR FOR ORAL TREATMENT OF VARICELLA-ZOSTER VIRUS INFECTIONS IN CHILDREN WITH CANCER

E. DE CLERCQ[1], Y. BENOIT[2], G. LAUREYS[2] and M.J. DELBEKE[2]
[1]Rega Institute for Medical Research, University of Leuven, B-3000 Leuven, Belgium and [2]Department of Pediatrics, University of Ghent, B-9000 Ghent, Belgium.

(_E_)-5-(2-Bromovinyl)-2'-deoxyuridine (BVDU) is a highly potent and selective antiherpes agent (1). It is particularly effective against herpes simplex virus type 1 (HSV-1), varicella-zoster virus (VZV), suid herpesvirus type 1 (SHV-1), bovid herpesvirus type 1 (BHV-1) and simian varicella virus (SVV). In cell culture BVDU inhibits these viruses at a concentration of $\leqslant$ 0.01 µg/ml, that is a concentration which is at least 5000 times lower than the minimum concentration required to affect normal cell growth or metabolism. The prime determinant in the antiviral potency and selectivity of BVDU is the (_E_)-5-(2-bromovinyl) substituent at C-5 of the uracil ring. The _E_ ("Entgegen") configuration (or "upwards" position of bromine) is an essential feature in the antiviral activity, since the _Z_- ("Zusammen") isomer of BVDU with the bromine in the "downwards" position is about 100-fold less potent against HSV-1 than the _E_-isomer.

Herpes simplex virus type 2 (HSV-2) is markedly less sensitive to the inhibitory effects of BVDU than HSV-1. BVDU inhibits HSV-2 at a concentration of 1 - 10 µg/ml, that is 100 - 1000 times higher than the concentration required for the inhibition of HSV-1 replication. The differential sensitivity of HSV-1 and HSV-2 towards BVDU points to the usefulness of the drug as a probe for the identification of type 1 and type 2 HSV strains in clinical isolates, and BVDU is now widely used for this purpose.

The biochemical aspects of the mechanism of action of BVDU and other nucleoside analogues have been reviewed recently (2). The selective antiherpes activity of BVDU primarily depends on a specific phosphorylation by the virus-induced dThd (2'-deoxythymidine) kinase which converts the compound successively to its 5'-monophosphate (BVDUMP) and 5'-diphosphate (BVDUDP). Further phosphorylation of BVDUDP by a cellular kinase which has yet to be identified, yields BVDU 5'-triphosphate (BVDUTP) which can act as either inhibitor or substrate of the viral DNA polymerase. Since BVDU is specifically phosphorylated in the virus-infected cell, its incorporation into DNA will essentially be confined to the virus-infected cell, and within the HSV-1-infected cell, it is preferentially incorporated into viral DNA rather than cellular DNA.

A particular problem with BVDU is that, like all other 5-substituted 2'-deoxyuridines, it serves as an efficient substrate for pyrimidine nucleoside phosphorylases such as dThd phosphorylase (3) and Urd (uridine) phosphorylase, which cleave the N-glycosidic linkage of BVDU and thereby release the free pyrimidine base (E)-5-(2-bromovinyl)uracil (BVU). Due to this phosphorolytic cleavage, BVDU is rapidly cleared from the plasma, i.e. within 2-3 hours following its intraperitoneal administration to rats (4). In contrast with BVDU, BVU is cleared very slowly from the plasma where it is still detectable 24 hours after an intraperitoneal injection of BVDU.

The reason for the persistence of BVU in the plasma is that BVU, in contrast with other 5-substituted uracils, does not act as substrate for dihydrothymine dehydrogenase, which is responsible for the first step in the degradative pathway of pyrimidines (5). Injection of dUrd, dThd or any other 5-substituted dUrd (5-X-dUrd) at 3 hours after the injection of BVDU, that is at a time when BVDU has disappeared completely from the circulation, results in the re-apparition of BVDU in the plasma (4). This regeneration is apparently accomplished by a deoxyribosyl transfer catalyzed by pyrimidine nucleoside phosphorylases : BVU + 5-X-dUrd → BVDU + 5-X-uracil. This is a unique example of the regeneration of an active antiviral drug from its inactive metabolite in vivo. Other antiviral drugs such as adenine arabinoside (ara-A) and cytosine arabinoside (ara-C), cannot be reconverted to their active form after they have been catabolized to their metabolites, hypoxanthine arabinoside (ara-Hx) and uracil arabinoside (ara-U) respectively.

Not only can the phosphorolytic cleavage of BVDU to BVU be reversed, it can also be inhibited, i.e. by previous administration of 6-aminothymine, an inhibitor of pyrimidine nucleoside phosphorylases (5); and even totally prevented if the sugar moiety of BVDU is replaced by a cyclopentane ring (6). The resulting C-BVDU, or carbocyclic analogue of BVDU, is completely resistant to degradation by dThd phosphorylase and Urd phosphorylase (7), and in cell culture it is only slightly (about 5-fold) less potent against HSV-1 than BVDU. Further studies on the in vivo efficacy and pharmacokinetics of C-BVDU are warranted to assess its therapeutic potentials.

From a clinical viewpoint (8), BVDU has been pursued for the (i) topical treatment (0.1 % eye drops) of herpetic keratitis, (ii) systemic treatment (7.5 mg/kg/day for 5 days, orally) of mucocutaneous HSV-1 infections in immunocompromised patients (i.e. bone-marrow transplant recipients), (iii) systemic treatment (7.5 mg/kg/day for 5 days, orally) of severe herpes zoster in cancer patients, (iv) systemic treatment (7.5 mg/kg/day for 5 days, orally) of ophthalmic zoster in the elderly, and (v) systemic treatment (15 mg/kg/day for 5 days, orally) of VZV infections in children with cancer. These clinical studies have so far been conducted on an open (not placebo-controlled) basis and should therefore be interpreted with caution, but, as they stand, the results suggest that BVDU holds great promise for the treatment of HSV-1 and VZV infections.

Topical treatment of dendritic corneal ulcers, geographic corneal ulcers or stromal herpetic keratitis with BVDU 0.1 % eye drops led to a rapid resolution of the lesions, even in those patients that did not respond to other antiviral drugs such as idoxuridine (IDU), trifluridine (TFT), vidarabine (ara-A) or acyclovir (9). Similarly, combined treatment of BVDU 0.1 % eye drops with oral BVDU at 7.5 mg/kg/day for 5 days led to a prompt healing of keratouveitis and skin lesions in patients with ophthalmic zoster (9).

When BVDU was administered orally at 7.5 mg/kg/day for 5 days to cancer patients with severe localized or disseminated herpes zoster, progression of the infection, as based on the formation of new lesions, was arrested within 1-3 days of starting treatment (10), and a similar favorable response was noted in children with cancer who were treated with oral BVDU (at 15 mg/kg/day for 5 days) for an intercurrent varicella or zoster episode (11). Our experience with BVDU in the oral treatment of VZV infections in children with cancer is further documented in the present report.

From June 1980 to April 1984, 26 children with an intercurrent VZV infection and under antimitotic treatment for a malignant disorder were admitted to the University Hospital of Ghent. The diagnosis of varicella or zoster was based upon the presence of typical papulo-vesicular lesions. The diagnosis was confirmed by isolation of VZV from the vesicle fluid and/or a significant increase in the titer of specific VZV-antibodies following infection. BVDU was administered orally at 15 mg/kg body weight for 5 days, in 2 or 3 doses per day. Sixteen children had acute lymphoblastic leukemia (ALL) and 10 children had a malignant disease other than ALL : 5 of those had a malignant lymphoma, 4 children had a solid tumor and 1 child had histiocytosis X (type Hand-Schüller-Christian).

Fourteen of the 16 children with ALL were in complete remission at the moment of the VZV infection; 6 of these 14 were under polychemotherapy regimens and 8 were under maintenance therapy; 2 children were in active relapse while under polychemotherapy. Eight of the 16 children with ALL had varicella; the other eight had zoster. Seven of the 8 children had zoster in the craniocervical region. This localization seems to be related to radiotherapy of the skull. Five of the 8 children with ALL and varicella only had mucocutaneous lesions; the 3 other children also had signs of visceral or central nervous system (CNS) involvement. Three children had clinical and serological evidence of hepatitis; 2 of these 3 patients also had serious CNS problems with subcoma and convulsions. The 8 children with ALL and zoster had no signs of systemic involvement.

The duration of the lesions in the eight ALL patients with varicella ranged from 1 to 4 days (mean : 1.3). Upon BVDU treatment, new lesions ceased to develop within 2-7 days (mean : 4.0) and all children, including the 2 children with hepatitis and encephalitis and one child with pneumonitis, recovered completely.

The duration of the lesions in the eight ALL patients with zoster ranged from 1 to 9 days (mean : 3.3). Upon BVDU treatment new lesions ceased to develop within 1-5 days (mean : 2.6). All children, including the 2 children in relapse of their leukemia, recovered completely. One child had a recurrence of zoster more than 2 years after the first zoster episode. Oral BVDU was given again and the child recovered completely.

Of the 10 children with a malignant disease other than ALL, nine were in remission; 6 of these 9 children were under intensive chemotherapy. Six of the 10 children had varicella; the other four had zoster. None of these children had signs of visceral or CNS involvement.

The duration of the lesions in the six non-ALL patients with varicella ranged from 1 to 3 days (mean : 1.3). Upon BVDU treatment, new lesions ceased to develop within 3-4 days (mean : 3.3) and all children recovered completely.

The duration of the lesions in the four non-ALL patients with zoster ranged from 1 to 7 days (mean : 5.5). Upon BVDU treatment, new lesions ceased to develop within 1-3 days (mean : 2.0) and all four children recovered completely.

No toxic side effects could be attributed to BVDU treatment. Blood urea and creatinine were normal before, during and after treatment. Seven children had serum transaminase abnormalities before BVDU treatment was started. The serum transaminase levels normalized in all patients after BVDU treatment.

In conclusion, all twenty-six patients including those with visceral complications, recovered completely from their VZV infection without sequelae. Severe complications as often seen in patients with an hematopoietic malignancy were not encountered in any of the children treated with BVDU. BVDU seemed to arrest progress of the VZV infection and to promote rapid recovery. The treatment regimen was well tolerated by all children and no toxic side effects could be attributed to the drug. Unambiguous proof of the efficacy of BVDU has to be provided by double-blind controlled trials.

REFERENCES

1. De Clercq E (1984) J Antimicrob Chemother 14 (Suppl A):85-95
2. De Clercq E (1984) Biochem Pharmacol 14:2159-2169
3. Desgranges C, Razaka G, Rabaud M, Bricaud H, Balzarini J, De Clercq E (1983) Biochem Pharmacol 32:3583-3590
4. Desgranges C, Razaka G, Drouillet F, Bricaud H, Herdewijn P, De Clercq E (1984) Nucleic Acids Res 12:2081-2090
5. Desgranges C, Razaka G, Bricaud H, De Clercq E (1984) Biochem Pharmacol, submitted
6. Herdewijn P, De Clercq E, Balzarini J, Vanderhaeghe H (1984) J Med Chem, submitted
7. De Clercq E, Desgranges C, Herdewijn P, Sim IS, Walker RT (1984) Proceedings of the VIIIth International Symposium on Medicinal Chemistry, held in Uppsala, Sweden, August 27-31, 1984
8. De Clercq E (1984) Eur J Clin Microbiol 3:96-107
9. Maudgal PC, De Clercq E, Missotten L (1984) Antiviral Res, in press
10. Wildiers J, De Clercq E (1984) Eur J Cancer Clin Oncol 20:471-476
11. Benoit Y, Laureys G, Delbeke M-J, De Clercq E (1984) Eur J Pediatrics, in press

ANTIVIRAL ACTIVITIES OF SOME NEWER 2'-FLUORO-5-SUBSTITUTED ARABINOSYLPYRIMIDINE NUCLEOSIDES

J. J. FOX,* K. A. WATANABE,* R.F. SCHINAZI,[§] and C. LOPEZ*

Sloan Kettering Institute/Memorial Sloan-Kettering Cancer Center, NY, NY* and Emory University School of Medicine/Veterans Administration Medical Center, Atlanta, GA,[§] U.S.A.

Of several 2'-fluoro-5-substituted-arabinosylpyrimidine nucleosides synthesized in our laboratory (2), FIAC [2'-fluoro-5-iodo-ara-C] has demonstrated clinical efficacy against Herpesvirus infections in both Phase 1 (3) and Phase 2 (4) clinical trials in host compromised patients. The corresponding thymine analog [FMAU or 2'-fluoro-5-methyl-ara-U] was found to be more potent in mice infected with HSV-1 (5) or with HSV-2 (6) without toxicity at effective dose levels. FMAU was also found to be active in vitro and in vivo against P815 and L1210 leukemic cell lines resistant to cytosine arabinoside [Ara-C] (7,8). A Phase 1 trial of FMAU in patients with advanced cancer showed that drug-induced central nervous system dysfunction was the dose-limiting toxicity. Because of the potent and selective antiviral activity of FMAU, future trials using low doses of this drug in immunosuppressed patients with Herpesvirus infections are under consideration (9).

With FIAC and FMAU as lead compounds, we have extended our synthetic efforts to the preparation of various 2'-fluoro-ara-uracil (10) and -ara-cytosine (11) nucleoside analogs of the reported antiviral (12), 5-(E)-(2-bromovinyl)-2'-deoxyuridine [BVDU]. The 5-ethyl analogs of FMAU and of FMAC, namely FEAU and FEAC, were also synthesized (10,11).

The in vitro activities of these newer analogs against HSV (strain F) and against HSV-2 (strain G) are given in Table 1. It is noteworthy that the 2'-fluoro-5-halovinyl derivatives in both the uracil and cytosine series are about 4- to 20-fold more effective than BVDU against HSV-2. In these in vitro assays, the 5-iodovinyl analog of 2'-fluoro-ara-C was ~10-fold less cytotoxic to the host vero cells than FIAC.

With the 5-methyl- and 5-ethyl-substituted uracil nucleosides, FMAU and FEAU, both showed better therapeutic indices than the corresponding cytosine analogs, FMAC and FEAC. The 5-methyl-substituted analogs [FMAC and FMAU] were more effective but also more toxic than the corresponding ethyl analogs [FEAC and FEAU]. [We have found recently (13) that if the 5-alkyl substituents are extended to 3 carbon atoms or longer, the antiviral activity of the resultant compounds are severely diminished or completely abolished]. In these in vitro assays (Table 1), FEAU (though less potent than FMAU) was the least toxic and gave

TABLE 1.

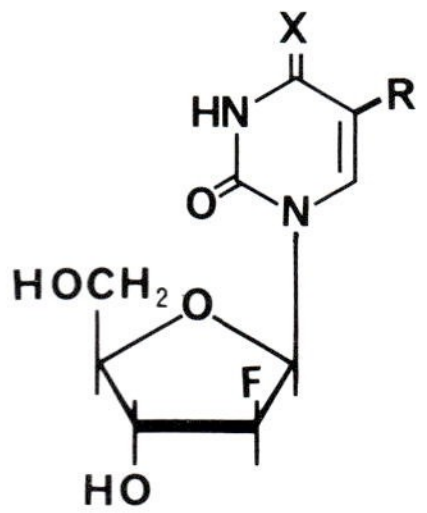

ANTIVIRAL ACTIVITY OF SOME 2'-FLUOROARABINOSYL PYRIMIDINE NUCLEOSIDES IN PLAQUE REDUCTION ASSAYS IN VERO CELLS

X	R	HSV-1 (F)*		HSV-2 (G)*			THER. INDEX (ID_{50}/ED_{90})	
		ED_{50} (μM)	ED_{90} (μM)	ED_{50} (μM)	ED_{90} (μM)	ID_{50} (μM)†	HSV-1	HSV-2
NH	FIAC	0.023	0.048	0.03	0.08	21.7	452	271
NH	FMAC	0.006	0.048	0.026	0.10	1.5	31	15
NH	FEAC	0.035	0.57	0.32	4.9	143	251	29
NH	(E)-CH-CHBr	0.068	0.52	0.037	4.5	23	44	5
NH	(E)-CH=CHI	0.088	0.74	0.027	2.3	>200	>270	>87
O	FMAU	0.010	0.042	0.023	0.09	2.8	67	31
O	FEAU	0.024	0.26	0.24	0.91	>200	>769	>220
O	(E)-CH=CHBr	0.067	0.47	0.13	0.73	101	215	138
O	(E)-CH=CHI	0.037	0.11	0.15	0.84	56	509	67
	BVDU	0.019	0.062	0.23	17.0	191	3081	11

*Correlation coefficient ≥ 0.86.

†Cytotoxic effect measured in rapidly dividing cells.

excellent therapeutic indices against HSV-1 and HSV-2.

Preliminary in vivo studies giving comparative antiviral effects of FEAU with FMAU and 5-ethyl-2'-deoxyuridine [EDU] in mice inoculated intracerebrally with HSV-2 are shown in Table 2. FEAU was active at 50 mg/kg per day and at doses of 100-200 mg/kg per day was highly effective in reducing mortality in these mice. At these dose levels no toxicity was observed. In normal mice, FEAU was nontoxic at doses of 800 mg/kg per day given twice daily for 4 days.

As shown in Table 2, EDU (which differs structurally from FEAU only by the absence of the 2'-fluoro substituent) is much less effective than FEAU in this HSV-2 system. This finding is consistent with our previous

TABLE 2.

COMPARATIVE ANTIVIRAL EFFECTS OF FEAU WITH FMAU AND EDU IN MICE INOCULATED INTRACEREBRALLY WITH HSV-2 (STRAIN G)

TREATMENT	DOSE* MG/KG/DAY	MDD**	% SURVIVORS
NEG CONTROL (NO VIRUS)		-	100
PBS (VIRUS CONTROL)		6.7	7
FEAU	10	9.4	8
"	50	11.8	25
"	100	11.0	72
"	200	(14)#	93
FMAU	0.5	9.4	67
EDU	800	7.6	13
"	1000	8.6	33

* Given 5 hr after intracerebral inoculation, dose schedule, twice a day for 4 days. 12-15 Animals used at each dose level.

** Calculated on Day 21.

\# Numbers in parentheses indicate death of a single animal.

observation (2) attesting to the importance of the 2'-fluoro substituent for anti-HSV activity exhibited by these arabinofuranosyl pyrimidine nucleosides.

It had been concluded previously (6) that FMAU was a most potent and selective antiviral compound for the treatment of mouse encephalitis caused by HSV-2 and therefore deserved consideration as a potential agent in human trials for the treatment of HSV encephalitis in neonates and adults. The preliminary data described herein for FEAU suggest that this compound may also be worthy of similar consideration.

REFERENCES

1. Supported in part by funds from The National Cancer Institute (Grant No. CA-08748, CA-18601 and CA-18856) and from The National Institute of Allergy and Infectious Diseases (Grant No. AI 18600) (R.F.S.) and The Veterans Administration (R.F.S.)

2. Watanabe KA, Reichman U, Hirota K, Lopez C, Fox JJ (1979) J Med Chem 22: 21-24

3. Young CW, Schneider R, Leyland-Jones B, Armstrong D, Tan CTC, Lopez C, Watanabe KA, Fox JJ, Philips FS (1983) Cancer Res 43:5006-5009

4. Leyland-Jones B, Donnelly H, Myskowski P, Donner A, Groshen S, Lopez C, Armstrong D, Young CW, Fox JJ (1983) AFCR Publications. Clin Res 31:369A

5. Fox JJ, Lopez C, Watanabe KA (1981) In: De las Heras FG (ed) Medicinal Chemistry Advances, Pergamon Press, New York, pp 27-40

6. Schinazi RF, Peters J, Sokol MK, Nahmias AJ (1983) Antimicrob Agents Chemother 24:95-103

7. Burchenal JH, Chou T-C, Lokys L, Smith RS, Watanabe KA, Su T-L, Fox JJ (1982) Cancer Res 42:2598-2600

8. Chou T-C, Burchenal JH, Schmid FA, Braun TJ, Su T-L, Watanabe KA, Fox JJ, Philips FS (1982) Cancer Res 42:3957-3963

9. Fanucchi MP, Leyland-Jones B, Young CW, Burchenal JH, Watanabe KA, Fox JJ (1985) Cancer Treat Rep (in press)

10. Watanabe KA, Su T-L, Reichman U, Greenberg N, Lopez C, Fox JJ (1984) J Med Chem 27:91-94

11. Perlman ME, Watanabe KA, Schinazi RF, Fox JJ (1985) J Med Chem (in press)

12. De Clercq E, Balzarini J, Descamps J, Huang GF, Torrence PF, Bergstrom DE, Jones AS, Serafinowski P, Verhelst G, Walker RT (1982) Mol Pharmacol 21:217-223

13. Watanabe KA, Su T-L, Schinazi RF, Fox JJ, unpublished results

Herpes Viruses and Virus Chemotherapy, R. Kono, editor

PRECLINICAL INVESTIGATIONS OF FIAU, AN ANTI-HERPES AGENT

C. McLAREN, M. S. CHEN, R. H. BARBHAIYA, R. A. BUROKER, F. B. OLESON
Bristol-Myers Company, Syracuse, New York 13221-4755

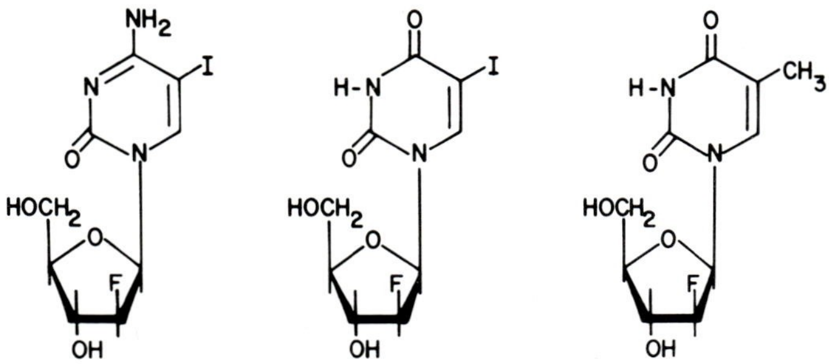

FIAC FIAU FMAU

FIAU, FIAC and FMAU were three of a series of nucleoside analogs prepared by Fox and Watanabe (1) that Bristol-Myers has examined as antivirals. The anti-herpes virus activity for these compounds (2) was confirmed in studies carried out in association with the NIAID Antiviral Substances Program contractors. A summary of these data (Table 1) shows similar activities of the compounds against herpes simplex 1 and 2, with greater activity against varicella zoster and cytomegaloviruses than with acyclovir.

TABLE 1
COMPARATIVE ANTIVIRAL ACTIVITY OF NUCLEOSIDE ANALOGS

	ID_{50} (mcg/ml)			
	FIAC	FIAU	FMAU	ACV
HSV-1	0.09	0.05	0.04	0.04
HSV-2	0.15	0.12	0.05	0.05
VZV	0.10	0.24	0.02	8.00
CMV	1.3	2.6	2.2	38

In vivo studies, principally those of Dr. E. Kern of the Antiviral Substances Program, showed that the protective activities of FIAC and FIAU were essentially the same in a number of models for HSV infections (i.p. and genital infections of mice or guinea pigs with either HSV-1 or HSV-2, with either p.o. or i.p. dosing of the test compound starting at varying times after infection). With both FIAC and FIAU treatment of a systemic HSV-2 infection of mice with 160 mg/kg/day for 5 days could be delayed as long as 48h p.i. and still produce a significant reduction in mortality. In such studies FMAU was effective at lower doses than were FIAU or FIAC.

The observation of CNS toxicity in man at 32 mg of FMAU/m^2/day by Memorial Sloan-Kettering Clinical Center workers reduced the priority of FMAU. Clinical studies of FIAC by the same group showed that after either oral or i.v. administration of FIAC, it was rapidly and almost totally deaminated to FIAU. These results, in conjunction with the equivalency in antiviral activities of FIAC and FIAU, led Bristol-Myers to choose FIAU as the compound for clinical development.

Pharmacokinetic studies with FIAU were performed in beagle dogs (Table 2). Oral absorption was good, with approximately 80% bioavailability after dosing with 10 mg/kg. The half-life was similar after both oral and intravenous administration.

TABLE 2
PHARMACOKINETICS OF FIAU IN BEAGLE DOGS* (10 mg/kg)

Route	Cmax (mcg/ml)	Tmax (hr)	AUC (mcg/ml/hr)	Half-life (hr)
i.v.	11.0	0.05	21.9	1.6
p.o.	10.8	0.33	18.71	1.7

*cross-over study with 3 animals

Toxicology studies were performed in mice, rats and monkeys. In acute single dose lethality studies, FIAU showed little toxicity after oral or intravenous dosing (oral LD_{50} = >3000 mg/kg rats; >1000 mg/kg monkeys; i.v. LD_{50} = >800 mg/kg rats; >1000 mg/kg monkeys).

Subsequent protracted dosing studies in rats and monkeys, however, showed significantly greater toxicity. The findings in animals dosed for four weeks, and residual toxicity observed after a six-week observation period, were of a late-onset type found with radiomimetic drugs and included myelosuppression and bone marrow depletion. Non-reversible cardiotoxicity occurred with higher doses of FIAU (Table 3).

TABLE 3

FIAU INTRAVENOUS TOXICOLOGY STUDIES (4 WEEKS DOSING - 6 WEEKS RECOVERY)

	Rats	Cynomolgus Monkeys
Doses (mg/kg/day)	500, 250, 50, 25, 10	150, 75, 25
Toxicity		
death	500	150, 75
myelosuppression		150, 75
lymphoid depletion	500, 250, 50	150, 75
bone marrow depletion	500	
enteropathy		150, 75
nephrotoxicity		150
testicular atrophy	500	
testicular giant cell		150
cardiotoxicity	500	150
Present after 6-wk recovery		
cardiac fibrosis	500, 250	150
decreased spermatogenesis	500	
No effect dose	25 mg/kg/day	25 mg/kg/day

In vitro confluent monolayers of Vero cells showed no measurable toxic effects following exposure to concentrations as high as 100 mcg/ml for 72 hr. However, Vero cells seeded at low densities ($2x10^4$ cells/ml) and in active growth phase, showed a 50% inhibition in growth after 72 hr incubation in the presence of 18 mcg/ml of FIAU drug. Only cultures exposed to less than the IC_{50} resumed normal growth after removal of the drug at 72 hr. This cytostatic effect is shown in Fig. 2.

CYTOTOXITY OF FIAU ON VERO CELLS

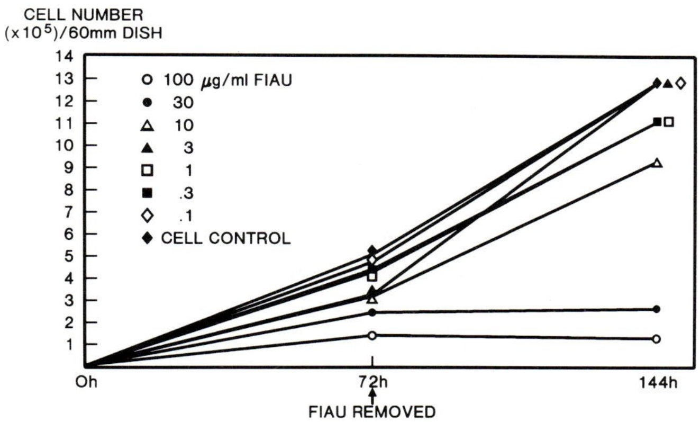

In most genetic toxicology studies FIAU and ACV gave similar results (Table 4). The results of the TK mouse lymphoma (mammalian gene mutation assay) were classed as inconclusive in that FIAU appeared to have a selective toxicity for the TK^+ cell population.

TABLE 4
FIAU GENETIC TOXICOLOGY STUDIES

Test	Endpoint	Results FIAU	ACV
Ames/ Salmonella	microbial gene mutation	Neg. (up to 3.5 mg/ml)	Neg. (up to 300 mg/ml)
Mouse lymphoma (TK)	mammalian gene mutation	inconclusive (0.1-6 mcg/ml)	Pos. (500-5000 mcg/ml)
Chinese hamster (HGPRT)	mammalian gene mutation	Neg. (7-7700 mcg/ml)	Neg. (16-4930 mcg/ml)
in vivo cytogenetics	chromosome aberrations	Neg. (100-1000 mg/kg)	Pos. (500 mg/kg)
BALB/c-3T3 in vitro transformation	neoplastic morphologic transformation	Pos. (0.1-1.0 mcg/ml)	Pos. (50 & 100 mcg/ml)

The mechanism of action of FIAU is dependent on viral thymidine kinase (TK). Kinetic studies (Table 5) showed that the initial phosphorylation of the fluorinated pyrimidines would occur more efficiently with viral rather than cellular TK, with FIAC having the lowest affinity for cellular TK.

TABLE 5

KINETIC CONSTANTS OF NUCLEOSIDE ANALOGS FOR VIRAL AND CELLULAR THYMIDINE KINASES

	Km(mcM)	Ki (mcM)				
Thymidine Kinase	Thd	FIAU	FMAU	FIAC	IUdR	ACV
Vero Cell	0.53	53	60	7080	0.38	4920[a]
HSV-1	0.14	0.14	0.18	0.11	0.11	45
HSV-2	0.68	0.95	1.40	2.42	0.25	180

[a]At saturating concentration of ACV, no inhibition could be detected.

The monophosphates of FIAU and FMAU had better affinities for cellular thymidylate kinase than for HSV thymidine/thymidylate kinases (Table 6). FIAC monophosphate (FIAC-MP), however, had poor affinity for either Vero or HSV enzymes and did not appear to be a substrate for any of the enzymes studied. Previous studies have shown that after exposure of cells to ^{14}C-FIAC, FIAU, not FIAC, was incorporated into cellular DNA (3). We have also found that FIAU-MP was the major component detected in such cells. Thus FIAC itself is unlikely to be the antiviral agent, but rather it is its deamination product FIAU which is converted to the inhibitory triphosphate.

TABLE 6

KINETIC CONSTANTS FOR THYMIDYLATE KINASE PURIFIED FROM VERO, HSV-1 AND HSV-2-INFECTED LMTK^{-} CELLS

Enzyme		Monophosphate Derivative (ki, mcM)			
Source	Thymidylate (Km,mcM)	FIAU	FMAU	FIAC	IUdR
Vero Cell	4.1	1.4	0.3	>900[a]	15.5
HSV-1	15.8	132	495	320[b]	13
HSV-2	77.0	114	195	1125[b]	NT[c]

[a]No inhibition could be detected at this concentration.
[b]Non-competitive inhibition against thymidylate.
[c]Not tested.

In summary, FIAU was chosen for clinical development over FIAC based on toxicological and mechanism of action studies. The findings of cardiotoxicity at high doses and dose-limiting myelosuppression are of concern and deserve further consideration.

REFERENCES

1. Watanabe KA, Reichman U, Hirota K, Lopez C, Fox JJ (1979) J Med Chem 23:21-24.
2. Lopez C, Watanabe KA, Fox JJ (1980) Antimicrob Agents Chemother 17:803-806.
3. Grant AJ, Feinberg A, Chou T, Watanabe KA, Fox JJ, Philips FS (1982) Biochem Pharmacol 31:1103-1108.

BROMOVINYL-ARABINOSYLURACIL (BV-ARAU) : ANTIVIRAL ACTIVITY AND PHARMACOLOGY

HARUHIKO MACHIDA, SHINJI SAKATA AND KENICHI SAITO
Research Laboratories, Yamasa Shoyu Co. Ltd., Choshi, Japan

INTRODUCTION

1-β-D-Arabinofuranosyl-*E*-5-(2-bromovinyl)uracil (BV-araU) was shown to be one of the most potent and selective inhibitors of replication of HSV-1 (1), which was originally synthesized in our laboratories in 1980 (2). Since BV-araU is one of thymidine analogues, one could expect its antiviral activity against the DNA viruses which induce viral specific thymidine kinase after infection, such as HSV and VZV. The structural formula of BV-araU (Fig. 1) is similar to that of *E*-5-(2-bromovinyl)-2'-deoxyuridine (BVDU). In BV-araU deoxyribose moiety of BVDU is replaced by arabinose. Thus, BV-araU might be considered to be a congener of BVDU. However, we have found some differences between BV-araU and BVDU in their antiviral activity and pharmacological action. We also compared BV-araU with other representative antiherpetic compounds for their in vitro antiviral activity.

MATERIALS AND METHODS

In vitro antiviral activity

Human embryonic lung fibroblast cells (HEL-F cells) were employed for in vitro studies on antiviral activity. A plaque reduction assay was employed for determination of both anti-HSV and anti-VZV activities. Three strains of each HSV-1 and HSV-2 and 10 strains of VZV were employed in this assay. Fifty per cent plaque depression dose (PD_{50}) was determined graphically. The PD_{50} values of the compounds are presented as the average of 2 to 4 separate experiments.

In vivo antiviral activity

Groups of 4-week-old male albino Jcl:ICR Swiss mice were infected intracerebrally with 6 LD_{50} of HSV-1. The infected mice were treated with drug twice daily for 4.5 days and observed daily for 3 weeks for death. The differences in mortality and the mean survival time of control and drug-treated groups were evaluated by χ square test with Yate correction and Student't *t*-test, respectively.

Determination of blood and urine drug concentrations

A single dose of 100 mg/kg of BV-araU or BVDU was administrated to groups of 3 adult Swiss mice. The mice were bled with a heparinized syringe at appropriate times after administration. The concentration of the test compounds in the plasma was determined by a high performance liquid chromatograph (HPLC) equipped with an anion-exchange resine, μBondapak C18. To examine urinary clearence of drug, the groups of 3 or 4 mice were housed in metabolism cages, and urines were collected. The concentration of drugs in urine was determined by HPLC.

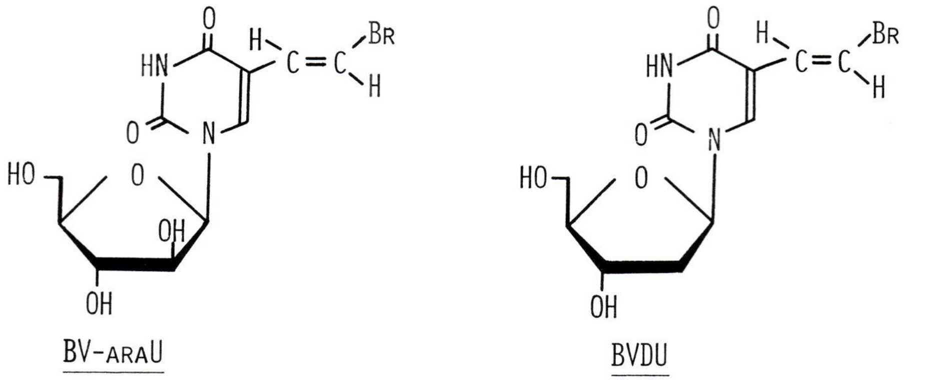

Fig. 1 Structural formula of BV-araU and BVDU

RESULTS

In vitro antiviral activity

For BV-araU and various other thymidine analogues, the PD_{50} values for both HSV-1 and HSV-2 were determined (Table 1). The anti-HSV-1 activity of BV-araU and its analogues was a little higher than that of ACV, and comparable to that of BVDU, FIAC and FMAU. However, FIAC, FMAU and ACV were highly active against HSV-2, whereas the halogenovinyl derivatives were not. In addition, BV-araU was highly effective against HSV isolates serologically identified to type 1.

Figure 2 shows the results of typical experiment on inhibition of plaque formation of VZV by BV-araU and BVDU. BV-araU inhibited plaque formation of all 10 strains tested more than 50% even at a concentration as low as 1 ng/ml. BVDU was also effective against VZV, but its PD_{50} values were 1 to 26 ng/ml, indicating that it was less active than BV-araU. FIAC and FMAU were relatively effective (comparable to BVDU), but ACV was much less active than these compounds (the PD_{50} values were 0.11 to 1.12 µg/ml).

In vivo antiviral activity

As shown previously (3), multiple intravenous (i.v.) doses of 50 or 200 mg/kg of BV-araU proved capable of increasing the mean survival time and decreasing the final mortality of the infected mice with statistical significance. Peroral (p.o.) treatment with BV-araU was also effective against the experimental encephalitis. The treatment with 12.5 or 25 mg/kg of BV-araU was effective in increasing the mean survival time, and that of 50 or 200 mg/kg was effective in both incerasing the mean survival time and decreasing the final mortality. Survivors per total in the two treated groups were 7/20 and 13/20, respectively, whereas it was 1/20 in the control group. The efficacy of oral and i.v. treatment with BV-araU was found to be comparable to that with BVDU.

TABLE I

ANTI-HSV ACTIVITY OF SEVERAL THYMIDINE ANALOGUES

Compound	50% plaque depression dose (μg/ml)					
	HSV-1			HSV-2		
	VR-3	CHR-3	MP	MS	UW-268	HG-52
BV-araU	0.010	0.014	0.006	7.3	11.7	26.3
CV-araU	0.018	0.022	0.017	19.5	8.4	26.6
IV-araU	0.014	0.016	0.005	4.3	4.2	18.0
BV-araUMP	0.013	0.011	0.005	15.0	15.1	26.9
IDU	0.28	0.40	0.66	1.95	6.1	6.2
BVDU	0.017	0.014	0.011	10.8	15.0	5.8
ACV	0.041	0.049	0.020	0.11	0.051	0.029
FIAC	0.013	0.015	0.008	0.019	0.011	0.023
FMAU	0.005	0.006	0.003	0.011	0.007	0.013

Blood concentration and urinary excretion in mice

The elimination half-life of BV-araU in blood of mice after either i.v. or p.o. administration was about 2.5 h. BV-araU was detected in the circulation of all mice as late as 8 h and 12 h after i.v. and p.o. administrations, respectively. When BVDU was administrated into mice, considerable amounts of BV-uracil, a metabolite of BVDU, were found in the plasma. The hafl-life of BVDU in the blood was 0.47 h and 1.74 h upon i.v. and p.o. administrations, respectively.

Urinary recoveries of BV-araU were about 60% and 28% after i.v. and p.o. adminstrations, respectively. Any identyfied metabolites were not found in the urine. In contrast with BV-araU, the urinary recovery of BVDU, including BV-uracil, was less than that of BV-araU. Only 28% of BVDU was recovered from 0 - 12 urines after i.v. administration. Neither BVDU nor BV-uracil was detected in the 12 - 24 urines. This rapid cxcretion confirms the rapid decrease of blood concentration of BVDU.

Toxicological study

In preliminary toxicological studies, BV-araU was found to exhibit little, if any, toxicity for mice and rats. Upon i.p. administration, the LD_{50} values of BV-araU for mice and rats were about 3,000 and more than 4,000 mg/kg, respectively. Upon other injection routes no lethal effect was observed at the limited administration doses (upon s.c. route; 5 g/kg and p.o. route; 10 g/kg). The LD_{50} value of BVDU upon i.p. administration for mice was estimated to be 1,466 mg/kg. This shows that BV-araU was significantly less toxic than BVDU. In addition, BV-araU did not exhibited mutagenicity against Bacillus subtilis. Mitomycin C, used as possitive control, showed mutagenicity in the same assay.

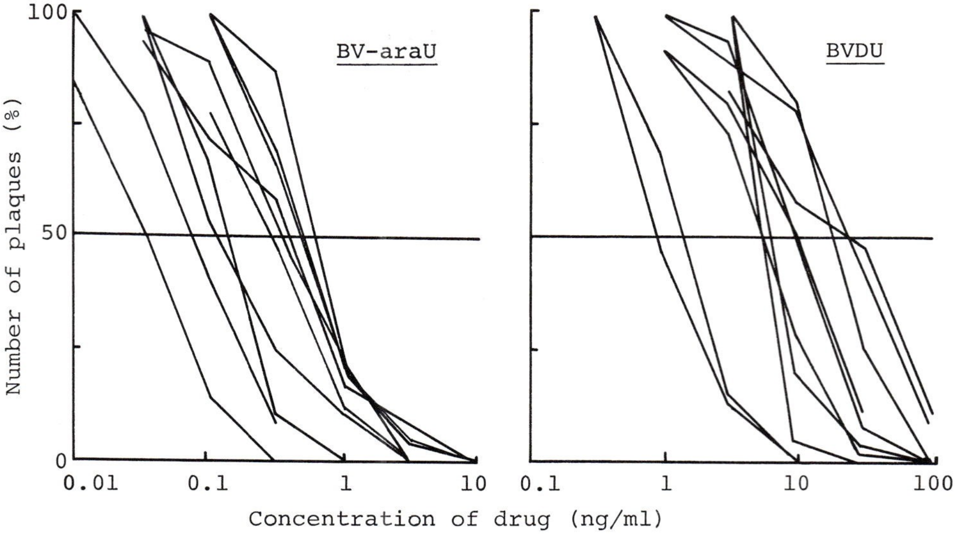

Fig. 2. Inhibition of plaque formation of VZV by BV-araU and BVDU

DISCUSSION

Antiviral activity of BV-araU against HSV was similar to that of BVDU. However, anti-VZV activity of BV-araU was considerably higher than that of BVDU, which was reported to be the most effective against experimental simian varicella (4). Dr. Soike and co-workers have found that intramuscular and p.o. treatments with BV-araU are highly effective in prevention of viremia in the simian varicella (5).

In the estimation of blood concentration and urinary excretion of BV-araU, we found that BV-uracil was detected neither in the plasma nor in the urine of mice into which BV-araU was administrated. BV-araU seems to be resistant to pyrimidine nucleoside phosphorylase. This contrasts with BVDU, because considerable amounts of BV-uracil was found in both the plasma and urine after administration of BVDU. As seen in rats (6), BV-uracil may be enzymatically produced from BVDU in mice.

REFERENCES

1. Machida H, Sakata S, Kuninaka A, Yoshino H (1981) Antimicrob Agents Chemoter 20:47-52
2. Sakata S, Shibuya S, Machida H, Yoshino H, Hirota K, Senda S, Ikeda K, Mizuno Y (1980) Nucleic Acids Res Symp Ser 8:s39-s42
3. Machida H, Sakata S (1984) Antiviral Res 4:135-141
4. Soike KF, Gibson S, Gerone PJ(1981) Antiviral Res 1:325-337
5. Soike KF, Baskin G, Cantrell C, Gerone P (1984) Antiviral Res, in press
6. Desgranges C, Razaka G, Drouillet F, Bricaud H, Herdewijn P, De Clercq E (1984) Nucleic Acids Res 12:2081-2090

© 1985 Elsevier Science Publishers B.V. (Biomedical Division)
Herpes Viruses and Virus Chemotherapy, R. Kono, editor

FOSCARNET AS A DRUG AGAINST CYTOMEGALOVIRUS

B. WAHREN[1], B. ÖBERG[2], M. WIKLUND[1], B. LÖNNQVIST[3], P. LJUNGMAN[1,3], O. RINGDÉN[4], J.O. LERNESTEDT[2] AND G. GAHRTON[3]

[1]Department of Virology, National Bacteriological Laboratory, Stockholm, [2]Department of Antiviral Chemotherapy, Astra Läkemedel, Södertälje, [3]Department of Medicine and [4]Transplantation Surgery, Huddinge Hospital, Huddinge (Sweden)

INTRODUCTION

Cytomegalovirus (CMV) infection constitutes one of the main problems during immunosuppression. The number of patients with such infections continue to increase due to the increasing use of immunosuppressive chemotherapy in transplantation and tumor therapy. The treatment of CMV infections has however been hampered by the lack of effective antiviral agents. Foscarnet (PFA, phosphonoformic acid) acts by preferentially inhibiting the synthesis of i.e. herpes viral nucleic acids (1). It is a non-competitive inhibitor due to a selective reversible affinity to the pyrophosphate-binding site on herpesvirus DNA polymerases (2). PFA is active in vitro and in vivo to herpes simplex virus (HSV) types 1 and 2, CMV, varicella-zoster and Epstein-Barr virus (1, 3). The inhibition of the HSV replication appears to be irreversible in cell culture, possibly due to inactivation of non-replicating virus (4). However, the inhibition of CMV in vitro is reversible after withdrawal of the drug, indicating a more stable genome (5), and this may be the case also in vivo. It would thus be important for the outcome of treatment that humoral and cell-mediated immunity are not affected by PFA.

Influence of PFA on lymphocyte activation

PFA in moderate (100 μM) and high (400 μM) doses was added in vitro to human lymphocytes for 3-6 days. ^{3}H-dTTP cellular incorporation (6) was only slightly diminished on day 3 and comparable to the medium control without PFA at 6 days (Table 1). Similarly, when PFA was added to lymphocyte cultures stimulated by the pokeweed mitogen (PWM, mainly stimulatory for B-cells) or phytohemagglutinin (PHA, T- and B-cells) no decrease in cellular DNA synthesis was noted.

CMV alone is known to activate T-cells of seropositive donors (6). In vivo however, CMV is immunosuppressive (10). In CMV seropositive donors, the lymphocyte activation by CMV ranged from 1.6 - 36-fold (mean 10-fold). However, CMV strongly reduced the PWM- and PHA-induced lymphocyte activation (Table 1). We therefore believe that CMV in vitro has a suppressive effect on the activation of the majority of T- and B-lymphocytes, although selectively CMV sensitized T-cells are stimulated. The role of PFA in this complex reaction remains uncertain. The result seen in Table 1 is a moderately diminished total lymphocyte activation (57-80% of the ^{3}H-incorporation value compared with CMV only).

TABLE 1. Influence of PFA on the lymphocyte activation by CMV and mitogens

Variable: Lymphocytes[1] incubated with		Variable for comparison	Mean lymphocyte ^{3}H-incorporation, %[2]: Day 3	Day 6
PFA	100 µM	Medium	68	88
	400 µM		74	146
PWM and PFA	100 µM	PWM	75	101
	400 µM		96	68
PHA and PFA	100 µM	PHA	100	81
	400 µM		102	83
CMV and PWM		PWM	28	59
CMV and PHA		PHA	36	62
CMV and PFA	100 µM	CMV[3]	57	80
	400 µM		60	59

1) Lymphocyte donors were 10 healthy persons; 8 of whom were seropositive. All cultures were made in triplicate.

2) Significantly decreased values (Student's t-test) are underlined.

3) Only lymphocytes from CMV seropositive persons were used here.

Treatment with PFA of CMV infections in transplant recipients

Emergency treatment for virologically diagnosed serious CMV infections was given to 10 bone marrow (11 episodes; BMT) and 8 renal transplant recipients. 2% PFA solution was given i.v. with a bolus dose of 9 mg/kg, and a constant infusion of 0.04-0.22 mg/kg/min for 4-31 (mean 11) days. A clinical response with temperature decrease and normalization of laboratory findings was seen in 6/11 episodes in BMT recipients and 6/7 (one not evaluable) renal transplant recipients (67%). The final outcome (Figure 1) shows that 6/9 patients with CMV-associated pneumonitis succumbed, in some patients due to other complications.

In Table 2 a comparison is made between CMV isolation attempts from urine, blood and/or bone marrow. The isolation frequency of 12 untreated transplant recipients with a CMV infection was 40%, and CMV was isolated almost exclusively from the urine. When CMV is isolated from bone marrow or blood, the prognosis for the patient is worse (7). The frequency of CMV isolations from urine, blood and/or marrow decreased from 71% to 23% after PFA treatment of the 19 CMV episodes mentioned above.

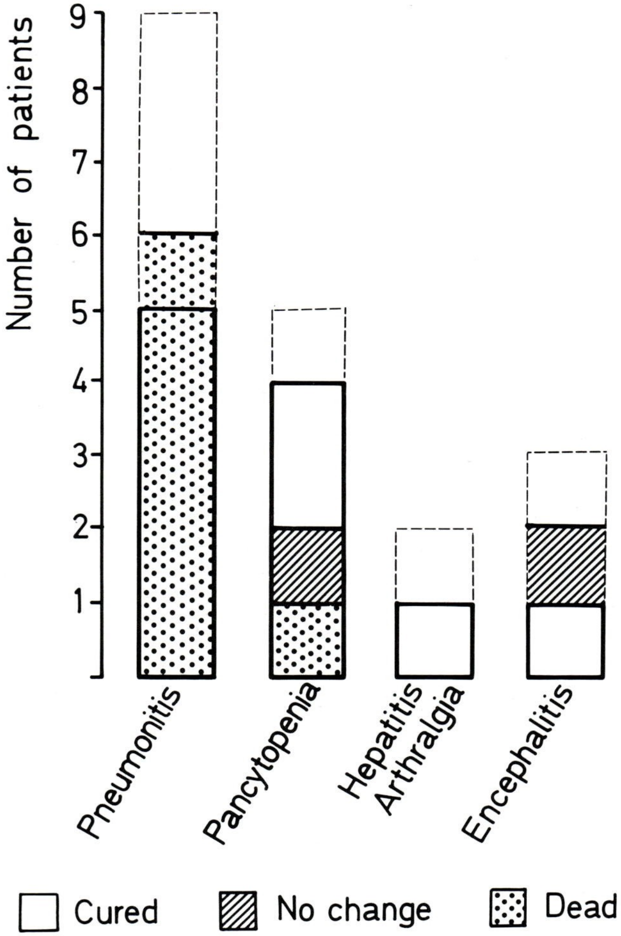

FIGURE 1. Outcome of therapy with PFA against CMV infections in recipients of bone marrow (-) and kidneys (--).

TABLE 2. CMV isolation and inhibitory concentrations (IC_{50}) of PFA in various patient groups.

Patient category	No. of CMV episodes	Frequency of CMV positive isolations	PFA treatment	IC_{50}, μM PFA mean (range)
Immunosuppressed	12	51/126 (40%)	No	197 (50-460)
Immunosuppressed	19	57/80 (71%)	Before	210 (100-600)
Immunosuppressed	19	25/55 (45%)	During	211 (50-430)
Immunosuppressed	19	18/79 (23%)	After	213 (50-400)
Non-immunosuppressed	16	16/16 (100%)	No	236 (50-450)

PFA sensitivity of CMV isolates before and after treatment

Herpesvirus isolates demonstrate a wide range of susceptibility to PFA (8, 9). No apparent difference was found in the range or mean of PFA sensitivities of CMV isolates from otherwise healthy individuals and patients who had received immunosuppressive treatment for transplantation (Table 2). More importantly, we found no PFA resistant CMV strains in isolates that were recovered 0-3 months after PFA treatment. The wide range of susceptibility to PFA can be noted in isolates from all the various patient groups.

CONCLUSIONS AND SUMMARY

The endogenous cellmediated reactivity to CMV was not significantly decreased by PFA. The slightly reduced lymphocyte activation after incubation with PFA and CMV is possibly due to the suppressive over-all effects of CMV. Intravenous PFA was used for treatment of 19 episodes of CMV infection in transplant recipients. Five BMT recipients with CMV pneumonitis succumbed, although clinical signs of improvement were observed during treatment. Four of six BMT recipients with other symptoms were cured. Six of eight renal transplant recipients were cured, three of these had CMV pneumonitis. Apart from one patient who experienced a reversible increase of liver enzymes, hallucinations and tremor coinciding with high (~1200 μM) plasma concentration of PFA the treatment was well tolerated. No CMV isolates obtained after therapy were resistant to the drug and future dosing to reach serum levels of 450 μM should be sufficient.

CMV infections in the immunocompromised patient seem to be susceptible to PFA treatment. This should probably be extended over a prolonged period of time to allow for immunological recovery after the CMV infection. Controlled trials are warranted to determine clinical efficacy.

ACKNOWLEDGEMENTS

The skilful technical assistance of Ms Siv Nordlund and Annelie Åkesson is gratefully acknowledged.

REFERENCES

1. Öberg B (1983) Pharmacol Ther 19:387
2. Eriksson B, Öberg B, Wahren B (1982) Biochim Biophys Acta 696:115
3. Eriksson B, Öberg B (1984) In: Antiviral Drugs and Interferon, Ed. Y Becker, Martinus Nijhoff Publ, Boston, pp. 127-142
4. Schnürer J, Öberg B (1981) Arch Virol 68:203
5. Wahren B, Öberg B (1980) Intervirol 14:7
6. Wahren B, Robèrt K-H, Nordlund S (1981) Scand J Immunol 13:581
7. Wahren B, Linde A, Sundqvist V-A, Ljungman P, Lönnqvist B, Ringdén O (1984) Transplantation, in press
8. Svennerholm B, Vahlne A, Lycke E (1979) Proc Soc Exp Biol Med 61:115
9. Wahren B, Wahren P, Harmenberg J, Sundqvist V-A (1983) J Virol Meth 6:271
10. Carney WP, Rubin RH, Hoffman RA, Hansen WP, Healey K, Hirsch MS (1981) 126:2114.

© 1985 Elsevier Science Publishers B.V. (Biomedical Division)
Herpes Viruses and Virus Chemotherapy, R. Kono, editor

PRE-CLINICAL EVALUATION OF 9-(1,3-dihydroxy-2-propoxymethyl)guanine: ANTIVIRAL ACTIVITY AND MECHANISM OF ACTION OF DHPG.

T.R. MATTHEWS*, D.F. SMEE, E.B. FRASER-SMITH, R.E. BOEHME.
Syntex Research
Palo Alto, Calif. 94304

INTRODUCTION

The acyclic nucleoside 9-(1,3-dihydroxy-2-propoxymethyl)guanine, DHPG, has been found to have broad spectrum in vitro activity against herpes viruses pathogenic to man. For example, using plaque reduction assay, 50 percent inhibition of HSV-1 or HSV-2 thymidine kinase-positive strains is accomplished with 0.12-2.4 μM DHPG (1, 2, 3). This level of activity is nearly identical to that of acyclovir (ACV). Likewise, Dr. Y. Bryson has found that clinical strains of VZV are inhibited by similar concentrations of DHPG and ACV (ID_{50} ~30 μM) (personal communication). DHPG inhibits human cytomegalovirus plaque formation by 50 percent at concentrations of $\leq$10 μM, in contrast to equivalent ACV activities at $\geq$70 μM (3, 4, 5). Finally, Epstein-Barr virus (EBV) genome replication is inhibited by 50 percent using 1 μM DHPG (6, 7).

Metabolism of DHPG in the HSV infected cell is similar to that of ACV. Once the monophosphate of DHPG is formed by the viral thymidine kinase, further conversion to the di- and triphosphate is done by host cellular enzymes. Phosphorylations of DHPG by HSV thymidine kinase and cellular guanylate kinase occur 50-500-fold more rapidly than comparable reactions with ACV (as expressed by the Vmax/Km ratios). Conversion from the diphosphate to the triphosphate is catalyzed by several enzymes and occurs at similar rates for DHPG and ACV (8, 9). The resulting triphosphate of DHPG metabolism is believed to be the active form of this compound which inhibits viral DNA synthesis. In this action, both DHPG-TP and ACV-TP preferentially inhibit viral DNA synthesis relative to that of host by 25-fold (2). A primary mechanism for this effect is believed to be competitive inhibition of viral DNA polymerase. DHPG-TP yields inhibition constants for HSV and CMV-specified polymerases of 40 nM and 22 nM, respectively. DHPG-TP is also incorporated into HSV DNA, resulting in inhibition of viral chain elongation (10, 11).

In vivo studies of DHPG using a murine encephalitis model and HSV-2 guinea pig vaginal infection model confirm the potent anti-HSV-2 activity of this compound. Of particular interest is the observation that although DHPG and ACV have nearly identical activity against HSV-2 in vitro, DHPG is nearly 80-fold more active in the encephalitis model. The oral fifty percent effective dose (ED_{50}) for DHPG is 7-10 mg/kg/day when treatment is started

24 hr post-infection. ACV, on the other hand, has an ED_{50} of >500 mg/kg/day. This difference was found using single or multiple daily dosing (2).

Such great differences in in vivo potency between DHPG and ACV are not explained by differences in adsorption, distribution, metabolism or pharmacokinetics in the treated animal. Likewise, cellular anabolism of both compounds is unlikely to provide the answer. For example, it is known that DHPG is more rapidly phosphorylated to the triphosphate in the HSV-1 infected cell than ACV, but triphosphate accumulation of the two nucleosides was similar in HSV-2 infected cells. Less ACV triphosphate may be needed to inhibit virus replication since this compound is a better inhibitor of HSV-1 DNA polymerase than DHPG triphosphate.

A possible answer of the superior in vivo potency of DHPG may rest in the manner in which the viral infected cell catabolizes and excretes the compound. When DHPG is removed from HSV infected cells, 60-70 percent of DHPG-TP is still present 24 hr later. In contrast, ACV-TP undergoes rapid breakdown in and excretion from the infected cell after drug removal (9). It is interesting to note that the catabolism of DHPG-TP in the uninfected cell is similar to that of ACV-TP in the infected cell. Vero cells exposed to 50 μM DHPG contained 1.29 picomoles/10^6 cells after 6 hours. Two hours after removal of DHPG, 80 percent of DHPG-TP was catabolized and by 12 hrs 98 percent was gone. This rapid catabolism of DHPG-TP in the uninfected cell is consistent with the observation that intracellular concentrations of DHPG-TP in the uninfected cell remained constant during a four day continous exposure to DHPG (9).

The question has not been completely resolved as to why DHPG requires phosphorylation by a viral-specified thymidine kinase to exhibit anti-HSV activity and yet is inhibitory to HCMV which lacks this specific enzyme. What has been observed is that a small degree of phosphorylation of DHPG can occur by cellular enzymes in uninfected cells. In HCMV-infected cells, an 8 to 10-fold increase in DHPG phosphorylation occurs, which is consistant with other observations that HCMV infection will stimulate many host enzyme activities.

Of significance, especially for the treatment of herpes infections of the immunocompromised host, is the potent enhancement of activity that results when DHPG and alpha, beta, or gamma interferons are used together (12, 13, 14, 15). Using the murine HSV-2 encephalitis model, animals infected for 24 hr were dosed once a day for 5 days with DHPG by subcutaneous route and 30 minutes later interferon was given intraperitoneally. Under these conditions, the ED_{50} of DHPG is reduced 10-fold. This effect is achieved witn doses of interferon which lack *in vivo* activity. Of interest is the fact that while both alpha and beta interferons had good *in vitro* activity the activity of gamma interferon was low. Yet, gamma interferon was active by itself *in vivo*. This suggests that the synergistic interaction between gamma interferon and DHPG as well as the activity of gamma interferon alone may be related to the immunological effects of this interferon as well as the direct action at the infective site.

From the results of these pre-clinical laboratory studies it is concluded that DHPG has sufficient *in vivo* potency and selectivity to be seriously considered for clinical study. Likewise the synergy between DHPG and interferon offers a unique combination for increasing success, especially in the immuno-compromised host.

REFERENCES

1. Smith, K.O., K.S. Galloway, W.L. Kennell, K.K. Ogilvie, and B.K. Radatus. 1982. A new nucleoside analog. 9-[[2-hydroxy-1-(hydroxymethyl)ethoxy] methyl]guanine, highly active *in vitro* against herpes simplex virus types 1 and 2. *Antimicrob. Agents Chemother.* 22(1):55-61.

2. Ashton, W.T., J.D. Karkas, A.K. Field, and R.L. Tolman. 1982. Activation by thymidine kinase and potent antiherpetic activity of 2'-nor-2'-deoxyguanosine (2' NDG). Biochem. and Biophys. Res. Commun. 108(4):1716-1721.

3. Smee, D.F., J.C. Martin, J.P.H. Verheyden, and T.R. Matthews. 1983. Anti-herpes activity of the acyclic nucleoside 9-(1,3-dihydroxy-2-propoxymethyl)guanine. Antimicrob. Agents Chemother. 23(5):676-682.

4. Field, A.K., M.E. Davies, C. DeWitt, H.C. Perry, R. Liou, J. Germershausen, J.D. Karkas, W.T. Ashton, D.B.R. Johnston, and R.L. Tolman. 1983. 9-([2-hydroxy-1-(hydroxymethyl)ethoxy]methyl)guanine: a selective inhibitor of herpes group virus replication. Proc. Natl. Acad. Sci. USA. 80(13):4139-43.

5. Mar, E.C., Y.C. Cheng, and E.S. Huang. 1983. Effect of 9-(1,3-dihydroxy-2-propoxymethyl)guanine on human cytomegalovirus replication *in vitro*. Antimicrob. Agents Chemother. 24(4):518-521.

6. Cheng, Y.C., E.S. Huang, J.C. Lin, E.C. Mar, J.S. Pagano, G.E. Dutschman, and S.P. Grill. 1983. Unique spectrum of activity of 9-[(1,3-dihydroxy-2-propoxy)methyl]guanine against herpesviruses *in vitro* and its mode of action against herpes simplex virus type 1. *Proc. Natl.* Acad. Sci. USA. 80(9):2767-70.

7. Lin, Jung-Chung, M. Carolyn Smith, and Joseph S. Pagano. 1984. Prolonged Inhibitory Effect of 9-(1,3-Dihydroxy-2-Propoxymethyl)Guanine Against Replication of Epstein-Barr Virus. J. of Virology. 50(1):50-55.

8. Boehme, R.E. 1984. Phosphorylation of the antiviral precursor 9-(1,3-dihydroxy-2-propoxymethyl)guanine monophosphate by guanylate kinase isozymes. J. Biol. Chem. In Press, October.

9. Smee, D.F., R. Boehme, M. Chernow, B.P. Binko, and T.R. Matthews. 1984. Intracellular metabolism and enzymatic phosphorylation of 9-(1,3-dihydroxy-2-propoxymethyl)guanine and acyclovir in Herpes Simplex virus-infected and uninfected cells. Biochem. Pharmacol. In Press.

10. Frank, K.B., T.F. Chiou, and Y.C. Cheng. 1984. Interaction of herpes simplex virus-induced DNA polymerase with 9-(1,3-dihydroxy-2-propoxymethyl) guanine triphosphate. J. Bio. Chem. 259(3)1566-1569.

11. Mar, E.C., J.F. Chiou, Y.C. Cheng and E.S. Huang. Inhibition of cellular DNA Polymerase alpha and human cytomegalovirus-induced DNA polymerase by the triphosphates of 9-(2-hydroxyethoxymethyl)guanine and 9-(1,3-dihydroxy-2-propoxymethyl)guanine. J. Virology. Submitted 1984.

12. Eppstein, D.A., and V.Y. Marsh. 1984. Potent synergistic inhibition of herpes simplex virus-2 by 9-[(1,3-dihydroxy-2-propoxy)methyl]guanine in combination with recombinant interferons. Biochem. and Biophys. Res. Commun. 120(1):66-73.

13. Fraser-Smith, E.B., D.A. Eppstein, Y.V. Marsh, and T.R. Matthews. 1984. Enhanced efficacy of the acyclic nucleoside 9-(1,3-dihydroxy-2-propoxymethyl)guanine in combination with beta interferon against herpes simplex virus type two in mice. Antimicrob. Agents Chemother. 25(5):563-565.

14. Fraser-Smith, E.B., D.A. Eppstein, Y.V. Marsh, and T.R. Matthews. 1984. Enhanced efficacy of the acyclic nucleoside 9-(1,3-dihydroxy-2-propoxymethyl)guanine in combination with alpha-interferon against herpes simplex virus type two in mice. Antimicrob. Agents Chemother. In Press, December.

15. Fraser-Smith, E.B., D.A. Eppstein, Y.V. Marsh, and T.R. Matthews. 1984. Enhanced Efficacy of the acyclic nucleoside 9-(1,3-dihydroxy-2-propoxymethyl)guanine in combination with gamma interferon against herpes simplex virus type two in mice. Antiviral Res. In Press.

CARBOCYCLIC ARABINOFURANOSYLADENINE (CYCLARADINE): SYNTHESIS AND ANTIVIRAL EFFICACY

ROBERT VINCE, WILLIAM M. SHANNON⁺, AND TATTANAHALLI L. NAGABHUSHAN[‡]

University of Minnesota, College of Pharmacy, 308 Harvard St. SE, Minneapolis, MN 55455; ⁺Southern Research Institute, Birmingham, AL 35255; [‡]Schering-Plough Corporation, 60 Orange St., Bloomfield, NJ 07003.

Although much effort has been expended in the search for effective antiviral agents for use in the treatment of human herpes virus infections, only a relatively small number of such drugs have been uncovered to date. The two most effective antiherpes drugs are D-arabinofuranosyladenine (Ara-A) and 9-(2-hydroxyethoxymethyl)guanine (Acyclovir). Both drugs have serious drawbacks inherent in their molecular structural design that limit their use in the treatment of herpes simplex virus (HSV) infections, especially HSV-2 genital infections. The molecular features of the Ara-A molecule are compatible with the substrate requirements of the ubiquitous enzyme, adenosine deaminase, and it is generally accepted that the major liability in its effectiveness is rapid deamination to the much less active arabinosyl hypoxanthine (1). Clinical studies have demonstrated that acyclovir is of minimal benefit in the treatment of recurrent genital herpes (2). HSV strains that are deficient in their ability to code for thymidine kinase are resistant to the drug (3).

Cyclaridine is a novel nucleoside analog that is highly efficacious in the topical treatment of HSV-2 genital infections. It is a carbocyclic analog of Ara-A prepared from aristeromycin by chemical inversion of configuration at the 2'-hydroxyl group. Carbocyclic nucleosides are those analogs which have a methylene group replacing the oxygen atom of the carbohydrate ring. They lack the labile glycosidic linkage and are stable to cleavage by phosphorylases or hydrolases while retaining the potential for therapeutic useful interaction with other enzymes involved in nucleotide metabolism. In the case of cyclaradine, the exchange of methylene for oxygen also renders the compound inert to adenosine deaminase. Thus, as expected, the addition of the adenosine deaminase inhibitor, 2'-deoxycoformycin, to growing P-388 mouse lymphoid leukemia cells increased the toxicity of Ara-a 20-fold, while no increase in toxicity was observed with cyclaradine.

The significant therapeutic effect of cyclaradine against lethal HSV-1 infections in mice, after i.p. inocululation of virus, was readily demonstrated. Cyclaradine was found to be as effective as Ara-A in reducing mortality in the virus infected animals. Whereas 95% of the virus-infected control (untreated) mice died, the mean survival time of 8.4 days, systemic treatment with Ara-A reduced the mortality to 0 to 10% when the drug was administered i.p. at nontoxic doses once a day for 7 days starting 4 h after virus inoculation. Likewise, cyclaradine was also significantly effective ($P<0.0005$) in decreasing the mortality to 0 to 10% when administered i.p. to infected animals at nontoxic doses of between 112 and 450 mg/kg per day on the same treatment schedule.

Optimum derivatization and formulation of cyclaradine to the methyoxyacetate ester prodrug (cyclaradine-MA) yielded a new topically active antiherpes agent (Fig. 1).

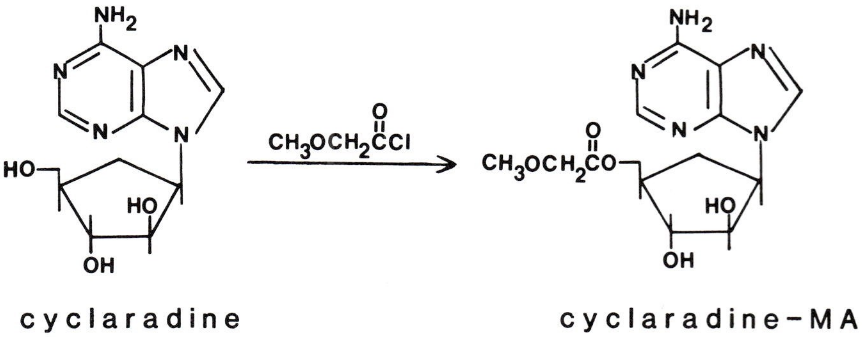

Fig. 1. Preparation of cyclaradine-MA

When administered intravaginally as 1 or 5 percent gels, cyclaradine-MA was found to significantly suppress lesion development (Fig. 2). The mean virus titers of the drug-treated groups were significantly below the mean virus titers of the control groups.

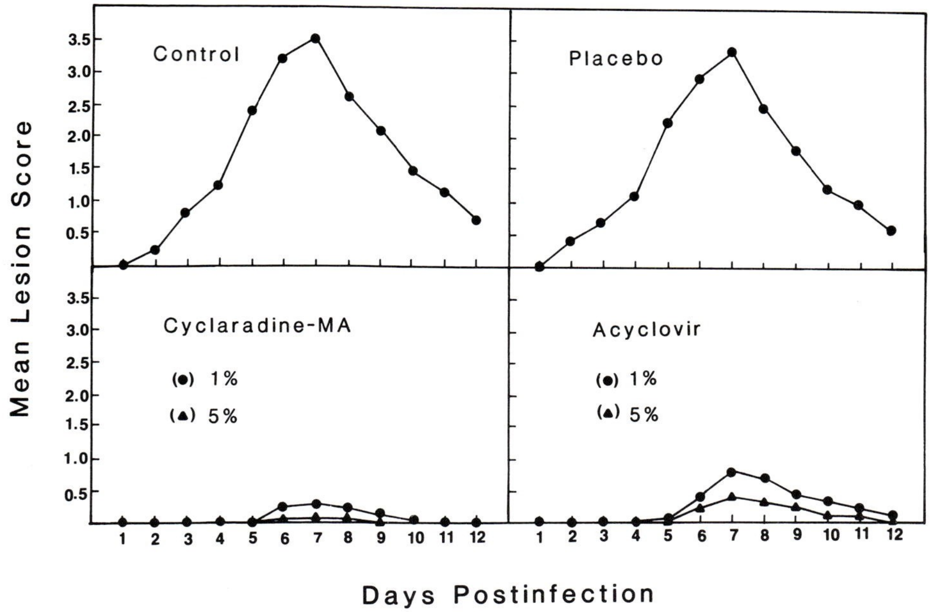

Fig. 2. Effect of topical treatment with cyclaradine-MA and acyclovir on the severity of HSV-2 genital lesions in guinea pigs. Hartley albino female guinea pigs were inoculated intravaginally with 10^5 median cell culture infectious doses of HSV-2 (strain MS) suspended in 0.1 ml of cell culture medium. All compounds were suspended in 0.4 percent agarose gel and administered intravaginally in a volume of 0.1 ml three times daily for 7 days starting 3 hours after infection. There were 20 animals in each control group and 10 in each drug-treated group. The placebo consisted of the 0.4 percent agarose gel alone. Lesions appearing on the external genitalia were scored on a scale of 0 to 4.

Intravaginal treatment of virus-infected guinea pigs with 1 and 5 percent gels of acyclovir also suppressed lesion development, but not as markedly as did cyclaradine-MA.

These results suggest that optimal derivatization and formulation of cyclaradine may result in a useful new antiherpes drug. The high antiviral activity and such other desirable features as hydrolytic stability, adenosine deaminase resistance, and low systemic toxicity, make cyclaradine and its derivatives excellent candidates for clinical trials against herpes virus infections.

REFERENCES

1. Buchanan JA, Hess F (1980) Pharmacol. Ther. 8:143; Shannon WM, Schabel FM, Jr. (1980) Ibid. 11:263; Galasso GJ (1981) Antivir. Res. 1:73.
2. Corey L, et al (1982) N. Engl. J. Med. 306:1313
3. Coen DM, Schaffer PA (1980) Proc. Natl. Acad. Sci. USA 77:2265; Field HJ, Darby G (1980) Antimicrob. Agents Chemother. 17:209; Schnipper LE, Crumpacker CS (198) Proc. Natl. Acad. Sci. USA 77:2270.

Herpes Viruses and Virus Chemotherapy, R. Kono, editor

SUSCEPTIBILITY OF SEVERAL CLINICAL ISOLATES OF VARICELLA-ZOSTER VIRUS TOWARDS ANTIHERPES DRUGS

S. SHIGETA[1], H. KAWAGUCHI[1], K. KONNO[1], T. YOKOTA[1] and E. DE CLERCQ[2]
[1]Department of Bacteriology, Fukushima Medical College, Fukushima 960, Japan and
[2]Rega Institute for Medical Research, Katholieke Universiteit Leuven, B-3000 Leuven, Belgium.

INTRODUCTION

We have previously examined several newly developed antiherpes compounds for their inhibitory effects on focus formation by varicella-zoster virus (VZV) in vitro (1). Among these compounds, bromovinyldeoxyuridine (BVDU) and bromovinyl-arabinofuranosyluracil (BVaraU) emerged as the most potent and most selective inhibitors of VZV. In the present study, we examined several clinical isolates of VZV for their susceptibility towards 8 antiherpes compounds.

MATERIALS AND METHODS

Viruses. Twenty-five isolates of VZV were obtained from 11 varicella and 14 herpes zoster patients during 1981 to 1984. All VZV isolates were submitted to the susceptibility tests following 2 or 3 passages in cultured human embryonic fibroblasts (HEF). Cell-free virus was prepared as described by Schmidt and Lennette (2) and stored at -80°C until used.

Compounds. The antiherpes compounds and their abbreviations are as follows : iododeoxyuridine (IDU), adenine arabinoside (ara-A), acycloguanosine (ACV), dihydroxypropoxymethylguanine (DHPG), bromovinyldeoxyuridine (BVDU), bromovinylarabinofuranosyluracil (BVaraU), carbocyclic bromovinyldeoxyuridine (C-BVDU) and phosphonoformic acid (PFA).

Antiviral assay. HEF were seeded in multi-well trays containing 1.6 cm-diameter wells. After 3 days incubation, when the cells formed a monolayer, 30 to 50 plaque forming units of VZV were inoculated and varying concentrations of the compounds were added immediately thereafter. Three monolayers were used for each dilution of the compounds and at 3 days after virus infection the foci were enumerated microscopically. The ID_{50} value of each compound was determined as the concentration of the compound required to reduce the number of foci to 50 % of that in the control cell cultures.

Assay of thymidine kinase (TK) activity. TK activity was assayed in vitro following the same procedure as that described by Hackstadt et al. (3). For the fractionation of the enzyme extract, 5 % polyacrylamide slab gel electrophoresis was used. The enzyme extract was applied to a polyacrylamide gel column, electrophoresed for 4 h at 4°C at a constant current of 50 mV. After electrophoresis, the gels were sliced into 2 mm sections and the amount of TK activity was determined in each slice.

RESULTS

Susceptibility of 25 clinical VZV isolates of VSV towards antiherpes agents. ID_{50} values of eight antiherpes compounds against 25 clinical VZV isolates were determined and the distribution of the ID_{50} values for each compound is illustrated in Fig. 1. The average ID_{50} of each compound and its standard deviation (SD) are also shown. The shadowed areas in Fig. 1 comprise the range of 2 SD values. This includes 95.4 % of the individual values. The Ito strain showed a surprisingly high resistance to IDU, and was therefore not included in the calculation of the average ID_{50} value of IDU. Of all eight compounds tested, BVaraU was the most potent, followed by BVDU. C-BVDU was about 5 times less potent than BVDU. The bromovinyl derivatives exceeded all other antiviral agents in potency : BVaraU and BVDU were active in the nanogram/ml concentration range, whereas ACV, araA, DHPG and PFA were active in the microgram/ml concentration range.

Characteristics of IDU resistant (Ito) strain of VZV. We further examined the IDU-resistant (Ito) strain of VZV for its susceptibility to other antiherpes drugs, i.e. bromodeoxyuridine (BDU), iodovinyldeoxyuridine (IVDU), iododeoxycy-

Fig 1. Susceptibility of Clinical Strains of VZV

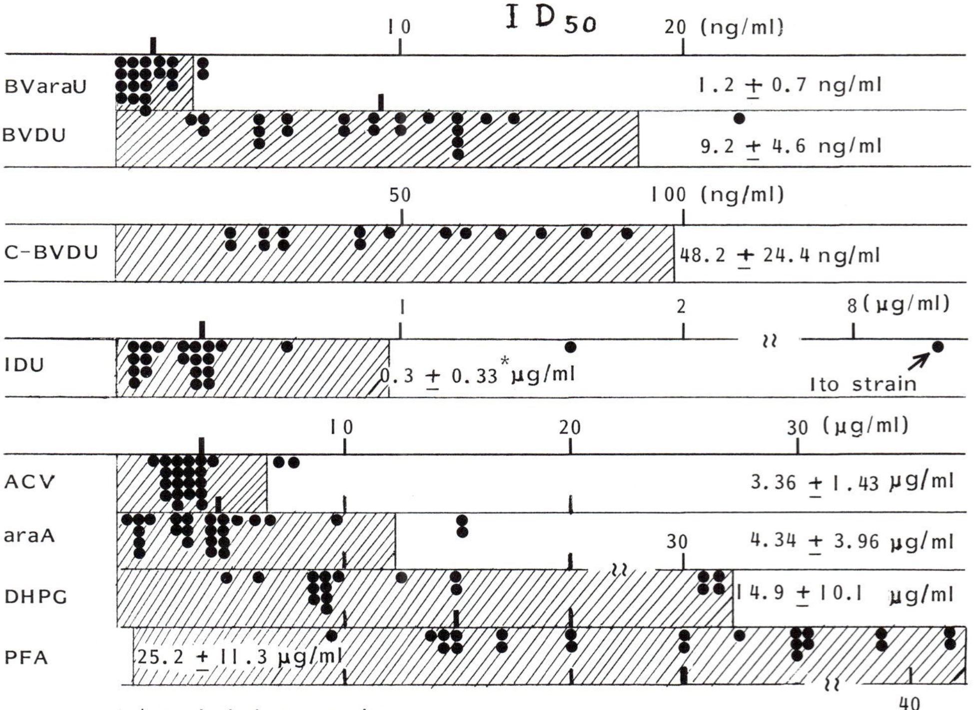

* excluded Ito strain

tidine (IDC) and bromovinyldeoxycytidine (BVDC). Table 1 shows the ID_{50} of several antiherpes compounds for the Ito strain, as compared to their average ID_{50} for the other VZV strains. The ID_{50} of IDU and BDU for the Ito strain were 8.3 and 9.2 μg/ml, respectively; this is 25 to 28 times greater than the ID_{50} for the other VZV strains. However, the ID_{50} values of the other nucleoside analogues (BVDU, IVDU, BVaraU, IDC, BVDC and ACV) for the Ito strain were quite similar to their ID_{50} values for the other VZV strains.

Table 1. ID_{50} of nucleoside analogues for the Ito strain (μg/ml)

Compound	Ito strain	Average of TK^+ VZV
IDU	8.3	0.3
BDU	9.2*	0.37*
BVDU	0.003	0.009
IVDU	0.001*	0.0015*
BVaraU	0.001	0.0012
IDC	1.7*	1.3*
BVDC	0.002*	0.02*
ACV	3.9	3.4

*Data taken from reference 1.

Thymidine kinase activity of Ito strain. Monolayers of a human breast cancer cell line were infected with either TK-positive VZV (Kanno strain), TK-negative VZV (Kanno-Kohmura strain) or VZV Ito strain. The characteristics of the former 2 VZV strains have been reported previously (1,4). Figure 2 demonstrates the fractionation of TK activity in VZV-infected cells and mock-infected cells. Viral TK activity (Rm = 0.48) was found in the cells infected with the Kanno (TK^+) or Ito strain but was not found in the cells infected with Kanno-Kohmura (TK^-) or in mock-infected cells. Similar results were obtained using HEF cells infected with VZV.

DISCUSSION

The clinical use of antiherpes compounds may lead to a selection of drug-resistant virus strains. We examined the susceptibility to antiherpes drugs of 25 clinical isolates of VZV. For each compound one or two VZV isolates were found which exceeded two standard deviations of ID_{50}. Among these isolates the Ito strain showed particularly high resistance towards IDU and BDU but similar susceptiblity to the other nucleoside analogues which are all known to be phosphorylated by the VZV TK. We have demonstrated that the Ito strain is fully effective in inducing TK activity in human breast cancer as well as HEF cells. It is not clear yet why the Ito strain is selectively resistant to IDU and BDU. Possibly, the TK encoded by the Ito strain differs from the other VZV strains in substrate affinity for IDU and BDU. The emergence of such virus mutants with altered substrate specificity has previously been reported for herpes simplex virus strains resistant to ACV.

Fig 2. Fractionation of TK activity in VZV-infected human breast cancer cells

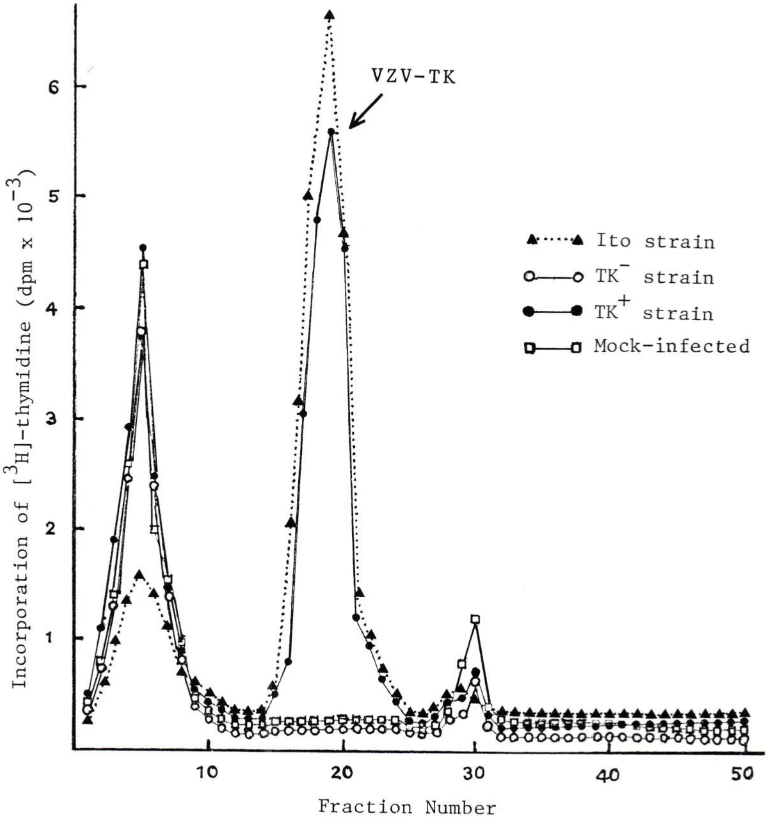

REFERENCES

1. Shigeta S, Yokota T, Iwabuchi T, Baba M, Konno K, Ogata M, De Clercq E (1983) J Infect Dis 147:576-584

2. Schmidt NJ, Lennette EH (1976) Infect Immun 14:709-715

3. Hackstadt T, Mallavia LP (1978) J Virol 25:510-517

4. Yokota T, Ogata M, Shigeta S (1983) Fukushima J Med Sci 29:101-111

5. Darby G, Field HJ, Salisbury SA (1981) Nature 289:81-83

Herpes Viruses and Virus Chemotherapy, R. Kono, editor

COMPARISON OF THE ANTIHERPETIC ACTIVITY OF ACV AND PFA IN CELL CULTURES AND GUINEA PIG SKIN INFECTION

Hong-shan Chen, Jing-he Li
Department of virology, Institute of Antibiotics, Chinese Academy of Medical Sciences, Tian-tan, Beijing, China

INTRODUCTION

ACV and PFA are two prospective antiherpetic agents showed therapiutic activities in laboratory and in clinics with different mode of action. ACV is a specific inhibitor of HSV-coded thymidine kinase(1) and PFA is an inhibitor of HSV-DNA polymerase(2), their antiviral effects in cell cultures and on guinea pig skin infections were compared in thir paper.

ANTIHERPETIC ACTIVITY IN CELL CULTURES.

Inhibition of HSV-I and II in 2-BS, vero and PRK cells.

ACV is more active than PFA in 2BS, vero and PRK cells, the ratio of IC_{50} between PFA/ACV were as high as 59.88-1250 (Table 1).The viruses cultivated in PRK and vero cells were more sensitive than those grown in 2BS cells.

TABLE 1

IC_{50} OF ACV AND PFA ON HSV-I,II INFECTION IN 2-BS, VERO AND PRK CELLS

Drugs	HSV-I			HSV-II		
	2BS	Vero	PRK	2BS	Vero	PRK
ACV	1.67*	0.08	0.07	0.30	0.03	0.03
PFA	100	100	20	53.33	5.33	10
PFA/ACV	59.88	1250	307.69	177.67	177.77	333.33

* IC_{50}: 50% inhibition of HSV. CPE. in cell culture, (mcg/ml)

Effects of multiplicity of infection on the antiviral activity.

The antiherpetic activity of ACV against HSV-I and II was greatly affected by the multiplicity of virus infection in cell culture. 10-1000 mcg/ml of ACV completely inhibited HSV 1 $TCID_{50}$ infection but partly inhibited 10-100 $TCID_{50}$ infection. Antiviral activity of PFA was not easily influenced by the multiplicity of virus infection,100-200 mcg/ml completely inhibited 10-100 $TCID_{50}$ infection and also inhibited 50-75% to 1000 $TCID_{50}$ infection. (Fig. 1)

Inhibition of EBV-VCA in B_{95-8} cells.

The EBV-VCA in cultivated B_{95-8} cells were more sensitive to ACV than to PFA, lmcg/ml of ACV inhibited 50% of VCA, but for PFA, more than 30 mcg/ml was needed.

The results showed that ACV was more active than PFA on inhibition of HSV-I,

II and EBV-VCA in cell cultures, but it was not so effective on high multiplicity of infection than that of PFA.

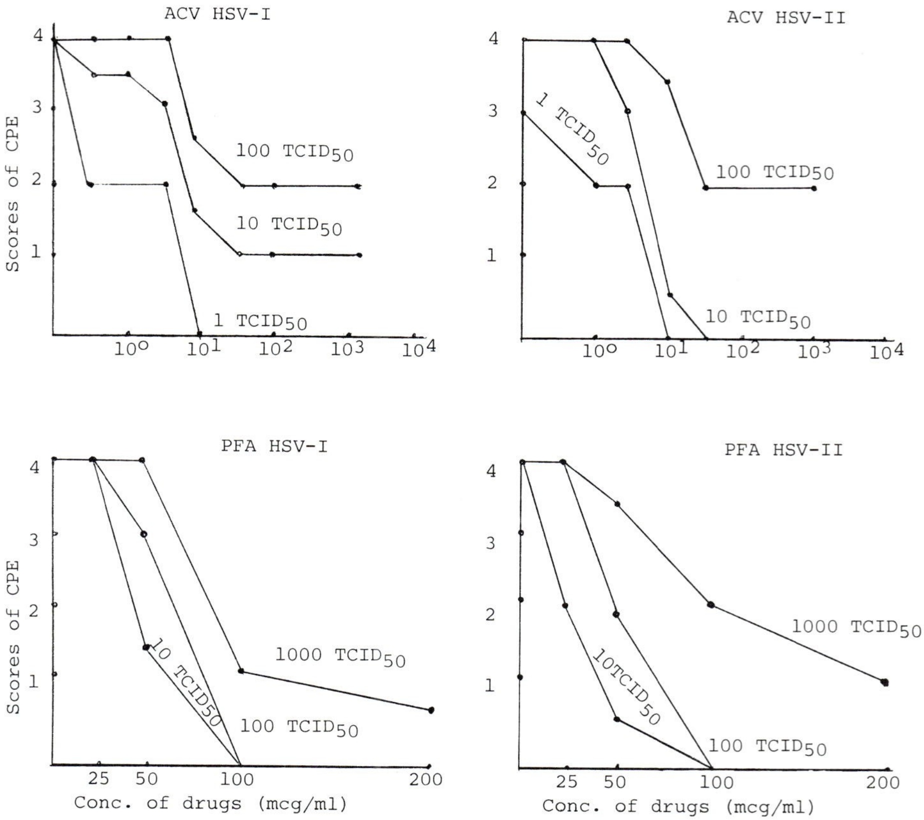

Fig. 1. Comparative inhibition of ACV and PFA against different multiplicity of HSV-I and II infection in 2BS calls

ANTIHERPETIC ACTIVITES IN GUINEA PIG SKIN INFECTION

Guinea pig skin infected with HSV-I were treated with ACV or PFA topically, various concentrations and different preparations were used in different regimens.

Influence of vehicals on the efficacy of topical treatment of ACV and PFA on guinea pig HSV-I skin infections (Table 2).

Aqeous solution. 0.1-1% of ACV or PFA, applied on guinea pig skin 24 hrs after infection b.i.d. for 3 days, showed that PFA had better effect than ACV on the 4th and 7th day of infection. 0.1% PFA inhibited 83.3% of skin lesion on 4th and 7th day after infection while 0.1% ACV could not inhibit the lesions at all. 1% PFA inhibted 91.7% of lesion but 1% ACV inhibited only 66.7% of the lesion.

Glycerin solution. 10% glycerin solution of both 1% ACV and PFA showed similar significant effect on HSV-I infected guinea skin when the drugs given

24 hrs after infection b.i.d. for 3 days, but PFA had better effect than that of ACV.

DMSO solution or cream. 1% PFA in 5% DMSO inhibited the skin lesion 58.33-66.67% on 4-7th day of infection when given 24 hrs after infection b.i.d. for 3 days, but was less effective than 10% glycerin-1% PFA. 3% ACV-10% DMSO cream given with the same regimen, the effect was just similar to that of 1% ACV-10% glycerin solution and was less effective than that of 1% PFA-5% DMSO.

TABLE II

THE INFLUENCE OF VEHICLES ON THE ANTIVIRAL ACTIVITIES OF ACV AND PFA ON HSV-I INFECTION OF GUINEA PIG SKIN.

Vehicles	Conc	% inhibition of lesion scores							
	Drug	PFA			ACV				
%	%	4	6	7	3	4	5	6	7
H_2O	0.1	83.3	83.3	75		0		0	
10% glycerin	1.0	91.7	97.7	66.6		66.7		66.7	
5% DMSO	1.0	75			54.5	46.2	28.6	28.6	37.5
10% DMSO cream	3.0	58.3			53.8	42.9	35.7	50.0	80.0

Influence of therapeutic regimens on the efficacy of ACV and PFA on HSV-I skin infection in guinea pigs (Fig. 2).

0.03% PFA (equivalent to 3 IC_{50} of PFA in HSV-infected cell culture) applied topically on HSV infected guinea pig skin. started 1.5 hrs post-infection, 7.i.d. for 2½ days (totally 17 times) controlled the lesions very well, but 0.01-0.1% ACV (equivalent to 10-100 IC_{50} of ACV in cell culture) applied with the same regimen gave no significant effect (fig. 2a).

2% PFA applied on HSV infected guinea pig skin, 24 hrs after infection b.i. d. for 3 days, gave very significant effect, but 3% ACV -10% DMSO cream applied with the same regimen gave no significant effect (Fig. 2b and 2c).

Increasing the doses of 3% ACV-10% DMSO cream to 5.i.d. for 7 days started 24 hrs postinfection, the result showed that the lesions were controlled similar to that of 2% PFA b.i.d. for 2 days. (Fig. 2d).

CONCLUSION AND DISCCUSION

ACV and PFA had different effects against HSV infection in cell cultures and on guinea pig skin. ACV was more effective against HSV-I, II and E-B virus infection than PFA in cell culture but PFA inhibited higher multiplicity of HSV infection than ACV there. 0.01-2% PFA applied topically on HSV-I guinea pig skin infection for 17 or 6 times within 2½-3 days respectively, inhibited the development of lesions, but 0.01-3% ACV gave no significent effect with the same regimen. Increasing the doses of 3% ACV-10% DMSO cream and prolonging the treatment enhanced the therapeutic effect. The difference of the effects of ACV and PFA in cell cultures and on guinea pig skin might be due to that ACV is competitive and PFA is non-competitive antiherpetic agent (3,4),it seemed not in relevent to the DMSO in the cream.

REFERENCES

1. Schaeffer HJ, Beauchamp L, de Miranda P, Elion GB, Baur DJ and Collins P (1978) Nature 272:583-585.

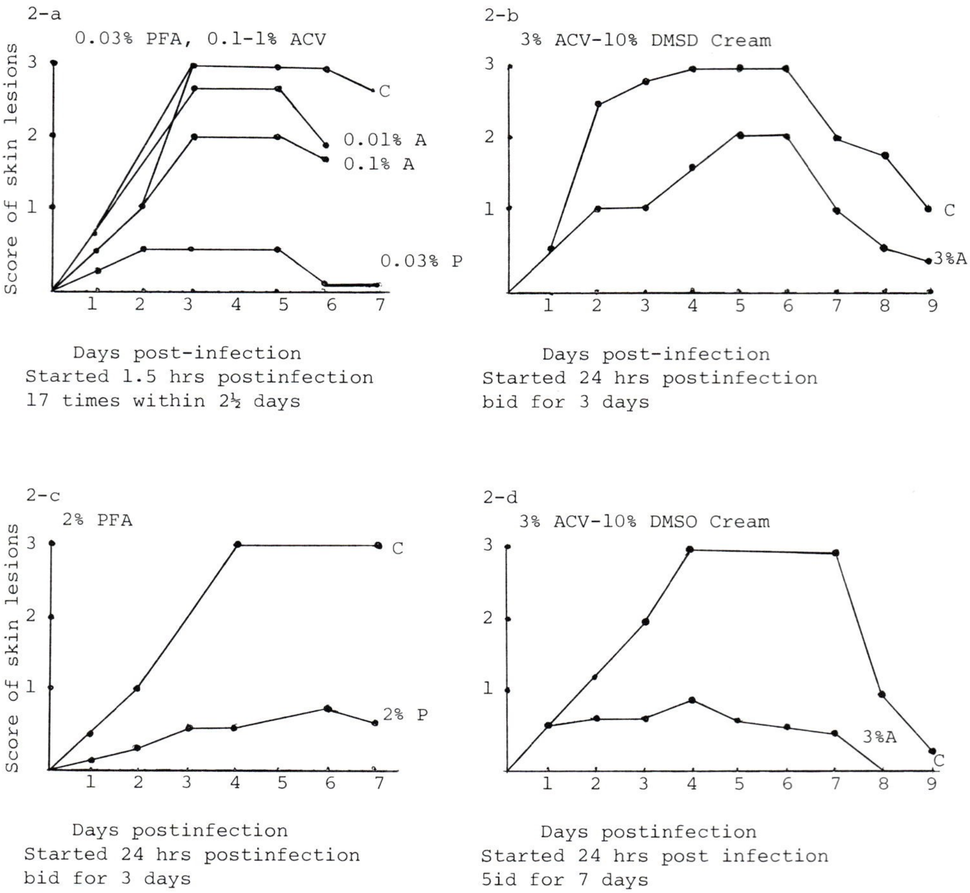

Fig. 2 Comparative effects of ACV and PFA on HSV-I infected guinea pig skin (A: ACV, P: PFA and C: Control)

2. Oberg B (1983) Pharmacol. Ther. 19:387-415.
3. Field HJ (1983) In: Proceedings of 13th International Congress of Chemotherapy. SY 50 part 18 pp. 1-8.
4. Spruance SL(1983) In: Proceedings of 13th International Congress of Chemotherapy. SY 50 part 18 pp. 12-22.

III CLINICAL EXPERIENCE WITH NEW ANTIHERPETIC COMPOUNDS

A. Ocular

Herpes Viruses and Virus Chemotherapy, R. Kono, editor

UPDATE ON ANTIVIRAL AGENTS: AN OVERVIEW OF OCULAR HERPES

HERBERT E. KAUFMAN

Department of Ophthalmology, LSU Eye Center, Louisiana State University Medical Center School of Medicine, New Orleans, Louisiana 70112, USA

VIRUS GENETICS DETERMINE DISEASE CHARACTERISTICS

Our understanding of the biology of herpesvirus in the causation of ocular disease has changed drastically in recent years. We have evidence from our laboratory that there are genetic differences between isolates of viruses from different patients, which determine the severity of ocular disease.[1] Some isolates without laboratory passage produce mild, almost trivial disease in rabbits, while others produce severe necrotizing stromal keratitis. Still others produce encephalitis and death. We have shown that even the shape of the dendritic ulcer on the cornea is determined by the viral genome, and recombinant studies, in collaboration with Dr. Bernard Roizman, have pinpointed the location on the genome where the morphology of the dendritic ulcer is determined.[2] Similarly, we have shown that stromal disease can be genetically determined and segregates independent of the factors that determine epithelial disease.

Ganglionic Colonization Prevents Superinfection

Further studies have indicated that in people, with few exceptions, multiple ganglia are colonized by herpes simplex virus type 1 (HSV-1), and all of the ganglia tend to be colonized by the same virus strain, as determined by DNA mapping.[3] Animal studies indicate that once the original virus, which can be an extremely mild avirulent virus, infects the ganglion, it is generally impossible to colonize that ganglion with even a highly neurovirulent virus or a superinfecting virus with a strong tendency to produce recurrent disease.[4] The only exceptions to this have been with the use of laboratory strains that produce minimal aberrant infections as opposed to regular wild strains, or when both eyes are infected at once, or when superinfection occurs shortly after the initial infection, before latency of the original strain has been established. In general, then, the colonization of the ganglion is determined by the first infecting virus, and the whole future of the patient's course with ocular herpetic disease is so determined.

Genetic Determination of Rate of Recurrence

Similarly in animals, if the two eyes are infected simultaneously by different virus strains with different rates of recurrence, it is clear that the virus that tends to recur more frequently will continue to do so, and that the eye infected with this virus will have frequent recurrences, and the eye infected with the virus with the lower rate of recurrence will have fewer recurrences -- all in the same animal with the same immunological status at the same time.[5]

Temperature and rate of recurrence. Some of our newest work, by Dr. Centifanto-Fitzgerald, indicates that the patients who have frequent recurrences of corneal herpes may harbor a virus strain that has an optimum growth temperature lower that of other virus strains. Since the corneal temperature is lower than the core body temperature, those who shed virus that grows better at the lower temperature have frequent corneal recurrences, while those who shed virus with a higher optimal growth temperature do not.[6] It is similarly attractive to hypothesize that a high temperature optimum favors recurrences triggered by fever, sun poisoning, etc., and that the shedding of virus in the tears and the saliva may require the appropriate temperature for colonization and clinical disease.

DRUG THERAPY OF OCULAR HERPETIC DISEASE

IDU, Ara-A, and Trifluridine

Drugs for the treatment of ocular herpes began with our introduction of iododeoxyuridine (IDU).[7] This drug is now more than 20 years old and is obsolete. Topical adenine arabinoside (Ara-A) is approximately as potent as IDU and significantly less potent than trifluorothymidine (trifluridine) and like IDU should probably be reserved for those cases that do not respond to more potent drugs.[8] Trifluridine seems to be the agent of choice for the topical treatment of epithelial herpes at present. In cases of dendritic ulcers, 97% of patients can be expected to be cured within two weeks.[9] Trifluridine appears significantly better than IDU or Ara-A, and also is more effective in the prevention of epithelial ulceration when corticosteroids must be used for the treatment of stromal disease.

Acyclovir

The newer thymidine-kinase selective drugs are exciting, but in ophthalmology it is not yet clear what they have to offer in the treatment of HSV-1 disease. It is clear that, so far, no drug or combination of drugs can eradicate virus from the ganglion and prevent the establishment of latency.

Acyclovir and stromal disease. Another possibility for these drugs would be the prevention or treatment of stromal disease, but their efficacy in this application is unclear. In the initial studies done by Burroughs-Wellcome comparing acyclovir with IDU, a small proportion of patients with dendritic ulcers went on to develop stromal disease in spite of therapy. The proportion was the same in both drug treatment groups.[10]

Poirier found that acyclovir penetrated into the anterior chamber[11] suggesting that, despite the results of the clinical study, there might be sufficient acyclovir in the stroma to be therapeutically active. We have also done an uncontrolled clinical study of patients with stromal disease, treated with both oral and topical acyclovir.[12] Although the serum levels of drug obtained were comparable to those found to produce prophylactic and therapeutic benefits in genital disease, there was no benefit in our patients, and the stromal disease generally appeared to follow the course that would be expected without antiviral treatment. Stromal disease was ameliorated by the addition of corticosteriods, with or without antivirals, but antiviral agents alone had no effect. In fact, even in a patient with virus in the stroma, seen by electron microscopy, the disease progressed during antiviral treatment, and surgery was required.

Acyclovir and recurrent disease. A third therapeutic possibility is the intriguing one that chronic administration of drug might prevent recurrences even if ganglionic latency is not eradicated. It is clear in the case of genital disease that the oral administration of acyclovir either prevents or drastically reduces recurrences as long as the drug is continued -- although there is no continuing effect after the drug is stopped.[13]

In rabbit studies in which both oral acyclovir and bromvinyldeoxyuridine were administered, we were unable either to reduce shedding or to reduce the clinical recurrence rate.[14] Although rabbits metabolize the drug more rapidly than humans and may not be an ideal model, the levels of drug were generally comparable to those found to be effective in human studies of genital disease. This question certainly requires further study, but so far, we have no reason to believe recurrences of ocular disease can be prevented.

Drug resistance and interferon. Acyclovir, and other drugs with similar mechanisms of action, tend to produce resistant virus. One person with a local resistant virus infection could presumably spread it to others and thereby create in the community a pool of resistant virus, even though the virus emerging from his own ganglion might remain sensitive. Whether this is a theoretical or an actual worry remains uncertain, but we must ask whether these drugs have enough of an advantage to warrant their use as primary drugs for topical administration when they are so valuable for systemic use. There is also the possible potentiation of the antiviral effect of both trifluridine and acyclovir by interferon. With interferon, it is possible not only that this effect may be potentiated to some extent, but also that the emergence of resistant virus may be reduced or eliminated; however, this remains unclear. Finally, there is the possibility that the chronic administration of interferon, rather than drugs, could prevent recurrences of herpes. I have carried out two studies in patients with human leukocyte interferon to try to suppress recurrences and have not been successful,[15] but it is always possible that higher concentrations of drug and more interferon might be effective.

In summary, the present status of the newer drugs remains uncertain. Their advantage over previous medication in the treatment of superficial ocular disease remains unclear, and much more work is required to determine if these drugs can prevent recurrences or treat stromal disease.

REFERENCES

1. Wander AH, Centifanto YM, Kaufman HE (1980) Arch Ophthalmol 98:1458-1461.
2. Centifanto-Fitzgerald YM, Yamaguchi T, Kaufman HE, Tognon M, Roizman B (1982) J Exp Med 155:475-489.
3. Lonsdale DM, Moira Brown S, Subak Sharpe JH, Warren KG, Koprowski H (1979) J Gen Virol 43:151-171.
4. Centifanto-Fitzgerald YM, Varnell ED, Kaufman HE (1982) Infect Immun 35:1125-1132.
5. Gerdes JC, Smith DS (1983) J Gen Virol 64:2441-2454.
6. Centifanto-Fitzgerald YM (In Press) In: O'Connor GR (ed) Advances in Immunology and Immunopathology of the Eye. Masson Publishing, USA, Inc., New York.
7. Kaufman HE, Nesburn AB, Maloney ED (1962) Arch Ophthalmol 67:583-591.
8. Dresner AJ, Seamans ML (1975) In: Pavan-Langston D, Buchanan RA, Alford CA Jr (eds) Adenine Arabinoside: An Antiviral Agent. Raven Press, New York.
9. Laibson PR, Arentsen JJ, Mazzanti WD, Eiferman RA (1977) Trans Am Ophthalmol Soc 75:316-324.
10. McCulley JP, Binder PS, Kaufman HE, O'Day DM, Poirier RH (1982) Ophthalmology 89:1195-1200.
11. Poirier RH, Kingham HD, deMiranda P, Annel M (1982) Arch Ophthalmol 100:1964-1967.
12. Sanitato JJ, Asbell PA, Varnell ED, Kissling GE, Kaufman HE (In Press) Am J Ophthalmol
13. Straus SE, Takiff HE, Seidlin M, Bachrach S, Lininger L, DiGiovanna JJ, Western KA, Smith HA, Lehrman SN, Creagh-Kirk T, Alling DW (1984) New Eng J Med 310:1545-1550.
14. Kaufman HE, Varnell ED, Centifanto-Fitzgerald YM, De Clercq E, Kissling GE (1983) Antimicrob Agents and Chemother 24:888-891.
15. Kaufman HE, Meyer RF, Laibson PR, Waltman SR, Nesburn AB, Shuster JJ (1976) J Infect Dis 133:A165-A168.

ACKNOWLEDGEMENTS

This work was supported in part by PHS grants EY02672 and EY02377 from the National Eye Institute, National Institutes of Health, Bethesda, Maryland.

Herpes Viruses and Virus Chemotherapy, R. Kono, editor

TREATMENT OF OCULAR HERPES BY NEW ANTIVIRAL AGENTS : IN PARTICULAR ACYCLOVIR (ACV) AND BROMOVINYLDEOXYURIDINE (BVDU)

P.C. MAUDGAL[1], E. DE CLERCQ[2] and L. MISSOTTEN[1]
[1]Department of Ophthalmology, Academic Hospital St. Rafaël, University of Leuven, Kapucijnenvoer 7, B-3000 Leuven, Belgium, and [2]Rega Institute for Medical Research, University of Leuven, Minderbroedersstraat 10, B-3000 Leuven, Belgium.

INTRODUCTION

Idoxuridine (IDU, 5-iodo-2'-deoxyuridine), vidarabine (Vira-A, 9-β-D-arabinofuranosyladenine), and trifluridine (trifluorothymidine, TFT, F_3T, 5-trifluoromethyl-2'-deoxyuridine) have been available for several years for the treatment of herpetic ocular infections. Recently, acyclovir [Zovirax®, ACV, 9-(2-hydroxyethoxymethyl)-guanine] eye ointment has been introduced in many countries. Several other antiherpes compounds have been developed and are currently under investigation for the topical and/or systemic therapy of herpes simplex virus type 1 (HSV-1), herpes simplex virus type 2 (HSV-2), and varicella-zoster virus (VZV) infections. The new antiherpes compounds include :

1. Glycyl-ACV [9-(2-glycyloxy)ethoxymethyl)guanine] (1)
2. DHPG [9-(1,3-dihydroxy-2-propoxymethyl)guanine, also known as BW759, BIOLF-62, and 2'-nor-2'-deoxyguanosine] (2,3)
3. BVDU [bromovinyldeoxyuridine, (E)-5-(2-bromovinyl)-2'-deoxyurudine] (4)
4. BVara-U [(E)-5-(2-bromovinyl)-1-β-D-arabinofuranosyluracil] (5)
5. FIAC [1-(2'-fluoro-2'-deoxy-β-D-arabinofuranosyl)-5-iodocytosine] (6,7)
6. FMAU [1-(2'-fluoro-2'-deoxy-β-D-arabinofuranosyl)-5-methyluracil] (7)
7. Cyclaradine (carbocyclic vidarabine) (8)
8. Foscarnet (phosphonoformate trisodium salt) (9,10)

Most of these compounds have been shown to exert a beneficial effect on experimental HSV-1 epithelial keratitis. ACV and BVDU have been tested for their efficacy in the treatment of epithelial keratitis, stromal disease and iritis in humans.

ACYCLOVIR

ACV is active against HSV-1, HSV-2 (11,12) and VZV (13). For the treatment of dendritic and geographic corneal ulcers, it is as effective as IDU (14,15), although the healing time of ulcers may be shorter with ACV treatment than with IDU treatment (16). Corneal ulcers clinically resistant to IDU or ara-A can be treated by topical ACV application (17,18).

Although there is evidence that topically applied ACV penetrates the intact cornea to attain antiviral concentrations in the aqueous (19), it is ineffective or only marginally effective in the treatment of experimental stromal keratitis

(20). In our experiments (unpublished data) significantly less severe stromal disease developed in the rabbits treated with ACV than in the placebo-treated group, but TFT produced significantly better healing than either ACV or placebo.

According to our clinical experience, 3 % ACV eye ointment applied five times a day exerted a satisfactory healing effect on dendritic keratitis, but some of these patients developed stromal disease which was refractory to ACV treatment. In patients who presented with stromal disease or iritis, ACV had only a marginal beneficial effect, whether it was combined with topical corticosteroids or not.

No serious toxic side effects have been observed with topical ACV treatment. Only reversible mild punctate staining of the bulbar conjunctiva has been noted upon topical ACV application (17).

Glycyl-ACV is a 30-fold more water-soluble ester derivative of ACV, and can be administered as 1-5 % eyedrops. It may be considered as a prodrug of ACV and its efficacy is similar to that of acyclovir (1). In rabbit experiments, 1 % glycyl-ACV eyedrops produced a significant healing of epithelial keratitis, stromal keratitis, and iritis. Yet, this beneficial effect was less pronounced than that obtained with 0.5 % BVDU eyedrops (21).

BROMOVINYLDEOXYURIDINE

BVDU is slightly more potent than ACV against HSV-1 (4), less active against HSV-2 (22), but markedly more effective against VZV (13).

BVDU has a significantly better healing effect than IDU in the treatment of experimental HSV-1 epithelial keratitis (23,24), whether both drugs are applied as ointments or eyedrops. It is also superior to TFT in the treatment of HSV-1 stromal keratitis (25) and iritis (26). When given to rabbits orally, at 10 mg or 100 mg per day, BVDU had a significant healing effect on iritis (26).

We have previously reported on the treatment of dendritic keratitis, geographic corneal ulcers and stromal keratitis by 0.1 % BVDU eyedrops (28,29). Till now, we have treated 69 patients with dendritic ulcers by 0.1 % BVDU eyedrops, and 66 of them were followed for an average period of 37 months. Thirty-four of these patients had been treated, albeit unsuccessfully, with IDU, TFT and/or Vira-A for their current episode. Those patients who had symptoms of less than one month duration healed within an average time of 8.3 days; those who had symptoms from one month to a year healed within 9 days, and those patients who had symptoms for more than one year healed within 12 days. Of the 66 patients, 40.5 % had had recurrences in the past; 30.3 % developed recurrences during the follow-up period.

Twenty-seven patients with geographic corneal ulcers have been treated with BVDU and followed for an average period of 33.6 months. Eighteen of them had not responded to IDU, TFT, and/or Vira-A treatment. One patient was also clinically resistant to Zovirax treatment. On BVDU treatment, all these patients healed within an average time of 12 days. The recurrence rate before BVDU therapy was 70 %; during the follow-up period after BVDU therapy it was reduced to 48 %.

Twenty-nine patients with stromal keratitis were treated with 0.1 % BVDU eyedrops, and 28 of them were followed for an average period of 29.5 months. Nineteen patients had not healed with IDU and/or TFT treatment. On BVDU treatment, all patients healed in about one month. Corticosteroid treatment was stopped in all patients at the time they were put on BVDU eyedrops. In a small number of patients corticosteroids had to be installed again if corneal edema persisted despite BVDU treatment. Most patients, however, responded to BVDU therapy alone. The recurrence rate before BVDU treatment was 72.4 %; after BVDU treatment it was reduced to 48.2 %.

Ophthalmic zoster patients were treated with oral BVDU capsules (3 x 125 mg/day for 5 days) combined with topical 0.1 % BVDU eyedrops (29,30). The formation of new skin lesions was arrested within 1-2 days and the existing lesions started to crust within 2-3 days. Skin lesions were completely healed within 6 to 12 days. Similarly, keratouveitis subsided rapidly. If the patient was admitted to therapy in the early phase of the disease, post-herpetic neuralgia did not develop. In other patients pain in the involved dermatome ceased during the therapy; but, in some patients, neuralgic pains re-appeared during the follow-up period.

Except for local hypersensitivity to topically applied BVDU in some patients, we did not observe any systemic or local toxic side effects of BVDU, whether the drug was administered by topical or oral route.

REFERENCES

1. Colla L, De Clercq E, Busson R, Vanderhaeghe H (1983) J Med Chem 26:602
2. Smith KO, Galloway KS, Kennell WL, Ogilvie KK, Radatus BK (1982) Antimicrob Agents Chemother 22:55
3. Ashton WT, Karkas JD, Field AK, Tolman RL (1982) Biochem Biophys Res Commun 108:1716
4. De Clercq E, Descamps J, De Somer P, Barr PJ, Jones AS, Walker RT (1979) Proc Natl Acad Sci USA 76:2947
5. Machida H, Sakata S, Kuninaka A, Yoshino H (1982) In: Shiota H, Cheng YC, Prusoff WH (eds) Herpesvirus. Clinical, Pharmacological and Basic Aspects. Excerpta Medica, Amsterdam, pp 165-174
6. Lopez C, Watanabe KA, Fox JJ (1980) Antimicrob Agents Chemother 17:803
7. Watanabe KA, Su TL, Klein RS, Chu CK, Matsuda A, Chun MW, Lopez C, Fox JJ (1983) J Med Chem 26:152
8. Vince R, Daluge S (1977) J Med Chem 20:612
9. Helgstrand E, Eriksson B, Johansson NG, Lannerö B, Larsson A, Misiorny A, Noren JO, Sjöberg B, Stenberg K, Stening G, Stridh S, Öberg B, Alenius S, Philipson L (1978) Science 201:819

10. Alenius S, Berg M, Broberg F, Eklind K, Lindborg B, Öberg B (1982) J Infect Dis 145:569

11. Elion GB, Furman PA, Fyfe JA, de Miranda P, Beauchamp L, Schaeffer HJ (1977) Proc Natl Acad Sci USA 74:5716

12. Schaeffer HJ, Beauchamp L, de Miranda P, Elion GB, Bauer DJ, Collins P (1978) Nature 272:583

13. Shigeta S, Yokota T, Iwabuchi T, Baba M, Konno K, Ogata M, De Clercq E (1983) J Infect Dis 147:576

14. Coster DJ, Wilhelmus KR, Michaud R, Jones BR (1980) Brit J Ophthalmol 64:763

15. Jones BR, Coster DJ, Michaud R, Wilhelmus KR (1981) In: Sundmacher R (ed) Herpetic Eye Diseases, JF Bergman Verlag, München, pp 318-322

16. Collum LMT, Benedict-Smith A, Hillary IB (1980) Brit J Ophthalmol 64:766

17. McGill J, Tormey P, Walker C (1981) In: Sundmacher R (ed) Herpetic Eye Diseases, JF Bergman Verlag, München, pp 318-322

18. Nesburn AB, Trousdale MD (1981) In: Sundmacher R (ed), Herpetic Eye Diseases, JF Bergman Verlag, München, pp 309-312

19. Poirier RH, Kingham JD, de Miranda P, Annel M (1982) Arch Ophthalmol 100:1964

20. Varnell ED, Kaufman HE (1981) In: Sundmacher R (ed), Herpetic Eye Diseases, JF Bergman Verlag, München, pp 303-308

21. Maudgal PC, De Clercq E, Descamps J, Missotten L (1984) Arch Ophthalmol 102: 140

22. De Clercq E, Descamps J, Verhelst G, Walker RT, Jones AS, Torrence PF, Shugar D (1980) J Infect Dis 141:563

23. Maudgal PC, De Clercq E, Descamps J, Missotten L, De Somer P, Busson R, Vanderhaeghe H, Verhelst G, Walker RT, Jones AS (1980) Antimicrob Agents Chemother 17:8

24. Maudgal PC, De Clercq E, Descamps J, Missotten L (1979) Bull Soc Belge Ophtalmol 186:109

25. Maudgal PC, De Clercq E, Descamps J, Missotten L, Wijnhoven J (1982) Arch Ophthalmol 100:653

26. Maudgal PC, Uyttebroeck W, De Clercq E, Missotten L (1982) Arch Ophthalmol 100:1337

27. Maudgal PC, Verbruggen AM, De Clercq E, Busson R, Bernaerts R, De Roo M, Ameye C, Missotten L (1984) Invest Ophthalmol Vis Sci : in press

28. Maudgal PC, Missotten L, De Clercq E, Descamps J, De Meuter E (1981) Albrecht von Graefes Arch Klin Exp Ophthalmol 216:261

29. Maudgal PC, De Clercq E, Missotten L (1984) Antiviral Res : in press

30. Maudgal PC, Dralands L, Lamberts L, De Clercq E, Descamps J, Missotten L (1981) Bull Soc Belge Ophtalmol 193:49

ANTIVIRAL DRUG COMBINATIONS FOR THE TREATMENT OF HERPETIC KERATITIS

J. COLIN
Department of ophthalmology, University of BREST, FRANCE.

INTRODUCTION

The synthesis of selective antivirals for herpes simplex virus has allowed successful treatment of most patients with herpetic keratitis. However some lesions do not respond well to them. Recently there has been considerable interest in evaluating combinations of antiviral agents, with different biochemical targets, as well as combinations of various antiviral agents with interferon with the hope of finding additive or even synergistic therapeutic effects. In such a case, smaller doses of each drug could be used, there by minimizing toxicity and the developpment of drug-resistant strains.

Sundmacher and cowerkers showed that high-titer Human Leukocyte interferon combined with Trifluorothymidine dramatically reduces the average healing time of herpetic superficial keratitis to about three days (HVS production is stopped significantly earlier if high titer Interferon is added to TFT).

This interferon effect is titre dependant. However a statistically significant effectiveness of 100^{6} 10 IU could not be verified.

De Koning et al followed the TFT-Interferon regime described by Sundmacher. Their criteria of healing were slightly different. None the less they arrived at exactly the same positive results.

Similar synergistic results have been obtained in controlled studies with ACV plus interferon. In two different studies Colin et al and De Koning et al treated patients with ACV plus HU-IFN and found that the mean healing time for established dendritic keratitis was significantly reduced, compared to healing times with ACV plus placebo. The advantage of this combination may be less danger of local toxicity and better antiviral activity in cases with concomittant deep herpetic disease.

First controlled clinical studies with E. Coli derived human inferon have shown that it is effective in such combinations, but slightly less effective than the natural leukocyte interferon.

Kaufman and Varnell have reported that tow drug combinations, TFT plus AVC and Vidarabine plus AVC, appeared to have an enhanced therapeutic effect, compared to the effect of each drug alone in the rabbit eye. Similar results were obtained in tissue culture.

We studied the therapeutic effect of 3 antiviral drug combinations in patients with superficial herpetic keratitis.

PATIENTS AND METHODS

Forty three patients with virologically verified herpetic keratitis were randomly treated with one of the following combinations : 3 % ACV ointment plus 1 % TFT drops, 3 % ACV ointment plus 3 % Vidarabine ointment, 1 % TFT drops plus 3 % Vidarabine ointment. Each drug was given three times daily.

DISTRIBUTION OF PATIENTS IN THE THREE TREATMENT GROUPS

		VIDARABINE PLUS TFT	VIDARABINE PLUS ACV	AVC PLUS TFT
NO OF PATIENTS		15	14	14
SEX	M	9	10	9
	F	6	4	3
AGE : 50 OR LESS		8	6	8
GREATER THAN 50		7	8	6
DURATIONS OF SYMPTOMS :				
1 WEEK		14	12	12
1-2 WEEKS		1	2	2
ULCER SIZE :				
SMALL DENDRITIC		9	10	9
LARGE DENDRITIC		6	4	5

We defined healing as the absence of fluorescein staining except for minor punctate stainings. The treatment was given for three more days after completion of healing.

RESULTS

15 patients were treated with Vidarabine - TFT combination. Treatment was discontinued in two cases because of severe corneal toxic reaction. The thirteen other patients healed in an average of 7.1 days.

14 patients were treated with Vidarabine - ACV combination. Treatment was discontinued in one case because of allergic reaction to ACV. The thirteen other patients healed in an average of 6.1 days.

14 patients were treated with the ACV - TFT combination. All patients healed in an average of 6.6 days.

The difference between the rates of healing in the three groups was not statistically significant

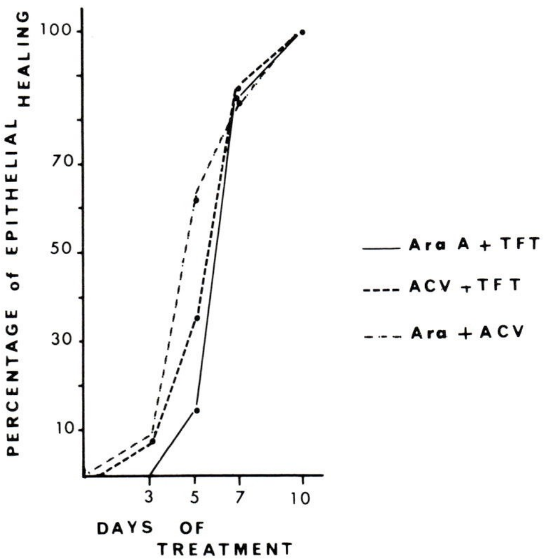

COMMENTS

In our study, the three antiviral drug combination were effective in the treatment of superficial herpetic keratitis. Each drug was given only three times daily. The mean healing were 7.1 days, 6.1 days and 6.6 days. These periods are very similar to those obtained with each antiviral drug alone used in previous studies. However a statiscally significant greater effectiveness of one of the combinations could not be verified, probably because of the limited distribution in each group.

Thus the tested combinations do not seem to offer advantages over the application of monosubstances in the treatment of dendritic keratitis. This result-although some what preliminary because of the limited number of patients in the study - is in striking contrast to the good results obtained with interferon - antiviral combinations in dendritic keratitis.

However more studies with combinations of synthetic antivirals are needed, especially with cases of deep herpetic keratitis where the interferon-antiviral combination offers no advantage.

REFERENCES

1. Colin J, Chastel C, Renard G, Cantell K Combination therapy for dendritic keratitis with human leukocyte interferon and Acyclovir. Am. J. Ophthalmol. 1983, 95, 346-348
2. De Koning E.W.J, Van Bijsterveld O.P, Cantell K Combination therapy for dendritic keratitis with human leukocyte interferon and Trifluorothymidine. Br. J. Ophthalmol. 1982, 66, 509-512
3. De Koning E.W.J, Van Bijsterveld O.P, Cantell K Combination therapy for dendritic keratitis with Acyclovir and -interferon. Arch.Ophthalmol. 1983, 101, 1866-1868
4. Kaufman H.E, Varnell E.D Antiviral chemotherapy. In : The role of viruses in human cancer, G. Giraldo and E. Beth, eds, Elsevier, In press.
5. Sundmacher R. Interferon in ocular viral diseases In: Gresser I. Ed., Interferon 4, pp 177-200, LONDON NEW-YORK, Academis Press 1982.

Herpes Viruses and Virus Chemotherapy, R. Kono, editor

PROBLEMS IN THE TREATMENT OF HERPETIC KERATITIS

HIROSHI SHIOTA

Department of Ophthalmology, Tokushima University
School of Medicine, Tokushima City 770, Japan

INTRODUCTION

Herpetic keratitis is one of the most difficult ocular infections to treat. Although there are good anti-herpes simplex virus(HSV) drugs, such as idoxuridine(IDU), adenine arabinoside(ara-A), trifluorothymidine(F_3T) and aciclovir(ACV), we still have various problems in the treatment of this disease. This paper deals with the following three problems: 1. Resistance or allergic reaction to antivirals, 2. Safe use of steroids, 3. Superinfections, particularly with fungi and *Pseudomonas aeruginosa*.

MATERIALS AND METHODS

1. Clinical treatment of ulcerative herpetic keratitis

Patients with ulcerative herpetic keratitis were examined in this study. Twenty patients received 3% ara-A ointment and twenty-three patients received 1% F_3T eye drops. Ninty-two patients were given 3% ACV ointment[1]. Treatments were given 5 times a day. The healing time of ulcers was assessed by the criteria of Laibson et al.[2].

2. Use of steroid in combination with human fibroblast interferon (Hu IFN-β)

Herpetic patients with stromal keratitis and keratoplasty were given dexamethasone eye drops in combination with Hu IFN-β eye drops. The appropriate concentrations of dexamethasone, ranging from 0.001% to 0.1%, were decided according to the severity of corneal edema and the drug was usually applied 4 times a day. Hu IFN-β eye drops were given initially at a titer of 10^5IU/ml 2 to 3 times a day and later at a titer of 10^6IU/ml 3 times a day. The effectiveness of the combination was evaluated as clinical improvement and no recurrence of ulcers.

3. Superinfections

1) Fungal superinfection

Two cases of simultaneous infection with fungus and HSV were confirmed by fungal isolation and a fluorescent antibody test for HSV.

2) *Pseudomonas aeruginosa* superinfection

Seven albino rabbits, the 101 strain of *P. aeruginosa* at 10^8/ml and the PH strain of HSV at 10^7pfu/ml were used. The right eyes of the 4 rabbits in the experimental group were inoculated with *P. aeruginosa* and their left eyes were inoculated with *P. aeruginosa* plus HSV. The right eyes of the three rabbits were inoculated with HSV and their left eyes were inoculated with vehicle. Nine sites of the cornea were inoculated by micro-trephination[3]. The eyes were observed with a photo-slit lamp for up to 14 days.

RESULTS

1. Clinical treatment of ulcerative herpetic keratitis

The results are summarized in Table I. As can be seen treatments with ara-A and F_3T were effective resulting in 90.0% and 91.3% cure, respectively. The two cases that did not respond to these drugs were cured on switch to F_3T and ara-A, respectively. For comparison the results of a survey done by the Association for Research in Infectious Diseases of the Eye, Japan, are shown indicating that ACV resulted in 88.0% cure[1].

TABLE I

EFFECTS OF ANTI-HSV DRUGS ON ULCERATIVE HERPETIC KERATITIS

Drug	No. of Eyes Cured/Treated	Healing Time (Days)
Ara-A	18/20(90.0%)	6.1
F_3T	21/23(91.3%)	6.0
ACV*	81/92(88.0%)	5.8

* Cited from ref. [1]

2. Use of steroid in combination with Hu IFN-β

1) Stromal herpetic keratitis

Fourteen cases were given Hu IFN-β drops at a titer of 10^5IU/ml. Good clinical improvement was seen in 9 cases and slight improvement in 5. Recurrence of ulcers was seen in 3 of 14 cases during the observation period of one month to 2 years. When 10^6IU/ml was used in 14 cases, good and slight improvements were seen in 11 and 3, respectively. Recurrence of ulcers was not seen during the observation period of one month to 2 years. These results are summarized in Table II .

TABLE II

COMBINED EFFECT OF HU IFN-β AND STEROID ON STROMAL HERPETIC KERATITIS

Titer of Hu IFN-β	Clinical Improvement		Recurrence of Ulcers
	Good	9	
10^5IU/ml	Slight	5	3/14(21.4%)
	None	0	
	Good	11	
10^6IU/ml	Slight	3	0/14(0%)
	None	0	

2) Herpetic keratitis after keratoplasty

Combined therapy with steroid and Hu IFN-β was started the day after keratoplasty in three cases and was continued for 3 months. When corneal edema was seen, steroid was applied under Hu IFN-β cover. In another case Hu IFN-β cover was not given just after keratoplasty, but it was given from the third time of steroid treatment after keratoplasty. Although steroid was applied, Hu IFN-β cover was given and no recurrence of ulcers was seen in any of the four cases during the observation period of 1 to 3 years.

3. Superinfections

1) Fungal superinfection

Two women of 25yrs. and 50 yrs. visited this hospital complaining of blurred vision and eye pain. They were diagnosed as having corneal ulcer, which was characterized by its geographic pattern, its opaque and uneven appearance, and the zigzag shape of its edge with intense corneal infiltration. *Acremonium sp.* and *Kabatiella sp.*, respectively, were isolated from these cases. Moreover a corneal scraping gave a positive reaction in a test with fluorescent antibody against HSV, indicating simultaneous infection with fungus and HSV. These two cases responded well to treatment with pimaricin and the anti-HSV drugs of ACV and IDU.

2) *P. aeruginosa* superinfection in rabbits

Eyes were examined 24 hours after inoculations. After *P. aeruginosa* inoculation, a few edematous sites with white infiltration in the cornea were seen, as shown in Fig. 1-a. After inoculation of *P. aeruginosa* plus HSV severe edema was seen with ring abscesses, as shown in Fig. 1-b. After inoculation of HSV fine ulcers were seen at some sites. After inoculation of vehicle only faint scars were seen. After 48 hours eyes inoculated with *P. aeruginosa* had also become edematous with ring abscesses, but those inoculated with *P. aeruginosa* and HSV showed much more severe clinical features with hypopyon. This tendency for eyes inoculated with *P. aeruginosa* and HSV to show more severe symptoms lasted until day 14. At 48 hours after HSV inoculation, dendritic ulcers without ring abscesses were seen at inoculated sites. These results show that *P. aeruginosa* and HSV had synergistic effects in causing severe keratitis.

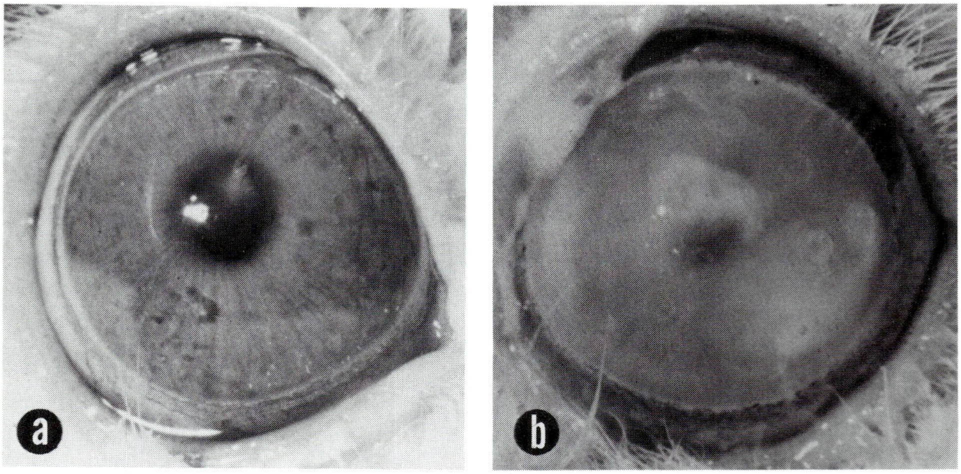

Fig. 1 (a)Right eye 24 hr after *P. aeruginosa* inoculation. (b)Left eye 24 hr after inoculation of *P. aeruginosa* plus HSV.

DISCUSSION

There are good anti-HSV drugs, such as IDU, ara-A, F_3T and ACV, available now for treatment of epithelial herpetic keratitis. Epithelial ulcers usually disappear within a week when treated with these drugs. However, some cases are irresponsive or allergic to these drugs. In the present study two cases did not respond to ara-A, but were cured when treatment was switched to F_3T. Conversely two cases that were irresponsive to F_3T were cured on switch to ara-A. McGill et al.[4] succeeded in curing 24 IDU-resistant cases by F_3T treatment. They also used F_3T eye drops on 8 cases that were allergic to IDU without subsequent development of hypersensitivity to F_3T. Kitano reported cure by switch to ACV of cases that were irresponsive to IDU[5]. Therefore, the problems of irresponsiveness and allergy can be overcome by using an alternative drug.

Another problem in herpetic keratitis is recurrence, the recurrence rate being reported to be 40% in 2 years[6]. The rate is even higher when steroid is applied. Nevertheless, steroid is useful in cases of severe stromal keratitis or keratoplasty. Therefore, steroids are usually used under antiviral cover. In such cases I have tried steroid treatment in combination with interferon, instead of ordinally antivirals. To my knowledge this is the first report on the safe and effective use of steroid in combination with interferon, or under interferon cover. When Hu IFN-β at 10^5IU/ml was used, 3 of 14 cases exhibited recurrence. However, when 10^6 IU/ml was used, no recurrence was seen in 14 cases. The number of cases reported here is not enough to allow definite conclusions, but the results clearly show a tendency. In our animal study with Hu IFN-β at 10^6IU/ml, three applications had a similar effect to ten applications[7]. Thus the use of eye drops of Hu IFN-β at 10^6IU/ml 3 times a day, is recommended when steroids must be used in herpetic keratitis.

Another problem in herpetic keratitis is superinfection, particularly with fungi and *Pseudomonas aeruginosa*. Fungal superinfection in herpetic keratitis has characteristic features: the ulcers are geographic, opaque and uneven, their edge is zigzag with intense corneal infiltration. Simultaneous infection with fungus and HSV should be suspected when corneal ulcers show these features. In such cases, treatment with anti-fungal and anti-HSV drugs is indicated. Ten of 49 cases (about 20%) of bacterial corneal ulcer in Japan were found to be due to *P. aeruginosa* infection [8], while 6 of 15 cases of superinfection of herpetic keratitis in America were found to be due to gram-negative rods which included *P. aeruginosa* [9]. Thus aminoglycosides are essential for treatment of these cases. On simultaneous infection of rabbit cornea, HSV and *P. aeruginosa* had synergistic effects in causing severe keratitis. Thus aminoglycosides besides anti-HSV drugs are recommended for treatment of ulcerative herpetic keratitis.

ACKNOWLEDGEMENT

I thank Toray Industries, Inc. for supplying Hu IFN-β eye drops.

REFERENCES

1. Shiota H (1982) Am J Med 73:307-310
2. Laibson PR, Hyndiuk R, Krachmer JH, Schultz RO (1975) Invest Ophthalmol 14:762-763
3. Jones BR, Al-Hussaini MK (1963) Trans Ophthalmol Soc UK 83:613-631
4. McGill J, Holt-Wilson AD, McKinnon JR, Williams HP, Jones BR (1974) Trans Ophthalmol Soc UK 94:342-352
5. Kitano S (1984) Presented at Int Symp on Pharmacol & Clin Approaches to Herpes Viruses & Virus Chemother, Jpn
6. Kaufman HE (1981) In: Nahmias AJ, Dowdle WR, Schinazi RF (eds) The Human Herpesviruses. Elsevier, New York-Oxford, pp 466-477
7. Shiota H, Yamane S (1982) In: Shiota H, Cheng YC, Prusoff WH (eds) Herpesvirus; Clinical, Pharmacological and Basic Aspects. Excerpta Medica, Amsterdam-Oxford-Princeton, pp 295-301
8. Tokuda H, Arimoto K, Oishi M, et al. (1982) Jpn Rev Clin Ophthalmol 76:1189-1202
9. Boisjoly HM, Pavan-Langston D, Kenyon KR, Baker AS (1983) Am J Ophthalmol 96:354-361

TREATMENT OF STROMAL HERPETIC KERATITIS BY PEPSIN-TREATED GAMMA-GLOBULIN

REIZO MANABE, YUICHI OHASHI, YOSHIKAZU SHIMOMURA
Department of Ophthalmology, Osaka University Medical School, Osaka 553, Japan

INTRODUCTION

With the great advance in antiviral drugs, epithelial herpetic keratitis is now well treated, however, the management of stromal herpetic keratitis has been an unsolved problem to us. Epithelial keratitis is caused by active proliferation of the virus in the corneal epithelium, whereas stromal keratitis is supposed to be the result of the host immune response to the virus or viral antigens present on the surface of infected keratocytes or endothelial cells (1,2). Therefore, the modalities of therapies for these two kinds of keratitis are clearly different. For the effective treatment of stromal keratitis, we must eliminate the virus as well as control the host immune response.

Pepsin-treated gamma-globulin (PTGG) which has been developed mainly for the therapy of immunocompromised patients lacks Fc portion of IgG. In other words, PTGG cannot mediate the immune reactions requiring the Fc portion of IgG, such as complement-dependent cytotoxicity (CDC) or antibody-dependent cellular cytotoxicity (ADCC) (3,4). Additionally PTGG solution has an extremely high level of divalent anti-herpes simplex virus (HSV) antibodies (3,4). Thus, PTGG is able to neutralize the virus as well as bind to the viral antigen on the cell surface. Postulated mechanism by which PTGG works against stromal herpetic keratitis is shown in Figure 1. HSV-specific PTGG bound to the cell surface viral antigen can block the binding between immunocompetent cells or native IgG and virus-infected

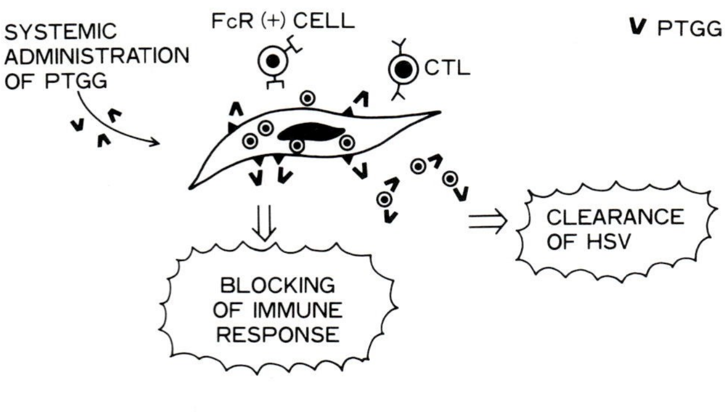

Fig. 1. Postulated effect of PTGG on stromal herpetic keratitis.

cells. As a result, PTGG inhibits CDC, ADCC, or cytolysis mediated by cytotoxic T lymphocytes as was demonstrated in in vitro experiments (4), and further development of the inflammation is suppressed as was proposed by Hoffman and Kappler (5). Moreover, PTGG can clear the virus from the site of the inflammation.

Based upon this theory, we investigated the efficacy of systemic PTGG-administration on the patients with stromal herpetic keratitis.

SUBJECTS AND METHODS

Patients

Included in this study were 34 patients with stromal herpetic keratitis who were followed up in the Corneal Service of our hospital from April, 1982 to March, 1984. All eyes were randomly divided into three groups and treated as follows: 17 eyes in Group 1 were treated with systemic administration of PTGG (2.5 g/day; Yamanouchi Pharmaceutical Co. Ltd., Japan) for 5 consecutive days plus subconjunctival injection of depot steroid (2 mg of dexamethasone/injection) twice a week; 11 eyes in Group 2 with subconjunctival steroid alone of the same schedule; 7 eyes in Group 3 with systemic PTGG alone for 5 days. All patients were covered with topical antivirals, antibiotics, and steroid.

Assessment of clinical findings

The patients with recurrent stromal keratitis were examined concerning the following clinical parameters on the day when the treatment was initiated and one week later.

Biomicroscopic observation

The degree of stromal edema and ciliary injection was assessed using a slit lamp.

Visual acuity

All patients were corrected for the best visual acuity.

RESULTS

In terms of the disease morbidity, the patients in Group 1 were improved most rapidly. Thus, one week after the initiation of the treatment, 7 out of 17 eyes (41%) in Group 1 showed marked reduction of stromal edema, whereas only 2 out of 11 eyes (18%) in Group 2 and 1 out of 7 eyes (14%) in Group 3 achieved improvement (Table I). Ciliary injection was subsided best in Group 1 as well. Visual acuity of all the groups of the patients was improved one week after the initiation of the treatment. There was no difference among three groups.

Focusing on the incidence of the recurrence during the period of 3 months after each treatment, it seems that less recurrence was observed in Group 3 (29%) which was treated with systemic PTGG alone for 5 days as compared with Group 1 (41%) and Group 2 (45%) (Table II).

TABLE I

CLINICAL EVALUATION OF THE DEGREE OF STROMAL EDEMA ONE WEEK AFTER THE TREATMENT

Group of Patients (Treatment)	Stromal Edema		
	Unchanged	Improved	Markedly Improved
1. (PTGG + ST)*	2/17 (12%)**	8/17 (47%)	7/17 (41%)
2. (ST)	3/11 (27%)	6/11 (56%)	2/11 (18%)
3. (PTGG)	0/7 (0%)	6/7 (86%)	1/7 (14%)

* PTGG = pepsin-treated gamma-globulin; ST = steroid.
** The number of patients categorized/examined.

TABLE II

THE INCIDENCE OF RECURRENCES FOLLOWING THE TREATMENT

Group of Patients	The Incidence of Recurrences*
1. (PTGG + ST)	7/17** (41%)
2. (ST)	5/11 (45%)
3. (PTGG)	2/7 (29%)

* The patients were followed up for 3 months after the treatments.
** The number of the patients with recurrence/examined.

DISCUSSION

Generally, steroid is the choice of the drug for the treatment of stromal herpetic keratitis. Although it brings about the rapid resolution of stromal edema as well as improvement of the visual acuity, the profound suppression of the local immunity resulted from the prolonged use of this potent drug is often harmful to the eye.

As mentioned earlier in this communication, PTGG is supposed to have two different actions on stromal keratitis; blocking the effector of immune responses and eliminating the virus. Since the working mechanisms of PTGG are different from those of steroids, we investigated in this trial whether PTGG treatment had any beneficial effect on stromal keratitis. From the biomicroscopic observation, the combined treatment with PTGG plus steroid gave the best result, suggesting that PTGG might work in synergy to steroid.

The interesting finding was that the less recurrence took place in the patients of Group 3 who had received PTGG treatment alone. This result is encouraging as well and the more controlled study for assessing the efficacy of PTGG is currently being carried out in our department. We believe that PTGG can be a good regimen in the therapy of stromal herpetic keratitis.

REFERENCES

1. Dawson CR, Togni B (1976) Surv Ophthalmol 21:121-135
2. Pavan-Langston D (1983) In: Thoft RA, Smolin G (eds) The Cornea. Little Brown and Company, Boston, pp 178-195
3. Melewicz F, Shore SL, Ades EW, Phillips DJ (1977) J Immunol 118:567-573
4. Ohashi Y, Sakaue Y, Hiraishi T, Hiraoka H, Kato S, Manabe R (1980) Folia Ophthalmol Jpn 31:1033-1038
5. Hoffman MK, Kappler JW (1978) Nature 272:64-65

POTENTIAL TREATMENTS FOR HERPES ZOSTER INFECTION

JAMES MCGILL*, PETER REES†, DAVID BRIGDEN†

*Southampton Eye Hospital, Southampton, Hants, England and †The Wellcome Research Laboratories, Beckenham, England

INTRODUCTION

In the assessment of the treatment of herpes zoster infection both the acute and chronic aspects of the disease must be taken into consideration. In the acute phase, treatment must be assessed in terms of the effect on pain and rash progression and resolution. In the long term, effects on post-herpetic neuralgia must be determined. Ocular involvement is an additional potential problem for patients with herpes zoster ophthalmicus.

HERPES ZOSTER SKIN RASH

Systemic steroids have been suggested as shortening the duration of post-herpetic neuralgia[1, 2] but they carry the risk of dissemination of the disease[3]. Systemic administration of adenine arabinoside has no significant effect on the disease process[8] and cytosine arabinoside was found to be inferior to placebo[9], depressing antibody formation and causing greater disease dissemination[10]. Idoxuridine in DMSO has been claimed to be of benefit[11] but a controlled study has shown it to have no significant benefit over DMSO alone in the treatment of the skin rash[12]. For these reasons many doctors have until now treated herpes zoster skin infection with supportive means only.

Acyclovir (ACV) has been shown _in vitro_ to have antiviral activity against the varicella zoster virus[13]. A placebo-controlled, double blind trial of intravenous ACV (5mg/kg t.i.d. for 5 days) was conducted in 40 patients with acute herpes zoster skin rash[16]. The ACV-treated patients fared significantly better than the placebo recipients in terms of the duration of new lesion formation and the times to loss of vesicles and full crusting (Table 1). Similar significant improvements in the resolution of the acute skin rash of herpes zoster have been reported in two other placebo controlled studies of intravenous ACV[14, 15]. In addition, Bean _et al._[15] have shown that ACV therapy significantly reduced the duration of virus shedding.

ACUTE PHASE PAIN AND POST-HERPETIC NEURALGIA

Both the acute phase pain and post-herpetic neuralgia associated with zoster can be severe, particularly in the elderly. In the study reported by McGill _et al._[16] there were fewer patients in the ACV group with increased pain or with pain remaining moderate or severe at the end of therapy when compared with the placebo group. Post-herpetic neuralgia, measured at 3 months, was also reduced in the ACV recipients but in neither case did the difference achieve statistical significance, probably as a result of the small numbers of patients included in the trial. In two other studies[14, 15], intravenous ACV was shown to significantly reduce the incidence of pain during the acute phase. In both cases, however, pain recurred or worsened in a number of patients following the end of treatment and no statistically significant differences in the incidence of post-herpetic neuralgia could be detected between the ACV and placebo groups at 1 to 3 months though trends in favour of ACV have again been reported[15]. The failure to achieve statistically significant reductions of post-herpetic neuralgia following ACV therapy may be related to the inclusion of a number of relatively young patients in these studies, resulting in a reduced incidence of post-herpetic neuralgia in both the ACV and placebo groups. Larger controlled studies, designed specifically to examine the influence of acute phase ACV therapy on the incidence of post-herpetic neuralgia are required.

OCULAR INVOLVEMENT

Ocular involvement of herpes zoster infection is serious, occurring in 50% to 60% of those with trigeminal involvement[4]. The disease process is sometimes prolonged, affecting all parts of the eye and leading to severe ocular damage and visual loss in many patients. The exact aetiology of the ocular lesions is obscure. Virus invasion may play a part in tissue damage since virus has been isolated from acute corneal epithelial ulcers and viral particles have been seen on the corneal stromal endothelium [5, 6]. Local immune and inflammatory mechanisms may also be important. Until now, most people have treated ocular herpes zoster involvement with topical steroids, though these can lead to the exacerbation and continuation of the disease process by enhancing virus replication and suppressing local immune or defence mechanisms. Topical steroid treatment may need to be continued for up to 18 months[7] and recurrences frequently occur either whilst on treatment or as the steroids are being withdrawn or stopped. Such recurrences can affect parts of the eye not initially involved and can lead to ocular damage (Tables 2 and 3).

In initial open studies using acyclovir ophthalmic ointment in acute herpes zoster kerato-uveitis, most patients had a quick resolution of their symptoms without any recurrence of their disease process[17]. This was in sharp contrast to the common clinical finding that patients treated with topical steroids required a prolonged course of treatment and suffered frequent recurrences. For this reason, a double blind trial was set up to compare topical steroids and acyclovir ophthalmic ointment in the treatment of acute herpes zoster kerato-uveitis[18]. Both drugs were administered 5 times daily until the clinical signs had resolved and were then weaned off over 4 to 6 weeks. Corneal epithelial disease resolved significantly faster in the acyclovir group but there was no significant difference in the resolution of stromal disease, uveitis or scleritis between the two groups. The initial treatment duration was similar for both groups of patients, but 12 of the 19 steroid recipients had a recurrence of their kerato-uveitis once treatment was stopped or was being weaned off. None of the 17 acyclovir recipients had a recurrence of their ocular symptoms and when total treatment durations were considered, the patients in the acyclovir group were seen to have fared significantly better than the steroid recipients (Table 4). The exact role of acyclovir, however, remains uncertain as this trial could have just exposed the adverse effects of steroids. Placebo controls could not be used in these patients as it was ethically not possible to treat with placebo a patient with a painful inflamed eye.

In an attempt to gain a broader impression of the usefulness of acyclovir, a retrospective analysis has been conducted[19] on all patients with acute herpes zoster ocular involvement presenting at Southampton Eye Hospital over the last four years and treated by a number of doctors. Retrospective analyses are not ideal but when the clinical outcomes of those patients treated, on an open basis, with either topical acyclovir, topical steroids or a combination of both were compared, a clear pattern emerged. Those treated with acyclovir fared appreciably better, with a quicker resolution of their epithelial or stromal disease and their uveitis settled on average in the same time as those treated with topical steroids. Herpes zoster kerato-uveitis was controlled by acyclovir alone in 51 out of 56 cases. In the first year after the onset of their infection the acyclovir treated patients had a significantly shorter course of treatment and there were no recurrences, compared with a 50% incidence in those treated with topical steroids, many of whom were still on treatment. With a longer follow-up period, 2 out of 56 patients treated with acyclovir had a recurrence of their kerato-uveitis (Table 5). A feature of topical steroid treatment of herpes zoster kerato-uveitis is that the eye whitens quickly. Acyclovir treated eyes do not do this, giving a false impression that the eye is not improving but the end point of the particular disease process e.g. uveitis, can be similar.

In patients with herpes zoster induced scleritis or in those with an acute limbal infiltration (i.e. sclerokeratitis) acyclovir ophthalmic ointment had little beneficial effect and in these cases topical steroids are indicated. Once topical steroids were added to the regime, however, they had to be weaned off slowly over 18 months to prevent recurrences. The addition of acyclovir to these patients conferred no beneficial effect in that they still need a prolonged course of treatment with frequent recurrences if the steroids are weaned off too quickly.

SUMMARY AND CONCLUSIONS

Intravenous acyclovir has been shown to be effective in treating the skin rash and in reducing the the pain associated with acute herpes zoster. Reductions in the incidence of post-herpetic neuralgia have been demonstrated following intravenous acyclovir therapy but have not achieved statistical significance. Intravenous therapy is restricted to those patients requiring hospitalisation and an effective out-patient therapy is urgently required. Controlled clinical trials are currently in progress to determine the efficacy of (high dose) oral acyclovir in the treatment of the acute phase of herpes zoster and its influence on post-herpetic neuralgia.

Ocular involvement can be a serious complication of trigeminal zoster and conventional treatment with steroids is not satisfactory because of the necessity for prolonged therapy and the high incidence of recurrences. Acyclovir ophthalmic ointment was found to be superior to steroids, with significant reductions in the duration of therapy and numbers of recurrences. Acyclovir alone was found to control herpes zoster kerato-uveitis in the majority of patients, without the need to add topical steroids. Further controlled studies are underway to determine the therapeutic role of acyclovir ophthalmic ointment in herpes zoster kerato-uveitis in patients with an acute skin rash and no ocular involvement or just slight conjunctival or corneal involvement.

TABLE 1

EFFECT OF ACYCLOVIR ON HERPES ZOSTER ACUTE SKIN RASH

	Median (Group Size)		p-value (Log Rank Analysis)
	Placebo	Acyclovir	
Days to formation of last new lesion	2.00 (20)	0.0 (17)	0.001
First day without vesicles	4.5 (20)	3.0 (17)	0.003
Days to full crusting	5.0 (20)	3.0 (17)	0.006

From: McGill et al 1983 (16)

TABLE 2

DEMONSTRATING THE HIGH INCIDENCE OF RECURRENCE OF HERPES ZOSTER OPHTHALMICUS WHEN TOPICAL STEROIDS ARE USED, EVEN IN COMBINATION WITH TOPICAL ACYCLOVIR

	Steroids	Steroids and Acyclovir
Number of patients	74	14
Recurrences on treatment	5 (2)	2 (1)
Recurrences as treatment was withdrawn	15 (8)	3 (3)
Recurrences after treatment was stopped	27	7

(numbers in brackets denote patients who had recurrences after treatment was stopped as well as recurrences on treatment)

TABLE 3

TO SHOW HOW PATIENTS TREATED WITH TOPICAL STEROIDS HAVE RECURRENCES AFFECTING PARTS OF THE EYE NOT INITIALLY INVOLVED (RETROSPECTIVE ANALYSIS)

Treatment Forms	Steroids	Acyclovir	Acyclovir and Steroids
Numbers of patients	74	56	14
% affecting new parts	16% (12)	3% (1)	29% (4)

TABLE 4

OUTCOME OF TREATMENT WITH EITHER TOPICAL ACYCLOVIR OR TOPICAL STEROIDS (BETNESOL) FIVE TIMES A DAY ON ACUTE HERPES ZOSTER OCULAR INVOLVEMENT

Group	Number	Number healed	Initial Treatment Duration (median days)	Number Disease Reappeared	Total treatment Duration (median days)
Acyclovir	17	16	75	0	75 (Range 17-144)
Steroids	19	18	68	12* (63%)	280** (Range 34-440)

*p<0.001 (Fisher's exact test, 2-tailed)

**p=0.002 (Mann-Whitney U test, 2-tailed)

From: McGill and Chapman, 1983 (18)

TABLE 5

SUMMARY OF A RETROSPECTIVE ANALYSIS OF 144 PATIENTS TREATED FOR ACUTE HERPES ZOSTER KERATO-UVEITIS

Therapy	Number of patients	Average Treatment Duration (days)	Total Recurrences	Recurrences after 1 year
Acyclovir	56	62.3	6% (2)	6% (2)
Steroids	74	200	50% (37)	5.4% (4)
Steroids + Acyclovir	14	197	57% (8)	7.1% (1)

REFERENCES

1. Elliott FA (1964) Lancet ii: 610-611.

2. Eaglstein WH, Kats R, Brown JA (1970) JAMA 211: 1681-1683

3. Rado JP, Tako J, Geder L, Jeney E (1965) Arch Intern Med 116: 329-335

4. Womack LW, Leisegang TJ (1983) Arch Ophthalmol 101: 42-45

5. Maudgal PC, Misotten L, de Clercq E, Descamps J (1980) Bull Soc belge Ophtal 190: 71-86

6. Hayashi K, Uchida Y, Ohshima M (1973) Am J Ophthalmol 75: 795-798

7. Marsh RJ (1976) Br J Hosp Med 15: 609-618

8. Marsh RJ, Laird R, Atkinson A, Steel A McD, Jones BR (1981) In: Sundmacher R, ed. Herpetische Augenerkrankungen. Munich: JR Bergmann Verlag pp. 449-454

9. Davis CM, Van Dersarl JV, Coltman CA (1973) JAMA 224: 122-123

10. Stevens DA, Jordan GW, Waddell TF, Merigan TC (1973) New Eng J Med 289: 873-878

11. Juel-Jensen BE, MacCallum FO, MacKenzie AMR, Pike MC (1970) Br Med J 4: 776-780

12. Wildenhoff KE, Ipsen J, Esmann V, Ingemann-Jensen J, Poulsen JH (1979) Scand J Infect Dis 11: 1-9

13. Crumpacker CS, Schnipper LE, Zaia JA, Levin MJ (1979) Antimicrobial Agents Chemother 15: 642-645

14. Peterslund NA, Seyer-Hansen K, Ipsen J, Esmann V, Schonheyder H, Juhl H (1981) Lancet ii: 827-30

15. Bean B, Braun C, Balfour HH (1982) Lancet ii: 118-121

16. McGill J, McDonald DR, Fall C, McKendrick GDW, Copplestone A (1983) J Infection 6: 157-161

17. McGill J (1981) Br J Ophthalmol 65: 542-545

18. McGill J, Chapman C (1983) Br J Ophthalmol 67: 746-750

19. McGill J, Manakian M (1984) in press.

THE PHARMACOLOGICAL CHARACTERIZATION OF HSV-1 OCULAR SHEDDING: INDUCTION AND ATTEMPTED BLOCKAGE

JAMES M. HILL, YOSHIKAZU SHIMOMURA, YASUNORI YAMAMOTO, AND LOUIS P. GANGAROSA
School of Medicine, Medical College of Georgia, Augusta, GA 30912

INTRODUCTION

HSV-1 infection is a leading cause of corneal disease and blindness. The most serious clinical problem is recurrence of the ocular lesions which can be progressively more severe with each episode. However, the mechanism which triggers recurrent HSV-1 infection is still unknown. The concept of latent infection of HSV-1 in neural tissues (trigeminal ganglion, sacral ganglion, superior cervical ganglion) is generally accepted. Reactivation of HSV-1 from latently infected tissues by administering epinephrine to rabbits has been reported (1-7). Recently, we reported that by supersensitizing the eye of a latently infected rabbit by iontophoresis of 6-hydroxydopamine (6-HD), one can reliably and with a high frequency induce HSV-1 shedding into the tear film by topical instillation of epinephrine (8). Using HSV-1 latently infected rabbits, we designed experiments to determine which adrenergic agonists can induce HSV-1 shedding into tear film and whether or not adrenergic antagonists would block the induced reactivation of the virus.

Methods

New Zealand albino rabbits (2.5-3.0 kg of body weight) were used for all experiments. The procedure of establishing latent infection was reported previously (8). All eyes had shed virus at least once spontaneously during post-inoculation days 20-39. These HSV-1 latently infected rabbits were used between 70-175 days post-inoculation. Iontophoresis of 1% 6-HD was performed using 0.75 mAmps for 3 min to the cornea to produce ocular adrenergic supersensitivity. The topical instillation of two drops (approximately 100 µl) of a 2% solution of an adrenergic agonist (epinephrine, norepinephrine, phenylephrine, clonidine and isoproterenol) was given 6 hours after iontophoresis and twice a day for the next 4 days. This produces HSV-1 shedding into tear films in 90-100% of the rabbit eyes. In other rabbits, iontophoresis of 0.01% epinephrine for 8 min at 0.8 mAmp was given once a day for 3 consecutive days. HSV-1 ocular shedding was detected and determined by using a previously reported eye swab procedure (8). The number of eyes in each experimental group was from 10-12. The specificity of HSV-1 in samples from ocular swabs was determined by a plaque-reduction assay on CV-1 cells with an HSV-1 hyperimmune rabbit antiserum. In addition, in four

(4) other experiments, an α-adrenergic antagonist (phentolamine, phenoxybenzamine, yohimbine, or thymoximine) was instilled 15 minutes before adrenergic agonist instillation.

Results

Table 1 displays the summary of each HSV-1 induction method. HSV-1 ocular shedding was detected in 40-60% of the eyes given epinephrine by topical application only or by 6-HD iontophoresis only, and the average duration of shedding for both groups was for only one day. HSV-1 ocular shedding occurred in 90-100% of the eyes and for a 3 day average duration when iontophoresis of 0.01% epinephrine was given for 3 consecutive days. Finally, the combined treatment of 1% 6-HD iontophoresis and topical application of 2% epinephrine resulted in HSV-1 shedding into the tear film in 90-100% of the eyes and the average duration was for 5 days.

TABLE 1. Induced HSV-1 Ocular Shedding

Method for Induction	Range of the Frequency of Shedding (%)	Average Duration of Shedding (days)
Iont. of 0.01% Epi. (3 times)	90 - 100	3.0
Iont. of 1.0% 6-HD (only once)	40 - 60	1.0
2% Epi. topically for 5 days (twice per day)	40 - 60	1.0
Iont. of 1.0% 6-HD once and 2% Epi. topically 5 days (9 treatments)	90 - 100	5.0

Ocular swabs were taken once a day for seven consecutive days beginning the day after the first treatment. Abbreviations are: Iont. = Iontophoresis; Epi. = Epinephrine; 6-HD = 6-hydroxydopamine

Table 2 displays the result of HSV-1 ocular shedding by the combined treatment of 1% 6-HD iontophoresis and other adrenergic agonists. As in Table 1, the combined treatment of 1% 6-HD by iontophoresis and 2% epinephrine topical instillation showed 100% frequency and the longest average duration of 5 days. With norepinephrine, HSV-1 shedding occurred in 70% of the eyes and for 2.5 days. With phenylephrine, there was shedding in 62% of the eyes and for 2.2 days.

With clonidine, the frequency was 38% but for only 1 day average duration. With 2% isoproterenol no HSV-1 ocular shedding was detected.

None of the α-adrenergic antagonists (phentolamine, yohimbine, phenoxybenzamine, or thymoximine) were able to significantly block the effects of 6-HD plus epinephrine on induced HSV-1 ocular shedding.

TABLE 2. The Effect of Adrenergic Agonists on HSV-1 Ocular Shedding

Agonist [2% solution]	Ocular receptor	Frequency of Shedding (%)	Average Duration of Shedding (days)
Epinephrine	α,β	100	5.0
Norepinephrine	α,β	70	2.5
Phenylephrine	α	62	2.2
Clonidine	α	38	1.0
Isoproterenol	β	0	0

Discussion

Previously, we reported that ocular instillation of epinephrine to adrenergically sensitized eyes induced HSV-1 ocular shedding in 100% eyes (8). Adrenergic supersensitivity was induced by iontophoresis of 1.0% 6-HD. In the present experiments the combined treatment of 1% 6-HD iontophoresis and topical instillation of 2% epinephrine resulted in the highest frequency and the longest average duration of HSV-1 shedding in tear film, confirming our previous report (8). In addition, further experiments were performed in rabbit eyes which were supersensitized by iontophoretic application of 6-HD and then given topical instillation of different adrenergic agonists which induced HSV-1 shedding in the tear film to varying degrees. Epinephrine and norepinephrine are thought to have an effect on both α- and β-adrenergic receptors in most tissues. Phenylephrine and clonidine which are thought to be more specific for α-receptor activation resulted in a lower frequency and shorter average duration of HSV-1 ocular shedding than epinephrine. Isoproterenol, the classical β-receptor agonist, resulted in no induction of HSV-1 shedding in tear film. These results implicate that an α-adrenergic receptor in ocular tissue is involved in the initial steps in the induction of HSV-1 reactivation, while β-adrenergic receptors may not be involved. However, the pretreatment with α-adrenergic antagonists (phentolamine, phenoxybenzamine, yohimbine, and thymoximine) have never shown any significant blockade of induced HSV-1 ocular shedding. We will make further efforts to define the role of the adrenergic relationship between the induction of HSV-1 ocular shedding and reactivation of the latent HSV-1 in the rabbit.

ACKNOWLEDGEMENTS

This study was supported by grant NEI-EY-04169. The authors wish to thank Mrs. Donna J. Lee, Mr. Earl Berman, and Mr. Michael Jones for technical assistance, and Mrs. Ida O. Thomas for secretarial assitance. This is contribution number 0871 from the Department of Cell and Molecular Biology, Medical College of Georgia, Augusta, Ga.

REFERENCES

1. Kwon BS, Gangarosa LP, Burch KD, deBack J, Hill JM (1981) Induction of ocular herpes simplex virus shedding by iontophoresis of epinephrine into rabbit cornea. Invest Ophthalmol Vis Sci 21:442-449.

2. Laibson PR, Kibrick S (1966) Reactivation of herpetic keratitis by epinephrine in rabbit. Arch Ophthalmol 75:254-260.

3. Laibson PR, Kibrick S (1967) Reactivation of herpetic keratitis in rabbit. II. Repeated reactivations in the same host. Arch Ophthalmol 77:244-248.

4. Kibrick S, Takahashi GH, Leibowitz HM, Laibson PR (1971) Local corticosteroid therapy and reactivation of herpetic keratitis. Arch Ophthalmol 86:694-698.

5. Schmidt JR, Rasmussen AF Jr. (1960) Activation of latent herpes simplex encephalitis by chemical means. J Infect Dis 106:154-158.

6. Kwon BS, Gangarosa LP, Green K, Hill JM (1982) Kinetics of ocular herpes simplex virus shedding induced by epinephrine iontophoresis. Invest Ophthalmol Vis Sci 22:818-821.

7. Hill JM, Kwon BS, Shimomura Y, Colborn GL, Yaghmai F, Gangarosa LP (1983) Herpes simplex virus recovery in neural tissues after ocular HSV shedding induced by epinephrine iontophoresis to the rabbit cornea. Invest Ophthalmol Vis Sci 24:243-247.

8. Shimomura Y, Gangarosa LP, Kataoka M, Hill JM (1984) HSV-1 shedding by iontophoresis of 6-hydroxydopamine followed by topical epinephrine. Invest Ophthalmol Vis Sci 24:1588-1594.

B. Cutaneous

TREATMENT OF RECURRENT OROFACIAL HERPES INFECTIONS: REVIEW OF CLINICAL TRIALS AND A STRATEGY FOR SUCCESSFUL THERAPY

SPOTSWOOD L. SPRUANCE AND DONNA J. FREEMAN

Department of Medicine and the Center for Infectious Diseases, Diagnostic Microbiology and Immunology, University of Utah School of Medicine, Salt Lake City, Utah, U.S.A.

Recurrent herpes simplex labialis is a mild but common illness which afflicts as many as 20-45% of the population at some point in their life. Treatment of uncomplicated herpes labialis in otherwise healthy subjects has been the subject of multiple clinical trials for 25 years, involving a wide variety of treatment modalities and routes of application. Unfortunately, studies with the majority of agents have generally been unrewarding. Typically, great enthusiasm was generated by an initial uncontrolled study only to be followed by disappointment when a proper double-blinded, placebo-controlled trial was performed. A summary of some of the agents studied is shown in Table 1. This brief review will not deal with the treatment of oral herpes in immunocompromised subjects or primary herpetic gingivostomatitis.

TABLE I
AGENTS STUDIED FOR THE TREATMENT OF HERPES LABIALIS

TOPICAL - NUCLEOSIDE ANALOGUES	TOPICAL - MISCELLANEOUS	ORAL
Acyclovir	Ether	Lysine
Adenine arabinoside	Chloroform	Levamisole
Adenine arabinoside monophosphate	Butylated hydroxytoluene	Lithium
	Epinephrine	Photodynamic inactivation
Cytosine arabinoside	Adenosine monophosphate	Inosine
Ethyldeoxyuridine	Heavy metals (zinc, borate)	Trimethoprim-sulfamethoxazole
Phosphonoformate	Kethoxal (3-ethoxy-2-oxobutyraldehyde)	
Iododeoxyuridine		Vitamins (bioflavinoids and ascorbic acid)

A few controlled studies of the treatment of herpes labialis have yielded positive results. Fiddian has reported a 25% shortening of the median healing time using topical 5% acyclovir in polyethylene glycol (Zovirax, Burroughs Wellcome Co.) (1). However, in a similar study involving a larger number of subjects, Spruance et al. observed no clinical benefit with topical 10% acyclovir in polyethylene glycol despite initiation of therapy in the erythema and prodromal stages of the illness (2). In a second report, Fiddian et al. treated 49 patients with recurrent herpes labialis with either topical 5% acyclovir in a new cream formulation or the vehicle control and observed a 33% shortening in the median time to healing (3). Other studies with the cream formulation of acyclovir are not as yet available.

TABLE 2

STRATEGY FOR SUCCESSFUL TREATMENT OF HERPES LABIALIS

1. Potent antiviral which acts intracellularly
2. Early start of treatment
3. Delivery of drug to infected cells

Table 2 shows a strategy for the development of successful treatments for herpes labialis. Many potent antivirals are available, some of which have been described at this symposium and which have been successfully used to treat other forms of herpes simplex virus infections. The second important element is early treatment. The rapid natural evolution of herpes labialis, hastened by humoral and cellular immune factors in the normal, non-immunocompromised host, provides only a brief therapeutic opportunity between the first signs or symptoms of the disease and the time point where clinical severity reaches a plateau and virus titers begin to decline. Treatment of the disease in the prodromal or erythema stage may be necessary to effect a major alteration in the course. Rapid clinical evolution may occur because the infection has a multifocal origin in the epidermis (4,5).

Drug delivery was stressed earlier in this symposium by Dr. Prusoff and is the major remaining problem in the development of effective chemotherapy for herpes labialis. While oral delivery of nucleoside antivirals may be feasible for selected cases, topical delivery of antivirals in otherwise healthy subjects is likely to be the treatment of choice in the future by virtue of cost, reduced toxicity or potential toxicity, and higher concentrations of antiviral in the target cells. It is important that topical antiviral preparations be capable of penetrating intact stratum corneum since the stratum corneum is likely normal in the early stages of the infection when treatment should be started.

Our laboratory has been involved in studies of the penetration of antiviral nucleosides through the stratum corneum of guinea pig and human skin. We have employed the Franz-type single-chambered diffusion apparatus in which a portion of skin is clamped across an opening in a glass chamber. The chamber contains normal saline which is stirred with a magnetic bar and a port in the side of the chamber allows withdrawal of samples to serially measure drug concentration. We have also used a modification of the Hubler guinea pig model of cutaneous HSV-1 infection to evaluate the therapeutic efficacy of different topical formulations. The use of minute punctures for inoculation of the skin and treatment for only 3 days during the early part of experimental lesion development create a therapeutic situation in which penetration of the test agent through the stratum corneum is a major determinant of the outcome (6).

We have been able to draw several important conclusions from our experimental studies of transcutaneous drug penetration. First, ACV in polyethylene glycol penetrates guinea pig skin at a very slow rate and has only a limited benefit in our animal model. Formulation of ACV in DMSO greatly increases skin penetration and the clinical response. Accordingly, we conclude that the marginal benefits to date of topical ACV ointment in recurrent human herpes labialis and genitalis do not indicate the therapeutic limits of topical therapy or of ACV, but rather reflect a failure of drug delivery. New topical formulations of ACV with better skin penetration could have exciting potential for human disease.

Second, studies with multiple nucleoside antivirals (ACV, BVDU, EDU, TFT and IDU) have shown that low rates of drug penetration, less than 0.2 microgram/cm^2-hr, are generally associated with only a small therapeutic response in the animal model, whereas good to excellent clinical results are achieved when penetration is enhanced to flux values of greater than 1 microgram/cm^2-hr. We are presently attempting to derive a mathematical term utilizing rates of skin penetration and in vitro antiviral inhibitory potency which will express the clinical potential of a topical antiviral formulation.

Third, we have found that penetration of human skin by trifluorothymidine in different vehicles appears to be qualitatively similar to the results obtained with the same formulations in guinea pig skin (7).

In addition to dimethylsulfoxide, a new agent is available for construction of topical antiviral formulations with penetration-enhancing qualities. 1-dodecylazacycloheptan-2-one (Azone, Nelson Research and Development) is a small, hydrophobic compound which has been reported to enhance the percutaneous penetration of a variety of compounds (8). We have shown that Azone can dramatically increase the penetration of trifluorothymidine thruogh guinea pig and human skin (7).

Finally, we have made the paradoxical observation that increasing concentrations of IDU in DMSO actually lead to a decrease in drug flux through the skin. When the final concentration of IDU was increased from 20 to 30%, the penetration of IDU through guinea pig skin fell from 15.5 to 7.3 mcg/cm^2-hr. This would appear to be due to dilution of DMSO and a decrease in the penetration-enhancing properties of the formulation. This observation indicates the value of in vitro penetration studies and offers a possible explanation for the conflicting reports of success with 20% IDU in DMSO (9) and failure with 30% IDU in DMSO (10) in the treatment of genital herpes.

REFERENCES

1. Fiddian, AP, L Ivanyi. 1983. Topical acyclovir in the management of recurrent herpes labialis. Brit. J. of Derm. 109:321-326.

2. Spruance, SL, CS Crumpacker, LE Schnipper, ER Kern, S Marlow, KA Arndt & JC Overall Jr. 1982. Early, patient-initiated treatment of herpes labialis with topical 10% acyclovir. Antimicrobial Agents and Chemotherapy. 25:553-555.

3. Fiddian, AP, JM Yeo, R Stubbings, D Dean. 1983. Successful treatment of herpes labialis with topical acyclovir. Brit. Med. J. 286:1699-1701.

4. Spruance, SL, G Wenerstrom. 1984. Pathogenesis of recurrent herpes simplex labialis: IV. Maturation of lesions within 8 hours after onset and implications for antiviral treatment. In press, Oral Surg. Oral Med. Oral Path.

5. Huff, JC, GG Krueger, JC Overall, J Copeland, S Spruance. 1981. The histopathologic evolution of recurrent herpes simlex labialis. J. of Amer. Acad. of Derm. 5(5):550-557.

6. Spruance, SL, MB McKeough & JR Cardinal. 1984. Penetration of guinea pig skin by acyclovir in different vehicles and correlation with the efficacy of topical therapy of experimental cutaneous herpes simplex virus infection. Antimicro. Agents Chemother. 25:10-15.

7. Spruance, SL, MB McKeough, K Sugibayashi, F Robertson, P Gaede, and DS Clark. 1984. Effect of Azone and propylene glycol on the skin penetration of trifluorothymidine and the efficacy of different topical formulations against cutaneous herpes simplex virus infection in guinea pigs. In press, Antimicrobial Agents and Chemotherapy.

8. Stoughton, RB. 1982. Enhanced percutaneous penetration with 1-dodecylaza-cycloheptan-2-one. Arch. Derm. 118:474-477.

9. Parker, JD. 1977. A double-blind trial of idoxuridine in recurrent genital herpes. J. Antimicro. Chemo. 3 (Supplement A):131-138.

10. Silvestri DL, L Corey & KK Holmes. 1982. Ineffectiveness of topical idoxuridine in dimethyl sulfoxide for therapy for genital herpes. J. Am. Med. Assoc. 248:953-959.

© 1985 Elsevier Science Publishers B.V. (Biomedical Division)
Herpes Viruses and Virus Chemotherapy, R. Kono, editor

EFFECT OF ARA-A AGAINST HERPES ZOSTER AS A COMPLICATION OF MALIGNANT TUMORS

MICHIHITO NIIMURA
Department of Dermatology, Jikei University School of Medicine, 19-18 Nishishimbashi 3-chome, Minato-ku, Tokyo 105 (Japan)

INTRODUCTION

Herpes zoster is usually a benign disease and spontaneous healing is the usual outcome. However, as a complication of malignancies, herpes zoster often has a poor prognosis and is apt to be associated with such sequelae as severe post-herpetic neuralgia. While there is no well established specific therapy for the disease at present, such an antiviral agent would be widely welcomed for priventing post herpetic neuralgia and other calamitous complications. Ara-A also called vidarabine, has potent antiviral activity against such DNA viruses as herpes simplex and varicella-zoster. Its anti-viral activity is thought to derive chiefly frcm its inhibition of viral DNA-dependent DNA polymerase.

MATERIALS AND METNODS

We made a multicenter, double-blind, controlled study of ara-A to establish its efficacy and safety in treating herpes zoster in patients with malignancies.

Because it was difficult to provide a placebo due to the poor solubility of ara-A in water and also because there was no adequate standard drug, the study was designed to evaluate the dose-response relation between a high dose preparation containing 300 mg of ara-A in each vial and a low dose preparation containing 50 mg of the drug in each vial. The bottles and syringes were kept covered with opaque materials at all times so that the different levels of drug could not be detected. The medications were administered in 500 ml of saline, intravenously, over 2 to 4 hours, daily, for five days.

The patients were enrolled in the study within five days of the onset of their skin lesions, and during the study period the use of nerve blocks and any other antiviral agents, such as interferon, gamma globlin, acyclovir, immune sera etc was prohibited.
In addition, no patients took any corticosteroid.

The patients were examined daily for the first five days, and then weekly for three weeks after therapy was discontinued. Skin lesions, such as erythema, vesicles and pustles, erosions and ulcers, crust formation and dissemination, as well as such neuralgic symptoms as pain numness and dyesthesia were carefully noted. Evaluation of each categories were global, and was rated each time at one of five levels: cured, markedly improved, improved, unchanged or worsened. Before and after treatment, laboratory examinations were performed. Viral cultures and anti-varicella-zoster antibobody titers were collected on each patient, confirming the clinical diagnosis.

RESULT

A total of 127 subjects, averaging 56 years of age, were enrolled, 61 assigned to the ara-A High and 66 assigned to the ara-A Low groups. For various reasons, 23 patients' data had to be excluded, though this did not alter the ratios in respect to age, sex or numbers of patients. Both group had similar types of underlying malignancies, severity of skin lesions and neurologic complications. While the general U-test analysis of each skin lesion showed no overall statistical difference between the two levels of the drug, 2 by 2 analyses at the each evaluation day revealed that there

TABLE 1. EVALUATION OF OVERALL IMPROVEMENT

Evaluation day	Group (Ara-A)	+++	++	+	-	x	Total	Unknown	Utest
1st day	High	8	22	10	3	5	48	3	N.S.
	Low	6	21	6	7	11	51	2	
3rd day	High	11	21	10	1	2	45	6	N.S.
	Low	8	22	3	6	8	47	6	
7th day	High	23	17	5	1	0	46	5	*
	Low	13	15	8	1	4	41	12	
14th day	High	32	9	1	0	0	42	9	*
	Low	22	13	4	1	1	42	12	
21st day	High	33	8	1	0	0	42	9	*
	Low	22	13	1	1	1	38	15	

+++: Markedly improved -: Unchanged N.S.: Not significant
++: Improved x: Aggravated * : P 0.05
-: Unchanged

was indeed statistical dermatologic improvement when comparing the results at first, third and seventh days after the end of therapy. This numerical analysis comfirmed the clinical impressions of the individual examiners. When neurological symptoms were included the global improvement, using U-test, showed statistical differences between the two groups at the seventh, fourteenth and twenty first days after the end of therapy. 2 by 2 analyses done on each week also confirmed the statistical validity of the above results. (Table 1.)

When the participating physicians were asked to rate the patients overall outcome, as to duration of the skin lesions, severity and sequelae of the disease, as well as possible side effects of the drug, the high dose group received a positive rating almost twice that of the low dose one. (Table 2.)

TABLE 2. EVALUATION OF OVERALL USEFULNESS

treatment group	+++	++	+	-	x	Total	U-test
Ara-A High	15	22	7	7	0	51	
(%)	(29)	(43)	(14)	(14)	(0)		*
Ara-A Low	12	10	17	14	0	53	
(%)	(23)	(19)	(32)	(26)	(0)		

+++: Markedly useful -: Useless * : P 0.05
++: Moderately useful x: Undesirable
+: Slightly useful

When the patients were stratified by age and in respect to the severity of the underlying disease, those sixty and over or the severely ill patients showed statistically greater improvement in the high dose group as versus the low dose one.

There was no significant difference in the incidence of side effects between the two groups. While there were laboratory abnormalities in these patients with cancer, there were no significant diferences between the two groups.

SUMMARY

A double blind study was made to assess the efficacy and safety of ara-A treatment for herpes zoster in cancer patients. The patients were rondomly divided into two groups: one group treated with high dose (300mg/day) of ara-A for five days and the other with a low dose (50mg/day) for five days.

Skin lesions improved in more patients of high dose group than in the low dose group at 1st, 3rd and 7th days after the end of treatment. The global improvement including skin lesions and neurologic symptomes indicated a trend to early improvement in the high dose group, compared with a low dose one. There were no significant difference in the overall safety rating between the high dose and low dose group. The average rating of global utility in the high dose group was significantly higher than in the low dose group.

We have drawn the conclusion that the treatment with ara-A, 300mg/day for five days, when initiated early, is useful as an antiviral therapy for herpes zoster in cancer patients.

Herpes Viruses and Virus Chemotherapy, R. Kono, editor

ACYCLOVIR CREAM - AN EFFECTIVE THERAPY FOR CUTANEOUS HERPES SIMPLEX INFECTIONS

S R KINGSLEY AND A P FIDDIAN

Department of Clinical Immunology and Chemotherapy, Wellcome Research Laboratories, Langley Court, Beckenham, Kent (England)

INTRODUCTION

Cutaneous infections caused by herpes simplex virus are extremely common, usually manifesting themselves as orofacial or genital lesions. Untreated primary HSV infections typically last an average of 2-3 weeks and thereafter the virus remains latent in the trigeminal or sacral ganglia. Symptomatic viral reactivation may subsequently be provoked by a number of factors, including fever, stress, sunburn, menses and underlying disease. The untreated recurrent infection typically lasts for an average of 1-2 weeks. Acyclovir (ACV; Zovirax[R]), has been used to treat both primary and recurrent HSV infections.

PROPERTIES OF ACV DERMAL PREPARATIONS

In general terms, the efficacy of an antiviral formulation will be affected by a). the antiviral activity of the drug, b) the natural history of the untreated disease and c) the time to onset of therapy. If the disease has a relatively short natural history then a drug effect will be difficult to ascertain, particularly if the start of therapy is delayed. Factors specific to topical preparations, such as the water or lipid solubility of the drug, and the skin penetrating properties of the drug and its vehicle, including their effects on the stratum corneum, also influence efficacy.

The two dermal formulations of ACV have different properties which may be related to differences in efficacy. ACV cream, which is licensed in the U.K. and many European countries for HSV infections of the skin (including initial and recurrent genital herpes and herpes labialis) is composed of 5% ACV in a base which contains propylene glycol (PG). PG aids the transdermal penetration of ACV by solubilising the drug in the vehicle. ACV ointment, which contains 5% ACV in polyethylene glycol, is licensed in the USA and Canada for the treatment of severe HSV infections of the skin, namely initial genital herpes and cutaneous HSV in the immunocompromised.

EFFECT OF TOPICAL FORMULATIONS ON CUTANEOUS HSV INFECTIONS IN ANIMALS

A number of in vivo studies have been conducted on experimental cutaneous herpes infections in guinea pigs and mice. ACV cream was found to be more effective than both ACV ointment and ACV in DMSO in the treatment of cutaneous HSV infections[1,2,3]. Four times daily application was found to be more effective than twice daily application for both formulations[1]. In addition, ACV cream was also found to provide effective prophylaxis against HSV when applied six times daily to the skin[4]. The greater effectiveness of the cream over the ointment was probably due to the better transdermal penetration properties of the former.

CLINICAL USE OF TOPICAL ACV

Both ACV cream and ointment have been shown to be highly effective in the treatment of severe cutaneous HSV infections. Table I contains details of the trials in which topical therapy has been used for the treatment of initial genital herpes. Both formulations led to a significant reduction in healing time and the duration of viral shedding.

TABLE I
CLINICAL EFFECTS OF TOPICAL ACV ON SEVERE CUTANEOUS HSV INFECTIONS

Ref.	Disease	Formulation	No. patients PCB/ACV	Healing times* PCB/ACV	p value	Viral shedding* PCB/ACV	p value
Whitley[5] et al., 1983	HSV in immuno-compromised	Ointment	29/30	21/15	<0.05	N/A	<0.001
Corey[6] et al., 1983	Initial genital herpes	Ointment	23/28	15/11	<0.05	5/2	<0.01
Thin[7] et al., 1983	Initial genital herpes	Ointment	22/18	13.5/9	<0.05	9/2	<0.05
Fiddian[8] et al., 1983a	Initial genital herpes	Ointment	36/34	13/9	0.001	8/3	<0.05
Kinghorn[9] et al., 1983	Initial genital herpes	Cream	22/27	14/8	<0.001	11/4	<0.001
Fiddian[8] et al., 1983a	Initial genital herpes	Cream	47/54	13/8	<0.001	9/3	<0.001

*median days N/A = not available

All studies, except for the Fiddian et al[8] ointment trial, also reported a significant drug-related decrease in the duration of symptoms (pain and itching) over placebo . As well as being effective in severe genital herpes, ACV ointment was also shown to be effective in other severe cutaneous HSV infections in the immunocompromised by reducing the duration of viral shedding, time to healing and time with pain[5] (see Table I).

Table II shows details of trials in which topical ACV was used for the treatment of recurrent genital herpes infections. In the two studies in which ACV cream was used, there was a significant reduction in healing time for both sexes. Use of ACV ointment was rather less effective, however, and a reduction in healing time was seen in only 2 of the 4 studies[10, 13]. In those studies where no reduction in healing time was found, the natural history of the disease (i.e. healing time in placebo-treated patients) was relatively short in comparison with the other ointment studies. This property of the infection would make a drug effect more difficult to demonstrate.

TABLE II

CLINICAL EFFECTS OF TOPICAL ACV ON RECURRENT GENITAL HERPES INFECTIONS

Author	Formulation	CIT/PIT* (sex - M/F)	No. patients PCB/ACV	Healing times† PCB/ACV	p value	Viral† shedding PCB/ACV	p value
Corey[10] et al., 1982	Ointment	CIT (M)	35/31	9.7/7.6	<0.05	2.2/1.0	<0.01
		CIT (F)	25/20	5.6/6.6	ns	1.1/0.4	<0.01
Reichman[11] et al., 1983	Ointment	CIT M	27/27	6.3/6.6	ns	3.2/2.0	<0.05
		CIT (F)	19/15	4.3/5.3	ns	1.2/1.6	ns
Luby[12] et al., 1984	Ointment	PIT (M)	91/85	6.6/6.5	ns	1.8/1.8	ns
		PIT (F)	71/62	4.3/4.7	ns	2.0/1.1	p<0.05
Lacey[13] et al., (in press)	Ointment	PIT (M)	17/16	9.5/6.0	<0.01	2/2	ns
		PIT (F)	7/8	7.0/4.5	<0.05	2/2	ns
Fiddian[8] et al., 1983a	Cream	PIT (M)	22/30	7.3/5.7	0.05	Δ71%/30%	<0.05
		PIT (F)	19/14	4.4/3.6	<0.05	Δ56%/17%	ns
Kinghorn[9] et al 1983	Cream	PIT (M)	12/14	8.9/5.8	<0.05	Δ73%/29%	<0.05
		PIT (F)	9/6	5.3/3.2	<0.01	Δ67%/33%	ns

*CIT = clinic-initiated therapy PIT = patient-initiated therapy
†mean or median days Δ percent patients with positive culture after day 0

All but one of the six studies[13] recorded significant reductions in viral shedding in at least one of the sexes. In one study, the non-significant findings in females were thought to be due to a delay in the start of therapy[11] while in another study they were probably influenced by the small group size[9]. The two cream studies showed that ACV led to a significant reduction in the duration of symptoms in both sexes, while the ointment was only seen to confer such benefit in one study (a reduction in the duration of pain in males[10]).

Table III details the results obtained from studies on herpes labialis. Since an untreated recurrent attack of herpes labialis can last for as little as 6 or 7 days, it was found that therapy needed to be started within the prodrome for a drug effect to be demonstrated. In the first two ointment studies[14, 15] therapy was clinician initiated usually once the lesion had advanced to the papule stage or beyond and this late onset of therapy is probably partly responsible for the treatment failure. In the three studies in which ointment application was patient initiated, the two in which the natural history of the disease (i.e. time to healing in placebo treated patients) was of relatively long duration showed either a significant reduction in time to healing[16] or a tendency towards a reduction in healing time[15]. In the third study, the natural history of the disease was so short that even frequent applications with a relatively high concentration (10%) of ACV in ointment had no apparent effect on the course of the disease[17].

TABLE III
CLINICAL EFFECT OF TOPICAL ACV ON HERPES LABIALIS

Author	Formulation	CIT/PIT* or Prophylaxis	No. patients PCB/ACV	Healing times PCB	Healing times ACV	p value
Spruance *et al*[14] 1982	Ointment	CIT	102/106	7.2	7.2	ns
Fiddian *et al*[15] 1983b	Ointment	CIT PIT	15/16 13/16	7 10	8 6	ns 0.1
Fiddian & Ivanyi 1983[16]	Ointment	PIT	16/15	8	6	<0.05
Spruance *et al*[17] 1984b	Ointment (10%)	PIT	36/33	5.2	6	ns
Fiddian *et al*[18] 1983c	Cream	PIT	40/34	6	4	0.01
van Vloten[19] *et al* 1983	Cream	PIT	31/29	6.6	5.4	0.05
Data on file (unpublished)	Cream	PIT	34/33	7.5	4.4	<0.05
Shaw (pers. comm)	Cream	PIT	38/34	10	9	ns

*CIT = clinic-initiated therapy PIT = patient-initiated therapy
† mean or median days

Of the 4 studies (all patient-initiated) in which ACV cream was used to treat herpes labialis, three showed a beneficial effect of the drug on the time to healing (Data on file; 18, 19). The fourth study showed no effect even though the natural history of the disease (i.e. the time to healing in the placebo patients) in this case was of relatively long duration (Shaw, pers. comm). However, patients had initially been followed during an untreated attack of herpes labialis and these infections had lasted for an average of 12 days. Thus it seemed as if, in this study, both the placebo (i.e. cream base containing propylene glycol) and the active cream had been effective in reducing the healing time of the lesions.

Data from one cream study[18] and one ointment study[16] suggested that use of the topical formulation may lead to an increase in the numbers of abortive lesions although the ointment data was not supported by Spruance et al[17].

The effect of topical ACV on the duration of symptoms was measured in four of the studies (two using ointment and two using cream). Although there was no significant reduction in the duration of pain or itching in any of the studies, all showed a tendency for ACV treated patients to have decreased duration of symptoms over placebo treated patients[14, 17, 18, 19].

ACV cream has also been used as prophylaxis against cold sores in patients who suffer frequent recurrences of these lesions (Gibson, pers. comm; 20) and, although four times daily application had some effect on recurrence rate (Gibson, pers. comm.) it is probable that oral prophylaxis will be more effective.

In conclusion, the data suggest that ACV cream may be a more effective therapy than acyclovir ointment, particularly for the treatment of cutaneous HSV infections with a relatively short natural history. The increased effectiveness of the cream is probably due to the presence of propylene glycol in the cream base which aids the transdermal penetration of the drug. Thus ACV cream is effective in both initial (severe) and recurrent (mild) infections while the ointment is only consistently effective in severe infection. In addition, there is some indication that in herpes labialis, ACV cream may increase abortive episodes of infection when therapy is started in the prodromal period and that frequent application of the formulation has some effect in preventing disease reactivation.

REFERENCES

1. Collins P and Oliver NM (1982) Am J Med 73 (suppl 1A): 96-99
2. Collins P and Oliver NM (1983) Poster presented to 2nd Int Acyclovir (Zovirax) Symposium, London, poster no. P-9
3. Spruance SL, McKeough MB and Cardinal JR (1984a) Antimicrob Agents Chemother 25: 10-15
4. Hill TJ, Blyth WA and Harbour DA (1982) Antiviral Res 2: 135-146
5. Whitley RJ, Barton NH, Levin M. et al. (1983) Abstracts of Int Congr Antimicrob Agents Chemother Las Vegas USA, Abst 563
6. Corey L, Benedetti J, Critchlow C et al (1983) J Antimicrob Chemother 12 (suppl B): 79-88
7. Thin RN, Nabarro JM, Parker JD and Fiddian AP (1983) Br J Vener Dis 59: 116-119
8. Fiddian AP, Kinghorn GR, Goldmeier D et al (1983a) J Antimicrob Chemother 12 (Suppl B): 67-77
9. Kinghorn GR, Turner EB, Barton IG et al (1983) Antiviral Research 3: 291-301
10. Corey L, Benedetti JK, Critchlow CW et al (1982) Am J Med 73 (suppl. 1A): 326-334
11. Reichman RC, Badger GJ, Guinan ME et al (1983) J Infect Dis 147: 336-340
12. Luby JP, Gnann JW, Alexander WJ et al (1984) J Infect Dis 150: 1-6
13. Lacey CJN, Meaden JD, Darville JM et al (1984) Eur J Sex Transm Dis (in press)
14. Spruance SL, Schnipper LE, Overall JC Jr. et al (1982) J Infect Dis 146: 85-90
15. Fiddian AP, Yeo JM and Clark AE (1983b) J Infect 6 (Suppl 1): 41-47
16. Fiddian AP and Ivanyi L (1983) Brit J Dermatol 109: 321-326
17. Spruance SL, Crumpacker CS, Schnipper LE et al (1984b) Antimicrob Agents Chemother 25: 553-555
18. Fiddian AP, Yeo JM, Stubbings R and Dean D (1983c) Br Med J 286: 1699-1701
19. van Vloten WA, Swart RNJ and Pot F. (1983) J Antimicrob Chemother 12 (suppl B): 89-93
20. Fawcett HA, Wansbrough-Jones MH, Clark AE and Leigh IM. Br Med J 287: 798-799

C. Genital

LONG TERM RECURRENCE RATES OF GENITAL HERPES INFECTIONS AFTER TREATMENT OF FIRST EPISODE GENITAL HERPES WITH ORAL ACYCLOVIR

GREGORY J. MERTZ, MD; JACKIE BENEDETTI, PhD; CATHY CRITCHLOW, MS and LAWRENCE COREY, MD

Departments of Medicine, Laboratory Medicine and Microbiology, University of Washington, Seattle, WA. Reprint requests to: Dr. Mertz, Department of Medicine, University of New Mexico School of Medicine, Albuquerque, NM 87131, USA

INTRODUCTION

Previous studies have shown topical, intravenous and oral acyclovir to be effective in shortening the course of first episode genital herpes simplex virus (HSV) infections (1-3). Long term followup revealed no significant differences between topical acyclovir and placebo recipients in the proportion of patients who subsequently had recurrences, the time to the first recurrence, or the rate of recurrence in the first year after treatment (2). In a small placebo controlled study of intravenous acyclovir therapy of first episode genital herpes infections, there was a trend suggesting that the time to first recurrence was delayed in acyclovir-treated patients (3). In a large placebo-controlled multicenter trial of oral acyclovir therapy of first episode genital herpes, there were no differences between acyclovir and placebo recipients in the time to first recurrence or the frequency of genital recurrences in the first year after treatment (1). In animal models, early initiation of therapy with topical or parenteral acyclovir therapy can reduce the frequency and number of latently infected ganglia (4-6). To evaluate whether treatment of first episode genital herpes with oral acyclovir may decrease the rate of recurrence of disease in the second year after treatment, we undertook an analysis of long term recurrence rates among patients enrolled in a double-blind, placebo-controlled trial of oral acyclovir therapy for the acute treatment of the first episode.

METHODS

Study design

Patients with first episode genital herpes infections who were seen within six days of the onset of lesions were randomly assigned capsules containing 200 mg of acyclovir or placebo and were instructed to take one capsule orally five times daily for ten days. After resolution of the first episode, the patients were followed by examination or telephone at monthly intervals for evidence of clinical recurrences. Patients were not informed of whether they received oral acyclovir or placebo therapy until six to 18 months after enrollment. All patients described in this report were treated and followed at the University of Washington.

Viral isolation

The method of viral isolation and typing and serologic assays have been described previously (1).

Statistical Analysis

Patients with first episodes of genital herpes were classified as having primary first episodes if the acute-phase serum lacked neutralizing antibody to both HSV-1 and -2 (titer $<1:4$). Patients whose acute phase serum revealed HSV neutralizing antibody with a titer of $\geq 1:8$ were classified as having nonprimary first episodes.

Chi-square and Wilcoxon tests were used to compare pretreatment demographic, clinical, and virologic data. The effect of treatment on the time to first recurrence was assessed by the log rank (Mantel-Cox) test, and rates of recurrence were compared by analysis of variance with repeated measures for each six month period.

RESULTS

Forty two acyclovir- and 42 placebo-treated patients were enrolled in the study. Eighty of the 84 patients completed therapy and were followed for more than 30 days after enrollment. Of the 42 acyclovir- and the 37 of 42 placebo-treated patients who completed therapy and were followed, 26 acyclovir- and 21 placebo-treated patients were female, and 16 acyclovir- and 17 placebo-treated patients were male. The number of acyclovir and placebo recipients with primary and nonprimary HSV-2 and primary HSV-1 infections who completed the initial course of treatment is shown in Table 1.

TABLE I.
NUMBER OF PATIENTS WITH HSV-2 AND HSV-1 INFECTIONS BY TREATMENT GROUP.

HSV-2 isolated	Acyclovir	Placebo
Primary	25	20
Nonprimary	4	9
HSV-1 isolated		
Primary	11	8

Time to First Recurrence

Among 29 acyclovir- and 29 placebo-treated patients with first episode genital HSV-2 infection, the median time to first recurrence was 68 days in both groups (p=0.56). Among 11 acyclovir- and 8 placebo-treated patients with first episode genital HSV-1 infection, the median times to the first recurrence were 164 and 174 days, respectively (p=0.37).

Long Term Recurrence Rates

Among the 25 acyclovir- and 20 placebo-treated patients who had primary genital HSV-2 infections, 13 acyclovir- and 12 placebo-treated patients were followed for more than 18 months. The recurrence rates for these patients are shown in Table 3.

TABLE 3.
MEAN (± Standard Deviation) NUMBER OF RECURRENCES PER 6 MONTH PERIOD AMONG PATIENTS WITH PRIMARY FIRST-EPISODE GENITAL HSV-2 INFECTIONS FOLLOWED MORE THAN 18 MONTHS.

Months After First Episode	Acyclovir Treated N=13	Placebo Treated N=12
0-6	2.4 ± 2.1	3.1 ± 2.2
7-12	2.9 ± 2.2	3.3 ± 2.3
13-18	2.7 ± 2.6	3.5 ± 3.0

There were no significant differences between the recurrence rates of acyclovir- and placebo-treated patients comparing each 6 month interval (p>0.22) nor were there any significant changes in recurrence rates over time in either group (p>0.71). Among 10 acyclovir- and 12 placebo-treated patients followed for over two years after their primary first episode HSV-2 infection, the recurrence rates were 3.60 and 3.08 recurrences, respectively, for the 6 month period from 19-24 months (p=0.56).

Discussion

Our analysis of long term recurrence rates suggests that recurrence rates of genital herpes do not change significantly in the second year after primary first episode genital HSV-2 infections in either acyclovir- or placebo-treated patients. Although the number of patients with primary genital HSV-2 infections followed for two or more years was small (10 acyclovir- and 12 placebo-treated patients), we observed no significant differences in the recurrence rates at six, 12, 18, or 24 months of follow up in our population. The mean number of recurrences in each six month period were slightly lower among acyclovir- as compared to placebo-treated patients, but the variation in recurrence rates was great and no significant differences emerged. Because of the small number of patients with long term followup and the risk of a type 2 error, we cannot exclude the possibility that there was a slight reduction in long term recurrence rates among acyclovir recipients. At present, however, our data suggests that whereas oral acyclovir is of clear clinical benefit in the treatment of first episode genital herpes infections, oral acyclovir therapy of first-episode genital herpes does not influence the time to first recurrence or short term recurrence rates (1) and does not appear to influence long term recurrence rates.

Acknowledgments: This study was supported by The National Institutes of Health grant AI-20381 and Venereal Diseases Research Foundation support for Dr. Mertz.

REFERENCES

1. Mertz GJ, Critchlow CW, Benedetti J, et al (1984) Double-blind placebo-controlled trial of oral acyclovir in first-episode genital herpes simplex virus infection. JAMA 252:1147-1151

2. Corey L, Nahmias AJ, Guinan ME, et al (1982) A trial of topical acyclovir in genital herpes infections. N Engl J Med 306:1313-1319

3. Corey L, Fife KH, Benedetti JK, et al (1983) Intravenous acyclovir for the treatment of primary genital herpes. Ann Int Med 98:914-921

4. Field HJ, De Clercq E (1981) Effects of oral treatment with acyclovir and bromovinyldeoxyuridine on the establishment and maintenance of latent herpes simplex virus infection in mice. J Gen Virol 56:259-265

5. Field HJ, Bell SE, Elion G, et al (1979) Effect of acycloguanosine treatment on acute and latent herpes simplex infections in mice. Antimicrob Agents Chemother 15:554-561

6. Pronovost AD, Lucia HL, Dann PR, et al (1982) Effect of acyclovir on genital herpes in guinea pigs. J Infect Dis 145:904-908

Herpes Viruses and Virus Chemotherapy, R. Kono, editor

CHANGING PATTERNS OF NEONATAL HERPES - AS AFFECTED BY ANTIVIRAL THERAPY AND OTHER FACTORS

A.J. NAHMIAS, M.D., H.L. KEYSERLING, M.D., AND R. WHITLEY, M.D.

Department of Pediatrics, Emory University School of Medicine, Atlanta, Georgia and Department of Pediatrics, University of Alabama, Birmingham, Alabama USA

The frequency, disease category and outcome of neonatal infection with herpes simplex virus type 2 and type 1 (HSV-2 and HSV-1) have changed over the past few years due to several influences, often counteracting each other. Some of the effects have been due to direct medical intervention, such as Cesarean section and antiviral therapy. However, the changes have also been a result of indirect effects that are cultural or medical in nature. The direct and indirect influences will be briefly outlined with particular reference to possible strategies (and their fallabilities) which might be contemplated for improved prevention in the future.

The prevalence of neonatal herpes has varied between countries and within each country. There should theoretically be an increase of neonatal herpes if an increase of genital herpes is noted. This appears to be the case in Finland and in Seattle, Washington. In the United Kingdom, however, there appears to have been no increase of neonatal herpes which would be expected to correspond with the alleged increase in genital herpes. In a lower socioeconomic hospital in Atlanta, there has been no increase in genital herpes nor in neonatal herpes over the past 20 years; the incidence of neonatal herpes has been around 1 in 3500 deliveries each year, similar to recent figures from Seattle. The discrepancies noted above are in large part due to problems, not only in reporting, but also in diagnosis.

There are many more neonatal cases of local CNS disease recognized in recent years in several regions. The diagnosis of this form of neonatal herpes is very difficult to make in the absence of the characteristic skin vesicles, which are present in less than half the cases. There have also been more cases of local skin, eye and/or mouth (SEM) neonatal HSV infections noted in the recent NIAID Collaborative Study. This is most likely due to the ability of current antivirals (Vidarabine or Acyclovir) to arrest the progression to more severe CNS or disseminated disease -- which would be expected to occur most likely in about three-quarters of untreated cases. There has been a universal decline of disseminated disease, involving the liver and other internal organs, in comparison to localized infections of the CNS or SEM. This is probably a result of the influence of transplacental antibodies in preventing most disseminated disease, without affecting as much local CNS or SEM infections. The likelihood of women developing primary genital infection in the last few weeks of pregnancy is much less today than that of having a recurrent genital infection, because the number of pregnant women having had genital herpes has increased. In a Health Maintenance Organization (HMO) middle class population in Atlanta, 10% of women at their first prenatal clinic visit gave a history of genital herpes, 4% in their consorts and an additional 20% had evidence of HSV-2 antibodies.

In our earlier reviews, primarily from literature reports which would tend to accentuate the more severe cases, the ratio of disseminated to local CNS to local SEM infections was 6:2:2. Since mortality and morbidity were high in the first two categories, the overall likelihood of infected babies surviving intact was about 20%. As the ratio of the disease categories currently seen in the U.S. is changing to 1:4:5, and as therapy is becoming more successful, about two-thirds of infected babies will now survive without sequelae. (Infection in premature cases, most often a result of maternal primary infections, are also declining from over 40% to around 20%).

On the one hand, then, an infection which maimed 4 of 5 babies is now maiming 1 out of 3. That is still too high and prevention would still be important. More recent data are suggesting that the risks of babies becoming infected in the U.S. are approximately as follows: 1 per 10,000 women in general; 1 per 1,000 women with a history of genital herpes; 1 per 20 women if the virus is recurring around the time of delivery, and probably 2 in 3, if not 3 in 4, if a primary genital infection is present. These new figures influence any potential approach to prophylaxis.

If indeed the present rate of a history of genital herpes in a pregnant woman or her partner is around 15% and that of HSV-2 antibodies 30% (and even higher in low socioeconomic populations), then the current policy of monitoring at 34 weeks by surveillance viral cultures is too costly-in relation to the 5% risk of infection in the neonate if the woman is shedding virus at the time of delivery with a 1% poor outcome in the treated neonate. Furthermore, cases resulting from asymptomatically infected women (at least 50%, if not 80%) would be missed by such monitoring. One alternative would be to administer an antiviral drug to all women with a positive history in herself and/or her contact, and possibly even to those with HSV-2 antibodies. (Even though several commercial kits are available to allegedly detect HSV-2 antibodies, their specificity is very questionable and would only add to the problem). We estimate that 3,000 women would have to be treated prophylactically, from 34 weeks gestation to delivery, in order to prevent one severe neonatal outcome. The problems of missing many cases are similar to those of viral monitoring noted above; in addition, however, there would be the possibilities of: (a) acute side-effects, particularly on the fetus if the drug is transmitted transplacentally or concentrates in the amniotic fluid; (b) modification of labor -- if non-compliant, the virus may reactivate at the worst time; (c) drug resistance; (d) immunosuppression; (e) the drug's mutagenicity or oncogenicity. We view such an approach then with great caution.

A second possible strategy would be to find a rapid laboratory test which would be used in every pregnant woman at labor and perform a C-section, if the test is positive. This test would have to be available 24 hours a day for 7 days a week in every hospital in the country. With such time demands, any test would be under extreme duress for specificity. Even with only a 5% false positive rate, we estimate that 300 unnecessary C-sections would be performed to prevent one bad outcome in a baby.

The only strategy which is potentially possible is to combine virus culture (or possibly rapid test, as here a few false positive results are not so crucial) with a prophylactic or therapeutic regimen. These might include hyperimmune globulin, for seronegative babies passing through an infected birth canal, and antivirals (we should learn within 6 months of the efficacy and toxicity of Acyclovir in comparison with Vidarabine).

Obviously, more research will be needed to arrive at the most rational and practical approach. At the international level, it is hard to predict: (a) the sexual patterns and contraceptive practices in different countries which will affect the rate of genital herpes, hence of neonatal herpes; (b) the prevalence of C-section deliveries which, if done for other than HSV indications at the increasing rate of 20% or over will protect, unbeknownst to all, cases of intrapartum infections, whether herpes, chlamydia, gonorrhea, or group B streptococci. Currently, at least one-quarter of cases of neonatal herpes resulting from primary infections could be prevented if pregnant women abstained from any form of sex - genital or oral - in the last month or two of pregnancy. Finally, other medical interventions on the acquisition or expression of genital herpes under active study will undoubtedly impact on our management of this problem. Having watched the changing patterns of neonatal herpes over the past 25 years, we can only view with some trepidation, if not some optimism, the next decade.

TREATMENT OF GENITAL HERPES SIMPLEX INFECTIONS WITH TOPICALLY ADMINISTERED ANTIVIRAL DRUGS

RICHARD C. REICHMAN, M.D.

University of Rochester School of Medicine, Infectious Diseases Unit, 601 Elmwood Avenue, P.O. Box MED, Rochester, New York 14642 (U.S.A.)

Topical treatment of genital herpes has the theoretical advantage of allowing delivery of antiviral compounds in high concentrations to sites of viral replication while minimizing chances of systemic toxicity. The development and evaluation of new topically administered antivirals and appropriate vehicles are areas of active investigation. Although several different antiviral compounds in topical formulations have been evaluated for the treatment of genital herpes, a limited number of these studies have been performed with attention to those problems known to be unique to clinical trials of treatments for cutaneous herpes simplex infections (1). The purpose of this paper is to review a limited number of recently completed and carefully performed investigations. The discussion will focus on studies of idoxuridine (IUDR) and acyclovir (ACV).

Studies of topically administered IUDR and ACV have evaluated the use of these compounds in both first episode and recurrent infections. In Table 1 are presented the results of a study of 30% IUDR in dimethyl sulfoxide (DMSO) for the treatment of primary genital herpes (2).

TABLE I.

EFFECTS OF 30% IDOXURIDINE IN DMSO IN THE TREATMENT OF PRIMARY GENITAL HERPES

	Idoxuridine (n=9)	Controls (n=23)
Virus shedding	2.6*	8.4
Time to crusting	5.3	4.4
Time to healing	19.6	17.9
Duration of pain	9.5	9.4
% with new lesions during treatment	78	78

Median recurrence time	39	30

* Mean number of days

Study medications were administered four times per day for seven days. Control groups received either DMSO alone or saline alone. No significant differences were noted between the two control groups, which are combined for purposes of analysis. There is a trend towards a decrease in duration of virus shedding among patients treated with IUDR in DMSO as compared to patients in the control groups (p=0.10). No other differences in measurements indicated were seen between patients who received IUDR and those who received a control preparation. Burning was a relatively common complaint among study participants and occurred in 56% of those receiving IUDR in DMSO, 43% of those receiving DMSO alone, and 25% of those who received saline. The effects of 5% ACV in polyethylene glycol (PEG) in the treatment of initial genital herpes are presented in Table II (3).

TABLE II.

EFFECTS OF 5% ACYCLOVIR IN POLYETHYLENE GLYCOL IN THE TREATMENT OF INITIAL GENITAL HERPES

	Acyclovir (n=18)	Placebo (n=22)	P Value
Virus shedding	2*	9	< .05
Time to crusting	5	7	< .05
Time to healing	9	13.5	< .05
Duration of pain	4	7	< .01
Duration of itching	2	6	< .01

* Median number of days

In this study, the duration of virus shedding and the duration of lesions were significantly less among patients who received ACV than among those treated with PEG alone. The duration of symptoms was also less among ACV recipients. The results of an analogous study of the same preparation are presented in Table III (4).

TABLE III.

EFFECTS OF 5% ACYCLOVIR IN POLYETHYLENE GLYCOL IN THE TREATMENT OF PRIMARY GENITAL HERPES

	Acyclovir	Placebo	P Value
Virus shedding	2.3*	5.6	< .001
Time to crusting	8.5	12.9	< .05
Time to healing	11.2	15.8	< .05
Duration of pain	5.2	7.0	< .05
Duration of itching	3.6	8.0	< .01
Days to recurrence	79	79	

* Mean number of days

In this study patients were seen within six days of the onset of lesions and treatment was administered 4 or 6 times per day for 7 days. A similar proportion of patients with disease caused by HSV-1 was observed in both groups. There was a significant difference between ACV and placebo recipients for each of the measurements indicated except for the time to subsequent recurrence, which was similar in both groups.

In Table IV, effects of 30% IUDR in DMSO in the treatment of recurrent genital herpes are presented (2).

TABLE IV.

EFFECTS OF 30% IDOXURIDINE IN DMSO IN THE TREATMENT OF RECURRENT GENITAL HERPES

	Idoxuridine (n=28)	DMSO (n=33)	Saline	P Value
Virus shedding	2.3*	3.3	3.8	< .05
Time to crusting	3.5	3.4	3.7	
Time to healing	10.2	8.8	10.7	
Duration of pain	3.3	3.9	3.6	
% with new lesions during treatment	32	24	45	

* Mean number of days

An antiviral effect was noted among study recipients who received IUDR in DMSO, but no other significant differences in indicated measurements of disease were seen among the three groups. Table V depicts the results of an investigation employing 5% ACV in PEG for treatment of recurrent genital herpes (5).

TABLE V.

EFFECTS OF 5% ACYCLOVIR IN POLYETHYLENE GLYCOL IN THE TREATMENT OF RECURRENT GENITAL HERPES

	Men		Women	
	Acyclovir	Placebo	Acyclovir	Placebo
Virus shedding	2.0*	3.2	1.6	1.2
Time to crusting	2.8	1.8	2.5	1.6
Time to healing	6.6	6.3	5.2	4.3
Duration of pain	3.4	4.9	2.7	3.4

* Mean number of days

Men who participated in this study and received ACV shed virus for a shorter period of time than did men who received PEG alone ($p < 0.05$). This antiviral effect was not detected in women, and no significant differences in other parameters indicated were observed.

To determine whether earlier initiation of therapy would produce more significant effects, a multi-centered study of patient initiated therapy employing 5% ACV in PEG was carried out (6). Three hundred nine patients were enrolled in this study and were treated six times per day for five days. A high percentage of participating patients had prodrome during the study, and therapy was initiated early in the treated episode. Results are presented in Table VI. Antiviral effects were demonstrated among women who particpated in this study ($p < 0.05$), but not among men. No significant differences in duration of lesions or symptoms were noted among study participants. An additional analysis of a subgroup of 100 patients treated within six hours of the onset of prodrome was also carried out. This additional analysis demonstrated no significant benefits among acyclovir recipients as compared to placebo recipients.

TABLE VI.

PATIENT-INITIATED TREATMENT OF RECURRENT GENITAL HERPES WITH 5% ACYCLOVIR IN POLYETHYLENE GLYCOL

	Men		Women	
	Acyclovir (n=85)	Placebo (n=91)	Acyclovir (n=62)	Placebo (n=71)
Virus shedding	1.8*	1.8	1.1	2.0
Time to crusting	2.6	2.7	1.5	1.5
Time to healing	6.5	6.6	4.7	4.3
Duration of pain, itching	3.7	3.8	5.4	4.4

* Mean number of days

In summary, treatment of genital herpes with topically administered drugs has the theoretical advantage of maximizing local concentrations of antivirals while minimizing systemic toxicity. Treatment of primary infections with 5% ACV in PEG produces both antiviral and clinical effects. However, beneficial effects from topical treatment of recurrent disease have been limited largely to decreases in the duration of virus shedding in subgroups of patients. More effective treatment of genital herpes with topically administered antivirals will probably require the use of improved drug formulations (7), rather than additional attempts to modify modes of administration of currently available preparations.

REFERENCES

1. Reichman RC (1983) Genital herpes simplex virus infections: Clinical trials and treatment. Proc. Intl. Cong. Chemother. 18:23-30.

2. Silvestri DL, Corey L, Holmes KK (1982) Ineffectiveness of topical idoxuridine in dimethyl sulfoxide for therapy for genital herpes. JAMA 248:953-959.

3. Thin RN, Nabarro JM, Parker JD, Fiddian AP (1983) Topical acyclovir in the treatment of initial genital herpes. Br J Vener Dis 59: 116-119.

4. Corey L, Benedetti JK, Critchlow CW, et al 91982) Double-blind controlled trial of topical acyclovir in genital herpes simplex virus infections. Amer J of Med 73(1A):326-334.

5. Reichman RC, Badger GJ, Guinan ME, et al (1983) Topically administered acyclovir in the treatment of recurrent herpes simplex genitalis: A

controlled trial. J of Infect Dis 147:336-340.

6. Luby JP, Gnann JW, Alexander WJ, et al (1984) A collaborative study of patient-initiated treatment of recurrent genital herpes with topical acyclovir or placebo. J of Infect Dis 150:1-6.

7. Spruance SL, McKeough MB, Cardinal JR (1984) Penetration of guinea pig skin by acyclovir in different vehicles and correlation with the efficacy of topical therapy of experimental cutaneous herpes simplex virus infection. Antimicrobial Agents and Chemotherapy 25:10-15.

D. Systemic

Herpes Viruses and Virus Chemotherapy, R. Kono, editor

THERAPEUTIC APPROACHES TO LIFE-THREATENING HERPES SIMPLEX AND VARICELLA-ZOSTER INFECTIONS IN THE IMMUNOCOMPROMISED HOST

RICHARD J. WHITLEY, M.D.

Departments of Pediatrics and Microbiology, University of Alabama School of Medicine, Suite #653/Children's Hospital Tower, Birmingham, Alabama, U.S.A.

The recognition of the utility of antiviral therapy is apparent for the treatment of herpes simplex virus (HSV) and varicella-zoster virus (VZV) infections in the immunocompromised host. Effective therapy of cytomegalovirus and Epstein-Barr virus infections in similar patient populations will likely be demonstrated in the next several years. This commentary will focus on the essential therapeutic endpoints required for proof of clinical usefulness of antiviral therapy in the treatment of VZV and HSV infections, particularly as it relates to altering the natural history of disease.

Varicella-zoster virus infections in the immunocompromised host are common. Frequencies of occurance vary from 5-15% percent per year for individuals with lymphoproliferative malignancies and bone marrow transplant recipients to 1.5-5.0% for renal transplant recipients and those with solid tumors. Four therapeutic endpoints have been unequivocally established for definition of usefulness as learned from double-blind, placebo-controlled investigations, particularly those performed to define the therapeutic index of vidarabine. First, therapy should accelerate the events of healing within the dermatome and prevent further skin extension. Acceleration of cessation of lesion formation, time to pustulation and scabbing will result in more prompt resolution of acute neuritis and a decrease in the frequency of post-herpetic neuralgia. To date only vidarabine, when parenterally administered, results in accelerated cutaneous healing in the immunocompromised host. Vidarabine therapy at a dosage of 10mg/kg/day given once daily as a continuous intravenous solution for five days will lead to a two day earlier time to pustulation and cessation of lesion formation.[1]

Although this difference might appear trivial, scabbing is accelerated for the median of the population by approximately ten days. Placebo-controlled trials such as this one also indicate healing occurred during the natural course of disease in nearly 70% of placebo recipients. This latter observation indicates that effective ambulatory therapy would be most desirable, thereby obviating the need for and costs associated with hospitalization.

Second, treatment should decrease, if not prevent, cutaneous dissemination, the indicator of blood-born spread of VZV and a harbinger of visceral complications.[1,2] The risk of cutaneous dissemination varies according to underlying disease and concomitant immunosuppressive therapy. Thus, patients with Hodgkin's disease or non-Hodgkin's lymphoma are at greater risk for cutaneous dissemination than patients who receive steroids to control such diseases as arthritis. Design of controlled trials, then, should take into consideration targeted populations in order to minimize patient risks. From recently completed controlled trials, both vidarabine and acyclovir[3] (15mg/kg/dose given every eight hours for seven days) will decrease the frequency of cutaneous dissemination.

Third, a major goal of therapy of VZV infections in the immunocompromised host should be prevention of death secondary to visceral organ involvement. Even with sophisticated biomedical support technology, mortality will still occur in 5-15% of patients, particularly those with varicella pneumonitis because of hemorrhagic necrosis of the lung. Therapeutic trials have demonstrated cutaneous dissemination can be prevented following parenteral administration of either vidarabine or acyclovir, and then, so also will the potential associated visceral complications.[1,3]

Finally, a fourth endpoint is the reduction of the pain of both acute neuritis associated with disease evolution in the dermatome, and post-herpetic neuralgia. This latter complication is especially debilitating for the elderly and/or when the ophthalmic branch of the trigeminal nerve is involved. As noted previously, acceleration of healing within the dermatome and prevention of progressive skin involvement correlates directly and statistically with resolution of pain and prevention of acute neuritis. To date, only vidarabine has a demonstrable effect on pain.[1]

Because of the cost associated with parenteral (vidarabine or acyclovir) in-hospital therapy, the risk of nosocomial infection, and unequivocal evidence of natural healing in the absence of therapy, ambulatory therapeutic regimens will be essential in the future. The development of oral medication such as acyclovir prodrugs, cyclaoradine, and the fluorinated pyrimidine analogs will likely lead to the next series of advances in the management of these infections.

The study of HSV infections in the immunocompromised host offers similar but not identical parameters for study. These infections are unusually severe and common in organ transplant recipients. As many as 40-70% of all organ transplant recipients whether heart, liver, kidney, or bone marrow will reactivate latent virus. Because of mandatory continuous immunosuppression to maintain graft function, the total time to healing for most patients will average five to seven weeks, a striking contrast to the normal host where healing is complete in ten days.[4] In contrast to VZV infections in the immunocompromised host, cutaneous dissemination and visceral complications are unusual, although an occasional case of HSV esophagitis will be encountered. More importantly, however, reactivated infection can be excruciatingly painful and disfiguring. Prolonged intra-oral disease can lead to nutritional deprivation unless alternatives for caloric supplementation are utilized. Thus, therapy should accelerate clearance of virus, crusting, and, ultimately, total healing. With healing accelerated, pain will resolve more promptly as previously demonstrated with therapy of localized shingles.

To date, only acyclovir when administered topically, orally or parenterally is useful for accelerating all events of healing.[4,5,6] Whether given intravenously or applied topically, treatment can accelerate healing by at least one week. Vidarabine influences certain parameters of healing but does not appear to provide the overall benefit of acyclovir for HSV infections in the immunocompromised host.

The recognition of subpopulations of patients at high risk for severe HSV infections has led to the demonstration of the utility of prophylaxis, as discussed elsewhere in this monograph. It is likely that such observations will be exploited and rather than treating the disease after it has occurred, novel drug delivery systems will be utilized (i.e. sustained release capsules or orally administered drugs targeted to specific sites).

REFERENCES

1. Whitley RJ, Soong SJ, Dolin R, Betts R, Linnemann C, Alford CA, and the NIAID Collaborative Antiviral Study Group (1982) Early vidarabine therapy to control the complications of herpes zoster in immunosuppressed patients. N Engl J Med 307:971-975.

2. Whitley RJ. (1984) Varicella-zoster virus infections. In: Galasso G, Buchanan R, Merigan T (eds) Antiviral Agents and Viral Diseases of Man, 2nd Edition. Raven Press Medical and Scientific Publishers, New York, pp 517-541.

3. Balfour HH, Bean B, Laskin OL, Ambinder RF, Meyers JD, Wade JC, Zaia JA, Aeppli D, Kirk LE, Segreti AC, Keeney RE, and the Burroughs Wellcome Collaborative Antiviral Study Group (1983) Acyclovir halts progression of herpes zoster in immunocompromised patients. N Engl J Med 307:1448-1453.

4. Whitley RJ, Spruance S, Hayden FG, Overall J, Alford CA, Gwaltney JM, Soong SJ, and the NIAID Collaborative Antiviral Study Group (1984) Vidarabine therapy of mucocutaneous herpes simplex virus infections in the immunocompromised host. J Infect Dis 149:1-8.

5. Meyers JD, Wade JC, Mitchell CD, Aral R, Lietman PS, Durack DT, Levin MJ, Segretti AC, Balfour HH. (1982) Multicenter collaborative trial of intravenous acyclovir for treatment of mucocutaneous herpes simplex virus infection in the immunocompromised host. Am J Med 73:229-236.

6. Wade JC, Newton B, McLaren C, Flournoy N, Keeney RE, and Meyers JD. (1982) Intravenous acyclovir to treat mucocutaneous herpes simplex virus infection after marrow transplantation. Ann Int Med 96:265-269.

9-(2-HYDROXYETHOXYMETHYL) GUANINE (ACYCLOVIR) FOR TREATMENT OF HERPES ZOSTER AND SIMPLEX INFECTION IN IMMUNOSUPPRESSED CHILDREN

ISAO SEKINE, TAKEO FUJIMOTO for Children's Cancer and Leukemia Study Group of JAPAN,
SHIRO SHIGETA, Department of Bacteriology, Fukushima Medical College, Fukushima, Japan

INTRODUCTION

Children with cancer tolerate many common viral infections with few or no sequelae.

On the other hand, serious viral infections in children with cancer are caused chiefly by the herpes group viruses including varicella zoster virus(1) and herpes simplex virus(2).

In 1978, Schaeffer(3) and his associates at Wellcome Research Laboratories in USA synthesized a specific anti-herpes agent, namely, acyclovir, which has been proved to be very effective against HSV(4), VZV(5) and EB virus(6) infections by many in vitro and clinical studies.

Systemic administrations of acyclovir have commonly been used thrice a day intermittent drip infusion method considering the plasma half life of the drug(7).

Kern(8) and Spector(9) reported that improved clinical efficacy and decreased side effects of the drug using continuous administration over 24 hrs against murine and human HSV infections, respectively. Pharmacokinetic studies of ACV performedby Elion(10) et al showed that intracellular ACV-TP tend to stay longer than non-phosphorylated ACV since ACV-TP can not penetrate the cell membrane.

Based on these findings, Children's Cancer and Leukemia Study Group of Japan carried out a clinical trial of ACV on immunocompromised children with herpes group infections using thrice a day intermittent, once a day continuous and once a day intermittent administration of ACV from April 1982 through April 1984.

SUBJECTS AND METHODS

The patients with either HSV or VZV infections were divided into 3 groups and ACV was administered by 3 different methods, that is, group A ; 5 mg / kg / dose thrice a day intermittent infusion over 1~2 hours, group B ; 15 mg / kg / dose once a day continuous infusion over 24 hrs and group C ; 5 mg / kg / dose once a day intermittent infusion over 1~2 hrs.

The duration of treatment was set as 10 days with minor changes according to the cessation of major symptoms of HSV or VZV infections.

Placebo group was not set up in this study mainly due to ethical reasons. However, the previous study done by the same study group was employed as a historical control.

The distribution of the patients into each group was tade by random table method.

Criteria to evaluate the clinical efficacy of ACV and severity of varicella were described in somewhere else(11). Statistical analysis was performed using Student's t test and Fisher's direct probability test.

RESULTS

A total of 69 immunocompromised patients with herpes group viral infection was enrolled into this study. The average ages of group A, B and C were 8.2, 8.7 and 6.6 years, respectivelyand no significant age differences were noted among the 3 groups (table I)

The clinical diagnosis of herpes group infection is described in table II and no significant differences were noted among the 3 group. The various immunocompromising underlying diseases and the number of patients with those disease in each groups are shown in table III and no statistical significance was noted among each groups. The time course relationship of major symptoms were examined and no statistical differences were noted among each groups regarding to the duration of fever, intensity of vesicle formation and intensity of scab formation.

The time course relationship of total cessation of new vesicle formation among patients with varicella on ACV is shown in Fig I. Varicella patients from group A and B were combined since group A and B showed no statistical differences in terms of efficacy and sideeffects of ACV (11). The figure showed some tendency that patients from group C took longer time

Fig. I

Varicella : Total Cessation of New Vesicle Formation

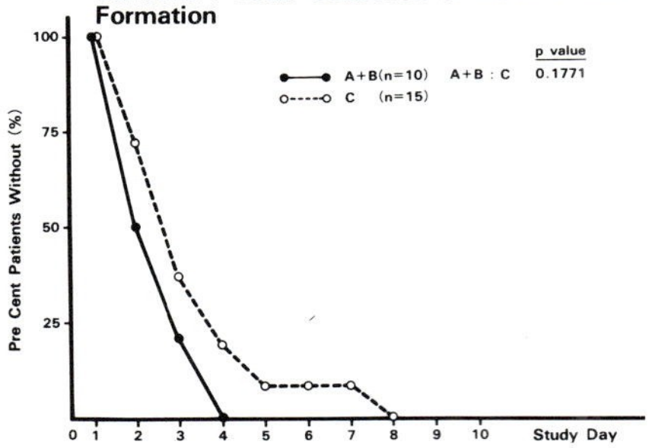

Table I

Background of A, B and C Group Patients

	A group	B group	C group
Number	25	23	21
Sex ratio (M : F)	14 : 11	11 : 12	15 : 6
Age(yr) 0~5	9	8	7
6~10	9	7	12
11~15	6	7	2
16~	1	1	0
Mean age(yr)*	8.2±4.8	8.7±6.9	6.6±3.1
Day of illness at the onset of ACV treatment(days)*	4.5±2.6	5.2±4.6	2.1±1.2
Body temp. prior to the onset of ACV treatment(℃)*	38.1±1.0	38.9±1.3	38.2±1.3
Initial blood counts*			
Total leukocytes ($\times 10^2/mm^3$)	47.6±29.4	45.5±24.1	31.1±21.5
Total lymphocytes($\times 10^2/mm^3$)	14.8±10.6	17.7±17.7	18.1±16.0

*mean±standard deviation

Table II

Clinical Diagnosis of Herpes Infection

Diagnosis	A group	B group	C group
VZV infections	21	18	20
Herpes zoster	16	11	4
Varicella	4	6	16
Varicella encephalitis	1	1	0
HSV infections	4	5	1
Herpetic gingivostomatitis	1	2	1
Kaposi's varicelliform eruption	1	2	0
Disseminated HSV infection	2	1	0

VZV : varicella zoster virus, HSV : herpes simplex virus

Table III

Underlying Diseases

	A group	B group	C group
Acute lymphoblastic leukemia	10 (2)*	7 (1)*	10
Acute myeloblastic leukemia	1 (0)	3 (2)	0
Adult T cell leukemia	0	1 (1)	0
Non Hodgkin's lymphoma	1 (1)	2 (1)	1
Rhabdomyosarcoma	1 (1)	3 (1)	0
Other solid tumors	3 (2)	2 (0)	2
Nephrotic syndrome	3 (3)	2 (2)	4
Atopic dermatitis (including hyper IgE syndrome)	2	2	0
Other immunocompromised status	4	2	4

*Number in parenthesis means the number of patients in relapse

Table IV

Efficasy of Acyclovir on Herpes Group Viral Infections

Clinical Diagnosis(group)		excellent	good	fair	poor	unknown
Herpes zoster	(A)	10	6	0	0	0
	(B)	10	1	0	0	0
	(C)	3	1	0	0	0
Varicella	(A)	3	1	0	0	0
	(B)	5	1	0	0	0
	(C)	12	0	0	4	0
Varicella encephalitis	(A)	1	0	0	0	0
	(B)	0	1	0	0	0
	(C)	0	0	0	0	0
HSV infections	(A)	2	1	1	0	0
	(B)	3	1	1	0	0
	(C)	1	0	0	0	0

Group A : n=25, Group B : n=23, Group C : n=21

to cease new vesicle formation but the difference between group A+B and group C was not significant (p=0.17).

The time course relationship of total scab formation among the patients with varicella was studied and no significant difference was noted between group A+B and group C.

The effective rates of group A, B and C were 96%, 91% and 81% respectively and no statistical differences were noted among each groups (table IV).

Howevere, the effective rates of varicella patients with acute leukemia from group A+B and C were 100% (7/7) and 62.5% (5/8) respectively, which showed a significant difference between the groups (p=0.026).

The comparative study of overall severity of varicella with acute leukemia between group A+B and historical control showed that the patients of control group took significantly severe courses of illness than those of group A+B (p=0.01). (table V).

The comparative study of overall severity of varicella with acute leukemia between group C and historical control showed that the control patients took significantly severecourses of illness than that of group C (p=0.04). (table VI).

The viral sheddings were noted up to 2 days in VZV infections and up to 1 day

Table V

Comparison of Clinical Symptoms between non-treated and ACV-treated Varicella

groups		case No.	case name	age	sex	clinical status of acute leukemia	onset of ACV treatment (day of illness)	varicella number	varicella nature	varicella duration (days)	fever duration (days)	fever max(℃)	complication	over all severity
non-treated group		1	S.N.	5	M	CR		(++)	giant	21	6	40	(−)	severe
		2	T.M.	6	M	CR		(++)	giant	11	10	40	(−)	severe
		3	T.O.	6	M	CR		(+)	medium	10	15	40.3	(−)	severe
		4	K.M.	4	M	CR		(++)	giant	7	3	39	(−)	intermediate
		5	H.A.	4	F	CR		(++)	giant	13	4	?	(−)	severe
		6	M.N.	4	M	PR		(++)	medium pustule	6	7	39.2	(−)	severe
		7	M.N.	7	F	CR		(++)	medium	8+α	—	—	(+)*	most serious (†)
ACV-treated group	(A)	1	T.S.	5	F	R	1	(±)	medium	9	3	39.0	(−)	mild
		2	K.Y.	3	M	CR	4	(+)	medium	12	7	40.0	(−)	severe
		3	T.M.	7	M	CR	5	(+)	medium	13	2	38.0	(−)	mild
	(B)	1	N.N.	4	F	R	3	(+)	medium	4	3	37.5	(−)	mild
		2	A.N.	4	M	CR	1	(±)	medium	4	3	40.2	(−)	mild
		3	N.S.	3	F	CR	1	(±)	medium	6	1	37.5	(−)	mild
		4	K.I.	3	M	CR	2	(±)	medium	9	1	37.5	(−)	mild

CR : complete remission
PR : pertial remission
R : relapse

* : renal and pulmonary hemorrhage

Table VI

Comparison of Clinical Symptoms between non-treated and ACV-treated Varicella

group	case No.	case name	age	sex	clinical status of acute leukemia	onset of ACV treament (day of illnest)	vesicle number	vesicle nature	vesicle duration (days)	fever duration (days)	fever max(℃)	complication	over all severity
ACV-treated group (C)	1	K.F.	4	F	R	1	(±)	medium	3	3	37	(−)	mild
	2	R.K.**	4	M	CR	2	(++)	medium	—	—	36.8	—	intermediate
	3	M.W.***	4	F	CR	1	(±)	medium	2	2	39	(−)	mild
	4	T.K.**	9	M	CR	2	(+)	medium	5	2	39	(−)	mild
	5	Y.S.	3	M	CR	1	(+)	medium	4	2	39	(−)	mild
	6	A.M.**	7	F	CR	2	(±)	medium	3	2	39	(−)	mild
	7	K.T.	14	M	CR	4	(++)	giant	(4)	(3)	40.9	(−)	severe
	8	S.S.***	7	M	CR	1	(+)	medium	(9)	(4)	39	relapsed varicella	severe

* : CR;complete remission, R;relapse
** : History of varicella in the past(+)
*** : History of live varicella vaccination(+)

Table VII

Result of Viral Culture from Vesicles

days of ACV treatment	group A VZV	group A HSV	group B VZV	group B HSV
−3∼0	8/13	1/3	5/12	2/2
1	0/2	1/1	0/2	
2	1/1	0/1	0/1	
3	0/0		0/1	
4	0/5		0/1	
5	0/3		0/4	
6∼	0/6		0/5	
total	9/14	1/3	5/12	2/2

numerator : No. of positive viral cultures
denominator : No. of patients with viral culture

in HSV infections in group A and up to 1 day in VZV infections and up to 1 day in HSV infections in group B after the initiation of ACV treatment. (table VII)

CONCLUSIONS

With above mentioned results, it was concluded that the ACV treatment with either intermittent once a day, thrice a day or continuous onse a day infusions were effective against HSV or VZV infections.

However, ACV dose of 5 mg / kg / dose×1 / day showed less effectiveness to compare with 15 mg / kg / day dose to suppress HSV or VZV infections in immunocompromised children.

REFERENCES

1. Feldman S, et al (1975) Pediatrics 56 : 388-397.
2. Muller SA, et al (1972) Am J Med 52 : 102-114.
3. Schaeffer HJ, et al (1978) Nature 272 : 583-585.
4. Meyers JD, et al (1982) Am J Med 73 (1A) : 229-235.
5. Prober CG, et al (1982) J Ped 101 : 622-625.
6. Pagano JS, et al (1983) J Antimicrob Chemother 12 : Suppl B, 113-121.
7. de Miranda P, et al (1983) J Antimicrob Chemother 12 : Suppl B, 29-37.
8. Kern ER, et al (1980) In : Int. Conference on Human Herpes Viruses. Emory Univ. Atlanta, 17～21 March.
9. Spector SA et al (1982) Am J Med 73 (1A) : 275-280.
10. Elion GB (1982) Am J Med 73 (1A) : 7-13.
11. Sekine I et al (1983) Rinsho Ketsueki 24 : 1260-1270.

THE USE OF ACYCLOVIR IN THE MANAGEMENT OF HERPES INFECTIONS IN THE IMMUNE COMPROMISED HOST

H. GRANT PRENTICE
Department of Haematology, Royal Free Hospital, Pond Street, London, NW3 2QG.

INTRODUCTION

In the patient with compromised immunity, attributable either to his disease or its treatment, reactivation of latent DNA viruses is a frequent event (1,2). Effective therapy of infection in the compromised (IC) host with reactivation of Herpes simplex (HSV) or Herpes zoster (VZV) with acyclovir (ACV) was reported in 1979 (3) and the role of ACV in the treatment of HSV in this setting was firmly established in a placebo controlled multicentre trial published in 1982 (4).

In four consecutive studies we have explored the role of ACV in the prevention of herpes virus recurrence in IC patients including pilot studies which will ultimately lead to long term prophylaxis for high risk groups.

PATIENTS, MATERIALS AND METHODS

In all studies only patients seropositive (≧1:8) for HSV have been entered.

Study 1. Twenty consecutive receipients of allogeneic bone marrow transplants (BMT) and 39 patients having chemotherapy (CT) for treatment of acute leukaemia (AL) were entered into a stratified (by treatment - BMT or CT) randomised double blind placebo controlled trial of ACV prophylaxis.

ACV or placebo was given by 1 hour IV infusion in 100mls of isotonic saline every 12 hours during the period of granulocytopenia ($<1 \times 10^9$/l). In those receiving ACV the dose was 5mg/kg.

Patients were observed for signs of herpes infection (HSV, VZV, EBV and CMV) and exhaustive samples were taken. These included urine samples, throat and perioral swabs twice weekly for HSV and CMV for viral cultures. In addition any possible viral lesion was sampled daily. Saliva specimens were taken weekly for EBV culture. HSV infection was confirmed only when the appropriate lesion was accompanied by isolation of the virus. CMV diagnosis was based on the typical clinical picture (e.g. hepatitis or pneumonitis) followed by at least a 4 fold rise in αCMV serological titre.

Blood levels of ACV and in-vitro sensitivity of Herpes virus isolates were routinely tested.

Study 2. Twenty consecutive HSV seropositive BMT recipients were given oral ACV 400mgs every 6 hours for 6 weeks after the day of transplantation in an open study. These patients were monitored for evidence of HSV/VZV and CMV infections as in Study 1 and pharmacokinetic profiles obtained.

Study 3. A well absorbed (in normal volunteers) ACV "prodrug" BW134U (diaminoacyclovir) was given in a dose of 400mg p.o. every 6 hours for one week to each of 7 consecutive HSV positive BMT recipients. The week of administration was randomly allocated within the first four weeks and during the other five weeks ACV was given as in Study 2. The same observations were made as in the preceding study but the emphasis was on the pharmacokinetic profile. This study was terminated prematurely because of the development of a more promising prodrug BWA515U and we proceeded to Study 4.

Study 4. BW515U is deoxyacyclovir a prodrug which was shown to be near 100% absorbed in normal volunteers.

Ten consecutive HSV seropositive BMT recipients have been treated in an open study with I.V. ACV 5mg/kg 12 hourly by 1 hour infusion for 2 weeks followed by BWA515U capsules 250mg 6 hourly for 1 week and then with oral ACV 400mg 6 hourly for up to 3 weeks. The same observations as in Studies 2 and 3 have been made and again particular emphasis has been placed on the pharmacokinetic profiles.

RESULTS

Study 1. HSV. In the marrow transplant recipients ACV provided total protection against HSV reactivation during the period of treatment. Five of ten BMT recipients experienced an HSV infection during this period ($p = 0.033$). The protective effect of ACV was confirmed in the log rank test for time to development of HSV infection ($p = 0.01$).

In the chemotherapy group two of 19 patients receiving ACV had HSV isolates. In the first the sample had been taken after 24 hours on trial and the lesion healed before the laboratory data was available. The second appeared in a patient who had two previous courses of treatment with ACV. By increasing the dose to 5mg/kg 8 hourly this lesion also resolved. The first isolate was fully sensitive to ACV but the second only partially sensitive (IC_{50} 5-9.5μmol/l). Ten of 20 patients receiving placebo developed HSV infections. Again the protective effect of ACV was significant ($p = 0.018$) including the log rank test ($p = 0.006$).

Other Herpes viruses (both groups).

No VZV infections were observed during the trial period. One CMV infection was proven, in a BMT patient receiving ACV. Extensive studies on EBV secretion gave inconclusive results (2).

Analysis of the number of days of fever showed a significant reduction in the ACV arm of the BMT group at all granulocyte counts, but this did not reach significance in the chemotherapy arm.

The duration of granulocytopenia was shorter in the patients receiving ACV in the BMT group compared with placebo and the cumulative frequency curves for the number of days with granulocytes $<1.0 \times 10^9/l$ is significantly less than the placebo arm ($p = 0.001$) when the patient with CMV is excluded from the analysis. Acquisition of HSV was closely correlated with prolonged granulocytopenia in the CT arm (t test $p = 0.019$).

The peak ACV level on day 14 was 26.3μM and at 12 hours was 0.3μM. All viral isolates from the placebo arms were fully sensitive.

The incidence of post trial herpes infections was high in both ACV and placebo arms in the BMT recipients.

Study 2 & 3. Twenty seven patients were entered to these studies but one withdrew because of nausea related to oral ACV therapy. 5 of 26 patients developed HSV infections (an oropharyngeal) of limited severity. The patient who withdrew also developed HSV and whilst receiving "therapeutic" I.V. ACV (5mg/kg 8 hourly) developed a fatal CMV infection. No VZV infections were observed.

There was no difference between the plasma level of ACV during the first four weeks between the ACV or BW134U groups. Only 6.3% of samples from patients receiving ACV had plasma ACV levels below the maximum ID_{50} of HSV isolated from the patients.

Only the patient who developed nausea and vomiting manifested any toxicity which appeared to be attributable to the drug.

Study 4. Analysis of Herpes infection is not yet available but preliminary pharmacokinetic profiles show a mean peak level (ACV) of approximately 17μM after 250mg oral BWA515U. This is well in excess of that expected with oral ACV (3 ± 1.5μM) at the higher dose of 400mg but not as high as that with I.V. ACV.

DISCUSSION

That recurrence of HSV infection can be prevented by I.V. ACV is now well established. This route of administration is satisfactory during the period of hospitalization. In Study 1 we saw a high rate of HSV, VZV and CMV reactivation in the BMT recipients which continued for many months.

Our aim in this group should logically be to prevent reactivation until the patients immunity has recovered sufficiently to allow them to safely handle these viruses. Oral ACV in Study 2 gave apparently adequate blood levels but was only partially effective in reducing the incidence of HSV reactivation. BW134U has been superseded by a very well absorbed ACV prodrug BWA515U (deoxyacyclovir) which we now propose to test in long term (? 6 months) prophylaxis in our seropositive marrow transplant recipients.

In addition to maintenance of the mucosal integrity by prevention of HSV reactivation we observed an unexpected benefit in that the time taken to granulocyte recovery was accelerated. We feel confident that this drug and its analogues given by I.V. infusion or orally lack toxicity and that the benefits we have demonstrated justify its use in prophylaxis during immunosuppression.

REFERENCES

1. Saral R, Burns WH, Laskin OL, Santos GW, Lietman PS (1981) Acyclovir prophylaxis of herpes-simplex-virus infections. A randomised, double-blind, controlled trial in bone-marrow-transplant recipients. New Engl J Med 305:63-67.
2. Hann IM, Prentice HG, Blacklock HA, Ross MGR, Brigden D, Rosling AE, Burke C, Crawford DH, Brumfitt W, Hoffbrand AV. Acyclovir prophylaxis of herpes virus infections in severely immunocompromised patients. A randomised double-blind trial. Brit Med J (In press).
3. Selby PJ, Jameson B, Watson JG et al (1979) Parenteral acyclovir therapy for herpes virus infections in man. Lancet ii:1267-1270.
4. Wade JC, Newton B, McLaren C, Flournoy N, Keeney RE, Meyers JD (1982) Intravenous acyclovir to treat mucocutaneous Herpes Simplex Virus infection after marrow transplantation: A double-blind trial. Ann Int Med 96:265-269.
5. Robbins G, Hann IM, Blacklock HA, Panjwani D, Ross M, Brigden D, Rees PJ, Collins P, Griffiths P, Hoffbrand AV, Prentice HG. Pharmacokinetics and prophylactic efficacy of oral acyclovir and its prodrug BW134U (In preparation).

TREATMENT WITH INTRAVENOUS ACYCLOVIR FOR HERPES GROUP VIRUS INFECTION IN CANCER CHILDREN

K.NISHIMURA*, T.AKABANE, J.AKATSUKA, F.BESSHO, T.FURUKAWA, T.ISE, A.ISHIKAWA, R.HOSOYA, R.KOIDE, H.KUDO, S.MATSUYAMA, H.MUCHI, T. NAGAO, S.NAKAZAWA, T.SHIDARA, N.TAGUCHI, I.TSUKIMOTO, Y.UEDA, M. USHIO, J.YADA, K.YAMADA, T.YOSHIKAWA

Tokyo Children's Leukemia Study Group (*Department of Pediatrics, St.Luke's International Hospital, 10-1, Akashicho, Chuoku), Tokyo 104, Japan

Acyclovir (ACV), an acyclic purine nucleoside analogue, has been introduced as a highly potent inhibitor of herpes simplex and varicella zoster viruses, and has extremely low toxicity for the normal host cells. We, Tokyo Children's Leukemia Study Group, have lately used ACV for the treatment of herpes group virus infection in the total of 94 children with cancer and some other diseases. This is, therefore, to report the result of our recent study.

MATERIAL AND METHODS

Ninety-four children, 1 month to 18 years old, 50 boys and 44 girls were treated with ACV in the period from April 1982 to Dec. 1983. Basic diseases and number of patients treated were as follows; 55 leukemia, 5 malignant lymphoma, 9 solid tumors, 5 autoimmune diseases, 4 nephrotic syndrome, 2 aplastic anemia, 1 histiocytosis and 13 others. As to the type of herpes group virus infection, chickenpox was 41, herpes zoster 39 and herpes simplex infection 14.

ACV was given 5 mg per Kg every 8 hours by IV drip over 1 hour for 5 consecutive days. Dosage was doubled to 10 mg per Kg every 8 hours when no improvement was seen after 3 days of infusion. Dosage was also modified according to serum creatinine level as follows; 5 mg per Kg every 12 hours when creatinine is 1.5 to 3.4 mg/dl, 5 mg per Kg every 24 hours when creatinine is 3.5 to 4.0 mg/dl and no administration when creatinine is higher than 4.0 mg/dl.

Effects were classified into excellent, good, fair, no effect and unclear. Excellent: no new rash within 3 days and crust formation within 5 days. Good: no new rash within 5 days and crust formation within 7 days. Fair: some effect less than above.

No other antiviral agents were used concurrently.

RESULTS

As to the total 94 cases, 24 showed excellent effect and 53 were good, effective rate being 82%.

As for chickenpox, the treatment was started at an average of 3 days after the onset. Defervescence took place in about 6 days, disappearance of vesicles in 6½ days. Two thirds of cancer children did not show significant rise of antibody titers. Out of 41 chicken pox, 11 showed excellent effect and 26 were good. Therefore, 90.2% were effective. Out of these cases, 31 were cancer children and among them 8 were excellent and 20 were good, effective rate being 90.3%.

As for herpes zoster, average age was 4 years older than chickenpox. The treatment was started at an average of 5 days after the onset. Vesicles disappeared in 7 days, crust formation began at 4 days and completed at 6.4 days and pain disappeared in less than 5 days. Serial determination of antibody titers generally showed good rise, suggesting one who can develop herpes zoster may have less immunosupression. As to the clinical effect for 39 herpes zoster children, excellent were 7 and good were 24, effective rate being 79.4%. Thirty of them were cancer children and their effective rate was 83.3%.

As for mucocutaneous herpes simplex, ACV was effective in 7 out of 10 cases and in 6(75%) out of 8 cancer children among them.

Probable adverse reactions observed are as follows; urticaria 2, transient elevation of transaminase 3, transient elevation of serum creatinine 1, vessel pain 1 and microhematuria 1. Laboratory data before, during and after the treatment showed no significant abnormalities.

Clinical Response

Type of viral infections	No.	Efficacy				
		Excellent	Good	Fair	None	Unclear
Chicken pox	41 (31)	11 (8)	26 (20)	1 (1)	0	3 (2)
Herpes zoster	39 (30)	7 (6)	24 (19)	4 (2)	0	4 (3)
Herpes-meningitis	1 (0)	0	0	0	0	1 (0)
Kaposi varicelli-form eruption	3 (0)	2 (0)	0	0	0	1 (0)
Herpes simplex (Stomatitis, Labialis, etc.)	10 (8)	4 (3)	3 (3)	1 (1)	1 (0)	1 (1)
Total	94 (69)	24(17) 25.5%(24.6%)	53(42) 56.4%(60.9%)	6(4)	1(0)	10(6)

( ) : Cancer children

Clinical effect for Chicken pox in children

Patient Details	No. of patients		41(31)
	Average days prior to ACV Rx		3. 00±1. 82(2. 87±1. 84)
	Average age (years)		5. 36±3. 22(5. 45±3. 06)
Clinical Results (days)	Days to normal BT	N =34	5. 88±3. 87
		n =26	6. 15±4. 25
	Days to disappearance of vesicles	N =34	6. 56±2. 56
		n =25	6. 64±2. 64
	Days to begin encrustation	N =36	3. 56±2. 14
		n =27	3. 74±2. 26
	Days to complete encrustation	N =36	6. 61±3. 16
		n =27	6. 70±3. 44
	Efficacy ratio	Excellent	11/41(26. 8%) : 8/31(25. 8%)
		Good	26/41(63. 4%) : 20/31(64. 5%)

(shaded) : All patients of C.P. (open) : Cancer patients

n : Cancer children

VZV antidody titer
in patients with chicken pox

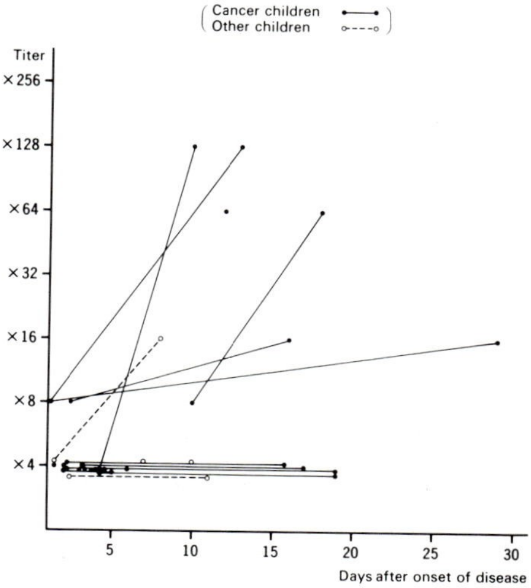

Clinical effect for Herpes zoster in children

Patient Details	No. of patients		39(30)
	Average days prior to ACV Rx		5. 05±3. 11(4. 87±3. 30)
	Average age(years)		9. 41±4. 46(9. 60±4. 41)
Clinical Results (days)	Days to disappearance of vesicle	N =30	6. 87±3. 25
		n =24	7. 04±2. 99
	Days to beginning of crusting	N =36	4. 14±2. 53
		n =27	4. 07±2. 64
	Days to complete crusting	N =36	6. 39±2. 84
		n =27	6. 37±3. 10
	Days to disappearance of pain	N =25	4. 92±2. 45
		n =18	4. 72±2. 44
	Efficacy ratio	Excellent	7/39(17. 9%) : 6/30(20. 0%)
		Good	24/39(61. 5%) : 19/30(63. 3%)

(shaded) : All patients H.Z. (open) : Cancer patients

n : Cancer children

VZV antibody titer
in patients with Herpes zoster

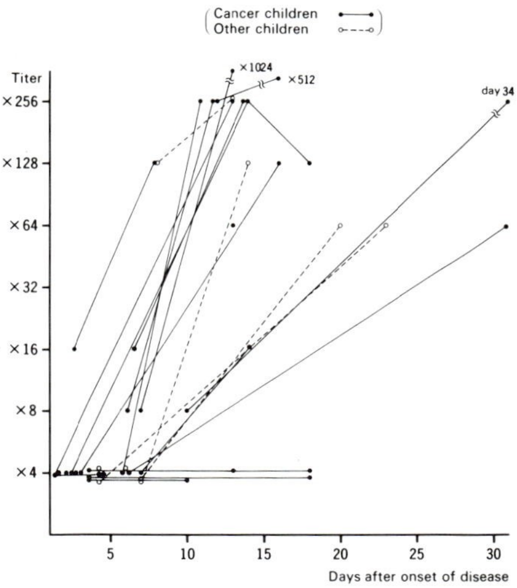

DISCUSSION

In immunocompromised children, chickenpox has been notorious for its very severe and often fatal course. We believe, therefore, evaluating the efficacy of this agent for chickenpox is most important in comparison with other form of herpes group virus infection. Hemorrhagic form of the disease and disseminated visceral lesions with avesicular skin rash and even with aexanthematous type have been well known (1,2). However, these serious form of the disease has been decreased markedly following introduction of ZIG and Ara-A into the treatment armament. The fact that ACV was effective in 90% of chickenpox in 41 children including 31 cancer cases in this study proved this drug to be a quite useful therapeutic agent, as reported in the American and European literatures (3). However, unless this drug is given slowly, its blood concentration rises too rapidly and crystalization may take place in renal tubules causing elevation of BUN and creatinine. In this study, no serious side effects were seen and medication did not have to be discontinued in any single case since ACV was given by IV drip over 1 hour period.

As to isolated virus, all strains of VZV were unfortunately lost by an accident. However, 4 strains of HSV remained alive and their sensitivity to ACV and to Ara-A were compared. Using human fibroblasts, minimum toxic concentration of ACV was found to be 100 gamma per ml and that of Ara-A 50 gamma. Minimum inhibitory concentration of ACV was only 0.8 gamma per ml and that of Ara-A 12.5 gamma. Thus their sensitivity to ACV was found to be significantly higher than to Ara-A and the safety margin of ACV is so wide being 0.8 to 100 gamma per ml.

CONCLUSIONS

1. ACV was effective in 90% of chickenpox, in 80% of herpes zoster and in 70% of mucocutaneous herpes simplex.

2. No serious adverse reactions were seen.

3. ACV can be used quite safely and effectively for herpes group virus infection, especially VZV infection, in immunocompromised children.

REFERENCES

1. Nishimura, K.: Leucémie et varicelle chez l'enfant. Méd. et Hyg. (Genève) 28:1520-1522, 1970

2. Nishimura, K.: Infection récurrente par le virus de la varicelle-zoster chez l'enfant. Méd. et Hyg. (Genève) 36:3257-3258, 1978

3. Fiddian, A.P., et al: Acyclovir: an update of the clinical applications of this antiherpes agent. Antiviral Research 4:99-117, 1984

IV HERPESVIRUS ASSOCIATED WITH CANCER

ASSOCIATION OF EPSTEIN-BARR VIRUS WITH NASOPHARYNGEAL CARCINOMA

JEN-YANG CHEN, MEI-YING LIU, R. PALMER BEASLEY* and CZAU-SIUNG YANG

Department of Bacteriology, College of Medicine, National Taiwan University and University of Washington Medical Research Unit*, Taipei, Taiwan 100, ROC

INTRODUCTION

The incidence of NPC in Taiwan is unusually high, namely the age-adjusted incidence rate is 5.2 per 100,000 population: 7.1 for males and 3.1 for females(1). A recent follow-up study of NPC showed that survival rate at 10 years could be as high as 77% if the treatment was initiated at stage 1 of the disease (2). Consequently, an early diagnosis is urgently needed for us to imporve the prognosis of the disease.

It is well established that NPC is closely related to Epstein-Barr Virus (EBV) (3-5). Among EBV-associated antibodies, the antibody against viral capsid antigen (anti-VCA) in IgA is a valuable marker for the early diagnosis as well as for prediction of the prognosis of NPC. In 1980 Cheng et al found an EBV-specific DNase in Raji cells superinfected with EBV and anti-EBV DNase antibody in NPC patients (6, 7). Chen et al demonstrated that serum anti-DNase activity in the stage 1 of NPC was as high as the other stages (8). Therefore, an attempt was made to see if this antibody can be used as a marker for the early diagnosis of the disease.

On the other hand we hardly obtained NPC biopsies large enough for our studies. So, since 1978 attempts have been made to transplant NPC biopsies to BALB/c (nu/nu) mice so that we can get sufficient amount of the specimens when we need. Up to now two biopsies have been successfully passaged in the nude mice for 6 years and a preliminary result of EBV DNA test in nude-mouse-passaged NPC tissues is also presented.

MATERIALS AND METHODS

Determination of anti-EBV DNase antibody

Serum specimens Twelve NPC and fifteen age- and sex-matched non-NPC serums were collected from a serum stock used for a prospective study of hepatocellular carcinoma at the University of Washington Medical Research Unit in Taipei.

Preparation of EBV DNase Well-grown P3HR1 cells (a Burkitt's lymphoma cell line) were cultivated in RPMI-1640 medium containing IUdR (60ug/ml) and 10% fetal bovine serum at 37°C for 3 days. After cultivating in IUdR-free medium for 2 more days, the cells were harvested and suspended in a buffer containing 10mM $MgCl_2$ β-mercaptoethanol and 50 mM tris-HCl, pH 8.0. The cell suspension was frozen and thawed 4 times and the supernatant (EBV DNase) was collected for enzyme assay. ^{14}C-labelled E. coli DNA was used as a substrate for testing the activity of the enzyme (8). One unit of DNase activity was defined as the amount of enzyme that converts 1.0 ug of the DNA to acid soluble nucloetides in 10 min at 37°C.

Antibody test A 0.05 unit of EBV DNase in 5 ul of the buffer described above was incubated with 5 ul of serum or buffer (control) at room temperature for 20 min. The enzyme activities in test and control groups were then tested. The anti-EBV DNase antibody activity in test serums was expressed as the units of DNase activity neutralized by 1 ml of serum (7).

Test for anti-VCA antibody in IgA Anti-VCA antibody titers were measured by the indirect immunofluorescence antibody technique as described previously (5).

Test for EBV DNA in nude-mouse-passaged NPC tissues

Transplantation of NPC biopsies to nude mice NPC biopsies obtained from the National Taiwan University Hospital were inoculated subcutaneously into 3-week-old BALB/c (nu/nu) mice within 3 hr after specimen collection. When transplanted tumor tissue grew to more than 5 mm in diameter, the tumors were removed for making touch smears for testing EBV-associated antigens, cell cultures and passages (9).

Detection of EBV DNA fragment in tumor tissues A cloned BamHI restriction endonuclease fragment W of EBV DNA, which was kindly supplied by Dr. J.L. Strominger of Harvard University, was used to transform E. coli X 1776. DNA extracted from transformed E. coli was cleaved with BamHI and subjected to agarose gel electrophoresis to obtain EBV DNA BamHI fragment (10). The fragment was labeled with ^{32}P by nick translation (11) to prepare BamHI fragment W probe.

DNA was extracted from nude-mouse-grown NPC tissues at different passages (12) and hybridized with EBV DNA BamHI fragment W by the spot hybridization technique (13).

RESULTS

Anti-EBV DNase antibody activity in NPC patients As shown in Table 1 four blood specimens (Nos. 1-4) were taken from patients before the diagnosis of NPC. Among them patients Nos. 2 and 3 showed significant levels of anti-DNase activity ($\geq$4 units of EBV DNase neutralized) 2 to 28 months before the diagnosis. Twelve of fifteen control serum specimens taken from patients died of non-NPC showed no anti-DNase activity and 3 specimens neutralized 0.4, 0.5 and 0.9 units of EBV DNase, respectively. Although clinical data of these patients were not available at the time of blood collection, the results strongly support the usefulness of this new marker for the early diagnosis of the disease. Among 4 remission cases low anti-DNase activity ($<$4 units) was observed in 3 patients (Nos. 7, 8 and 10), though No. 8 showed anti-VCA titers at 1:40 (a significant value). A recurrent case No. 12 revealed high anti-DNase activity and high anti-VCA titer (1:640) in IgA. The data suggest that this new marker might be also useful for prediction of the prognosis of NPC.

TABLE I

ANTI-EBV DNase ACTIVITY IN NPC PATIENTS

Patient	Date of Diag-nosis	Date of Death	Date of Blood Collec-tion	Months before/ after Diag-nosis	EBV DNase Units Neutra-lized	Anti-VCA Titer in IgA	Remark
1	6-77	6-78	6-76	-12	3.6	10	
2	12-78	10-79	3-78	-9	5.8	-	
3	6-80	9-80	2-78	-28	8.4	40	
			4-79	-14	8.8	160	
			4-80	-2	8.9	160	
4	11-79	8-81	6-77	-29	1.4	-	
5	1-71	7-79	4-77	+76	8.0	640	
6	10-73	3-78	10-76	+36	8.1	640	
7	1-75	1-80	1-77	+24	2.0	-	Remission
			1-78	+36	3.1	-	Remission
			1-79	+48	3.1	10	
8	6-76	12-79	3-77	+9	3.7	40	Remission
			3-78	+21	3.7	40	Remission
9	8-75	1-82	11-76	+15	5.7	160	Remission
10	5-76	7-81	8-77	+15	0.5	-	Remission
11	11-77	2-79	4-78	+5	7.5	160	After radio therapy
12	12-72	8-79	2-78	+62	7.5	640	Recurrence

Transplantation of NPC biopsies to nude mice During the past 6 years in total 176 histopathologically confirmed NPC specimens were inoculated into 3-week old nude mice. The rate of tumor-take by the mice was pretty low (8%) even if the mice were inoculated subcutaneously with a tumor-producing agent (TPA, 30 ng/ mouse) at the time of transplantation or irradiated with 500 rads ^{60}Co 2 days before biopsy inoculation.

Detection of EBV DNA BamHI fragment W in nude-mouse-passaged NPC Our previous studies showed the presence of EBV genome in nude-mouse-passaged NPC (7, 14). Recently, we have found sarcomas in nude mice inoculated with the cells derived from the in vitro cultures of nude-mouse-passaged NPC tissues. Therefore, an attempt was made to test EBV DNA in the sarcoma. As shown in Fig. 1, the 52nd and 63rd nude mouse passages of NPC 306 and the 58th passage of NPC 295 contained DNA homologous to EBV DNA BamHI fragment W but the 15th nude mouse passage of hepatoma J5 (J5-15) and two sarcomas, NPC 306-37C_1B_{33} and NPC 295 C_1B_{28}, did not. NPC 306-37C_1B_{33} and 295 C_1B_{28} had been passaged in nude mice 37 times and once respectively, cultivated in vitro once and then passaged in the mice 33 and 28 more times, separately. The above results indicate that these sarcoma cells were not derived from mouse fibroblasts transformed by NPC cells, because no EBV DNA fragment was detected in the sarcoma cells. More studies are needed to clarify the state of EBV DNA BamHI fragments in nude-mouse-grown NPC at different stages.

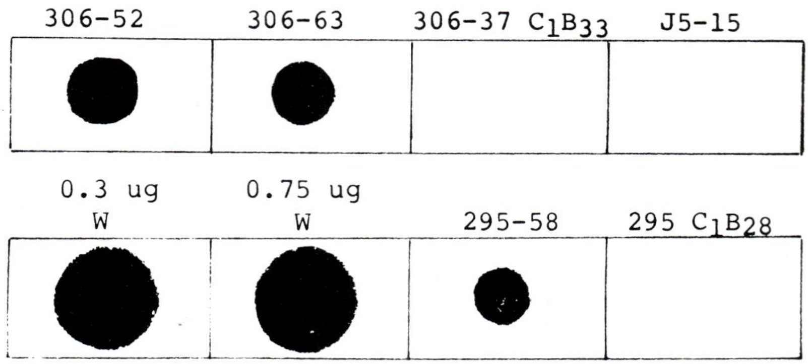

Fig. 1. Hybridization of DNA extracted from nude-mouse-passaged NPC with cloned EBV BamHI fragment W.

ACKNOWLEDGEMENTS

We wish to express our thanks to Dr. Lu-Yu Hwang for supplying clinical records of the patients and to Miss Li-Yong Chan for the nucleic acid hybridization test.

REFERENCES

1. Lin TM, Hsu MM, Chen KP, Chiang TC, Jung PF, Hirayama T (1971) Gann Monograph 10:137-144.
2. Hsu MM, Huang SC, Lynn TC, Hsieh T, Tu SM (1982) Otolaryngol Head Neck Surg 90:289-295.
3. Henle W, Henle G, Ho JHC, Burtin P, Cachin Y, Glifford P, De Schryver A, De Thé G, Diehl V, Klein G (1970) J Natl Cancer Inst 44:225-231.
4. Henle W, Ho JHC, Henle G, Kwan HC (1973) J Natl Cancer Inst 51:361-369.
5. Yang CS, Yang HM, Yeh YS, Lynn TC (1979) Comp Immun Microbiol Infect Dis 2: 167-175.
6. Cheng YC, Chen JY, Hoffmann PJ, Glaser R (1980) Virology 100:334-338.
7. Cheng YC, Chen JY, Glaser R, Henle W(1980)Proc Natl Acad Sci USA 77:6162-6165.
8. Chen JY, Liu MY, Lynn TC, Yang CS(1982) Chinese J Microbiol Immunol 15:255-261.
9. Yang CS, Hsu YV, Chan TK, Yeh YS, Chu CT, Tu SM (1982) J Formosan Med Assoc 81:882-891.
10. Skare J, Strominger JL (1980) Proc Natl Acad Sci 77:3860-3864.
11. Maniatis T, Jeffrey A, Kleid DG (1975) Proc Natl Acad Sci USA 72:1184-1188.
12. Blin N, Stafford DW (1976) Nucleic Acids Res 3:2303-2308.
13. Scotto J, Hadchouel M, Hery C, Yvart J, Tiollais P, Brechot C (1983) Hepatology 3:279-284.
14. Raab-Traub N, Hood R, Yang CS, Henry II B, Pagano JS (1983) J Virol 48:580-590.

EPSTEIN-BARR VIRUS-ACTIVATING AND TUMOR-PROMOTING NATURAL PRODUCTS: THEIR POSSIBLE ROLE IN CAUSATION OF BURKITT'S LYMPHOMA AND NASOPHARYNGEAL CARCINOMA

YOHEI ITO, HARUKUNI TOKUDA, HAJIME OHIGASHI AND KOICHI KOSHIMIZU

Department of Microbiology, Faculty of Medicine and Department of Food Sciences and Technology, Faculty of Agriculture, Kyoto University, Kyoto 606, Japan

INTRODUCTION

Many species of plants of Euphorbiaceae and Thymeleaeceae families are known to yield skin irritaing latex and chemical characteristics of such irritants have been definte to be the diterpene ester compounds based on skeltal structures of tigliane, daphnane, ingenane and others[1]. The chemical extracts of from these plants also have been known to exert effect of tumor-promotion[2] and, such capacity was shown to overlap with their Epstein-Barr virus(EBV)-activating potency[3]. Many plants of the two families, Euphorbiaceae in particular, are currently used as herbal drugs or folk remedies in many developing areas of the world, including the areas where the two EBV-associated diseases, Burkitt's lymphoma(BL) and nasopharyngeal carcinoma(NPC) are endemic[4,5]. Another aspect to view on the matter is the fact that plant such as Aleurites fordii (Chinese tung oil tree), a member of Euphorbiaceae, is seen growing and being grown for an industrial purpose to obtain tung oil, in southern provinces of China where NPC has the highest incident rate. The plant itself is also used as herbal drug[6]. In the present communication, attempts will be made to link the existence of these active substances and the two diseases, NPC and BL, with peculiar geographic distribution, hopefully to propose a theory for explaining their etiology and pecuriality.

MATERIALS AND METHODS

Cells and cell cultures

The human lymphoblastoid Raji cells, latently infected by EBV and carry multiple copies of EBV genomes were cultivated in RPMI 1640 medium containing 10% fetal calf serum, 100 units of penicillin and 250 ug/ml of streptomycin. The spontaneous rate of induction of EBV early antigen(EA) in our subline Raji was less than 0.01%.

Assay method

The synergistic assay method[3] was used throughout the study.

This assay method takes the advantages of a phenomenon[7] that when EBV genome-carrying nonproducer Raji cells are exposed to two inducing agents of different feature, such as short-chain fatty acids(n-butyrate) and tumor-promoting diterpene esters(TPA = 12-O-tetradecanoylphorbol-13-acetate), in the culture, the expression of EBV EA is enhanced synergistically up to approximately 30 to 40% of the total cell population. Using this as a marker, we can readily screen EBV-activating and possibly tumor-promoting principles or substances in environment or in nature. The results of this assay becomes available in 48 hr, whereas the promoter assay on mouse skin takes at least 4 to 6 weeks for a simple sample to be determined. The present method is much convenient and economical than the conventional assay procedure.

Extracts and compounds

The crude extracts from plant materials, soil samples and others were obtained by ether extraction. After then, the solvent was evapolated and the resultant residue was weighed and resolved in dimethylsulfoxide(DMSO) as a stock solution of 10 mg/ml and kept frozen till time of use. The purification procedures of the plant diterpene esters are described elsewhere[8].

RESULTS AND DISCUSSION

EBV-activating agents in nature

Employing the synergistic assay method for EBV activation in vitro we were able to identify over 50 products in our environment. They could be categolized into three major groups as follows: 1)Plant diterpene esters, 2)microbial indole alkaloids and 3) principles in human physiological fluids. Such active agents are listed in Table 1.

Plant diterpene esters The chemical structures of diterpene ester compounds have been determined by elaborate efforts of organic chemists of the world and, most, if not all, of such substances are reaily available in pure form. The major grouping of such compounds based on the skelton of tigliane, daphnane and ingenane has been referred to previously. In Figure 1, the core structures and some compounds which we have assayed for their EBV-activating potency is listed.

Microbial indole alkaloids The first indole alkaloid with strong skin irritating effect was isolated from mycelium of a strain of Streptomyces mediocidus and was designated as teleocidin B[9]. Later,

TABLE 1
EBV-ACTIVATING SUBSTANCES IN NATURE

Higher Plants	
Euphorbiaceae	Diterpene esters(TPA, HPA[8], HHPA[6])
Thymelaeaceae	Diterpene esters(Mezerein[3])
Soil Microbes	
Strepotomyces mediocidus	Indole alkaloids(teleocidin[9])
Streptoverticilluim blastmyceticum	Indole alkaloids(Indolactum)
Physiological Fluids	
Serum factor	Protein
Semen principle	Protein(?)

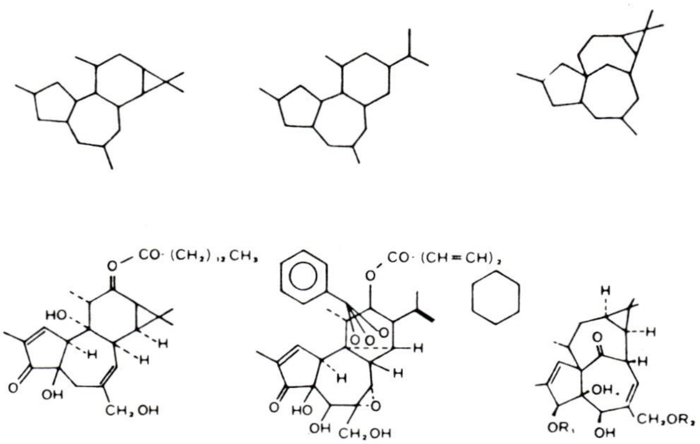

A B C

FIG. 1. Basic skeletal structures of three major plant diterpene esters with EBV-activating potency (typical compound shown below). A, Tigliane(TPA); B, Daphnane(Mezerein); C, Ingenane(Milliamin).

it was shown that the agent is a powerful tumor promoter[10] and also an efficient EBV activator. The comparison of such activity of teleocidin with one of the most powerful and efficient EBV activator TPA is listed in Table 2. Recently, we have screened about 3,000 strains of soil microbes for EBV EA-inducing activity and isolated a new series of compounds, indolactam, which is composed of nine-membered lactam ring and corresponds to the core structure of the teleocidins. The representative compounds of both groups, teleocidin B and indoluctam V, are illustrated in Figure 2.

Principles in physiological fluids These include serum factor[11] and semen principle[12]. The EBV-activating potency of some semen samples are almost as potent as that of TPA. The implication of these findings deserves further investigation.

Environmental EBV activators and BL and NPC

Many species of plants mostly of *Euphorbiaceae* family which contain EBV-activating diterpene esters are found in BL and NPC endemic area. This, however, not necessarily provide evidence for their linkage with the cause of diseases. For problem of how these active substances can gain access to the human system, the following route may be considered: 1) intake as herbal drugs, 2) inhaled as some volatile praction of plant oil (tung oil), 3) inhaled as pollen of flowers of the plant with active substance and 4) inhailing soil dusts from soil containig active principles released by the plants[13].

Another point in this theory is the synergestic action of the short-chain fatty acids produced *in vivo* by microbes of normal flora at the site where the malignacies are foreseen to emerge. The preceeding inflammation at the site may induce opportunistic propagation of indeginous microbes such as *Fusobacterium nucleatum*, a common bacteria in human nasal and oral cavities and, which is an efficient producer of butyric acid. Such bacterial products may act together with the exogenous promoter diterpene esters at the site of inflammation to activate the EBV genome in the B lymphocytes infiltrating in the tissue and, subsequently initiate the chain of event leading to the induction of malignant tumors, such as BL and/or NPC[14].

In *in vitro* observations, the EBV EA-induced lymphatic cells are usually destinated to death by expression of the early genes. On the other hand,it has been evidently demonstrated that such EA-expressing activated cells aquires capacity to readily fuse with cells of homologous and heterologous groups and transfer their activated genetic materials to the recipient cells[15]. This provides more convenient thoughts in explaning development of the diseases.

The malaria hypothesis for explaining the co-factor for BL is longstanding. From immunological aspects, the idea still deserves attention. However, despite the ubiquitous distribution of EBV, not all of the malaria infested area shows occurance of BL cases. It is

TABLE 2

EBV-ACTIVATING POTENCY OF TWO TUMOR PROMOTERS: TPA AND TELEOCIDIN B*

T P A (ng/ml)	100	20	10	5	2.5
EBV EA(%)	58.8	60.3	34.3	17.8	6.9
Teleocidin B (ng/ml)	100	20	10	5	2.5
EBV EA(%)	59.5	56.8	48.7	24.6	14.3

* Assayed by synergistic assay method[3] with 4 mM n-butyrate

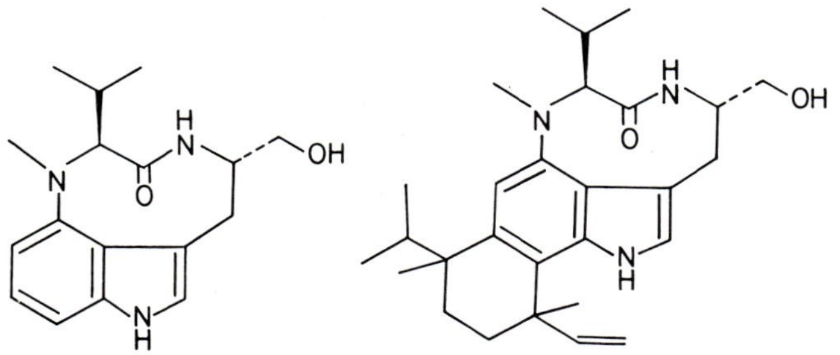

Indolcatam V Teleocidin B

FIG. 2. EBV-activating indole alkaloids.

obious that malaria has little to do with NPC. Our promoter and EBV-activating diterpene ester hypothesis does not contradict with that of malaria in BL area because many of these plants are being used as anti-malaria herbal drugs.

SUMMARY

The presence of EBV-activating and possibly tumor-promoting agents in the local environment of areas where two EBV-associated diseases, BL and NPC are endemic, was proposed as a new co-factor in explaning the etiology of the diseases. The supporting data, however, is still fragmentally and, much more studies have to be done to further clarify this important issue.

REFERENCES

1. Evans FJ, Schmidt RJ (1980) J. med. Plant Res. 38:291-316

2. Diamond L, O'Brien TG, Barid WM (1980) Advanc. Cancer Res. 32:1-74

3. Ito Y, Yanase S, Fujita J, Harayama T, Takashima M, Imanaka H (1981) Cancer Letters 13:29-37

4. Kokwaro JO (1976) In: Kokwaro JO (ed) Medicinal plants of East Africa. East Africa Literature Bureau, Nairobi, pp 85-100

5. Ito Y, Kishishita M, Morigaki T, Yanase S, Hirayama T (1981) Cancer Campaign 5:255-262

6. Ito Y, Yanase S, Tokuda H, Kishishita M, Ohigashi H, Hirota M, Koshimizu K (1983) Cancer Letters 18:87-95

7. Ito Y, Kawanishi M, Harayama T, Takabayashi S (1981) Cancer Letters 12:175-180

8. Ohigashi H, Ohtsuka T, Hirota M, Koshimizu K, Tokuda H, Ito Y (1983) Agric. Biol. Chem. 47:1617-1622

9. Takashima M, Sasaki H (1960) Bull. Agric. Chem. Soc. Jpn. 24:647-651

10. Fujiki H, Mori M, Nakayasu M, Terada M, Sugimura T, Moore RE (1981) Proc. Natl. Acad. Sci. USA 78:3872-3876

11. Bauer G, Höfler P, zur Hausen H (1982) Virology 121:184-194

12. Ito Y, Tokuda H, Morigaki T, Shimizu K, Kawana T, Sanada S, Yoshida O (1984) Cancer Letters 23:129-134

13. Ito Y, Ohigashi H, Koshimizu K, Zeng Y (1983) Cancer Letters 19:113-117

14. Hirayama T, Ito Y (1981) Prev. Med. 10:614-622

15. Bayliss GJ, Wolf H (1980) Nature 287:164

CURRENT STUDIES ON NASOPHARYNGEAL CARCINOMA (NPC) IN GUANGDONG PROVINCE, CHINA

PAN Qi-chao

Cancer Institute, Zhongshan Medical College, Dongfeng IV Road, Guangzhou, China

Recently, a monogragh, "Nasopharyngeal Carcinoma - Clinical and Laboratory Researches", edited by Drs. Li Chen-chuan, Pan Qi-chao and Chen Jian-jing, was published in Guangzhou. In this book are compiled the results of epidemiological, clinical and basic researches in the Tumor Hospital and Cancer Institute of the Zhongshan Medical College. Now, I would like to present briefly the results of current studies on NPC in Guangdong, China.

I. EPIDEMIOLOGICAL STUDIES

Guangdong is the highest risk area for NPC among all provinces in China with a standardized mortality rate of $6.47/10^5$ populations per year. It accounts for 13.74% of death of all malignancies. Among the 149,393 cases of malignancies collected in the Tumor Hospital, Zhongshan Medical College, from 1964 to 1981, there were 47,848 cases (32.04%) of NPC, ranking first among all cancers in this hospital, but according to the investigation of cancer deaths in the whole province, NPC ranks third next to liver and esophagus cancers. There is a geographical aggregation of NPC mortality in Guangdong province, being higher in counties and cities in the central part (Guangzhou city and Foshan district) and in the lower reaches of the West River (Shaoching district). Incidentally, higher mortality rate was shown also in people speaking Cantonese dialect than in those speaking South Fukein or Hakka dialect.

Since 1970 a cancer registry has been set up in Zhongshan county. From 1970-1979 the annual NPC mortality rates varied between $9.09-11.66/10^5$ with an average of $11.24/10^5$ (standardized mortality rate), consisting 20.42% of all malignancies. NPC mortality rate ranked second next to liver cancer. The average mortality rate was $16.25/10^5$ for male and $6.64/10^5$ for female with a M:F ratio of 2.45:1. The average standardized incidence rate was $14.18/10^5$, 20.45 for male and 8.33 for female, with the same M:F ratio as for mortality rate. Both mortality and incidence rates showed no significant change during these years. However, the proportion of early (stage I & II) NPC cases rose from 41.12% in 1970 to 68.18% in 1979, whereas the late (Stage III & IV) cases decreased from 58.88% in 1970 to 31.82% in 1979, this may be attributed to the propagation of knowledge of cancer prevention in this county.

Sihui county is the highest risk area for NPC among all counties in Guangdong province. For the years 1970-1980 the average standardized NPC mortality rate was $15.22/10^5$, $22.33/10^5$ for male and $10.88/10^5$ for female. The flutu-ation of the mortality rate each year ($13.06-19.55/10^5$) was not significant. For most of the years NPC mortality rates ranked first among all cancers, only in 3 years the rates dropped somewhat, lower than that for liver cancer in male. The average crude NPC incidence rate in 1971-1980 was $18.11/10^5$, $26.77/10^5$ for male and $10.93/10^5$ for female. By analyzing the geographical distribution of NPC mortality and incidence rates, we are able to spot a high risk zone (A) on the reaches of Longjiang River in the central part of the county. The incidence and mortality rate of zone A (23.48 and $21.39/10^5$, respectively) was significantly higher than those of its peripheral area —— zone B (15.10 and $13.43/10^5$, respectively).

II. ETIOLOGICAL STUDIES

1. Epstein-Barr virus is closely associated with NPC, and a high percentage of NPC patients have VCA-IgA antibodies in their sera. Li Wan-jun et al reported some of the findings in their clinical serological studies on NPC patients. Sera of 1006 pretreated NPC patients and 2114 controls were collected for VCA-IgA antibody detection by immunoenzymatic method. The positive rate of serum VCA-IgA ($\geq$ 1:10) in NPC cases was 90.9%, in head and neck cancers 6.0%, in other cancers 3.5%, in patients with nasopharyngeal hyperplastic lesions 5.1% and in normal subjects 0.6%. The GMT of these groups were 76.0, 3.0, 2.7, 2.8 and 2.6, respectively. The serum VCA-IgA titer of NPC patients rose with the size of metastatic cervical lymph nodes and clinical staging, thus the GMT of the patients with N_0 was 44.3, N_1 - 74.1, N_2 - 102.2, N_3 - 184.5 and the GMT of patients in

stage I was 32.8, stage II - 61.9, stage III - 90.6 and stage IV - 146.7.

Jian Shao-wen, Wu Yin-tang et al showed that the VCA-IgA positive rate in 294 NPC patients (89.8%) is very much higher compared with 15.3% in 118 cases with hyperplastic lesion of nasopharynx, and 7.5% in 40 normal persons. They found that the increasing of IgA antibody was concordent with the IgG antibody both are against VCA or EA in the same NPC patient. Luo Hui-ling et al studied the serum VCA-IgA of NPC patients treated by radiationtherapy. The GMT of VCA-IgA antibody in a group of 56 NPC cases dropped from 32.41 before treatment to 17.21 after treatment. However, among these 56 cases only 30 cases (52.6%) showed decreasing of their VCA-IgA titers (GMT from 96.16 to 15.17), 11 cases (19.6%) showed no change of the antibody titer. 15 cases (26.8%) even showed increasing of the antibody titer. Generally, patients showing decreasing titers had high VCA-IgA titers, which decreased with the regression of tumor, especially that of the cervical metastatic lymph nodes, after radiation.

Chen Jian-jing et al tested each sample of serum with 6 methods for the presence of EBV antibodies, namely EBNA, VCA-IgA (IF), VCA-IgA (IE), and they showed that there is a close relationship between anti VCA and EA antibodies (both IgA and IgG), but the anti-EBNA antibody level was not parallel to the anti-VCA or EA antibodies. They suggested that a comprehensive assay of multiple anti-EBV antibodies can increase the early detection rate and also eliminate the false negatives.

2. Epidemiological data and the results of some animal experiments indicated that some trace elements might possess carcinogenic activity. Since NPC has a charaoteristic geographical distribution, it is suspected that its etiology may have some association with the contents of trace elements in the environment. Huang Jia-chen et al reported a positive correlation (r = 0.59) existed between nickel contents in rice and drinking water and NPC mortality rates. Thus, the Ni contents of drinking water and rice had been found to be higher in high risk county Sihui (25.04 µg/L water, 0.26 mg/kg rice) than those in low risk county WuHua (9.36 µg/L water, 0.15 mg/kg rice).

The difference was statistically significant. It is interesting to find that the Ni content of normal human hair in Sihui county (2.18 μg/g) was higher than that found in Wuhua county (1.13 μg/g), and the Ni content of the hair of NPC patients (3.60 μg/g) in Sihui was even higher than that of normal person.

Ou Bao-xiang et al showed that NPC can be induced in rats by the promotion of Ni ($NiSO_4$ in drinking water or in intranasal gel) after the initiation of subthreshold dose of dinitroso-piperazine (DNP). One squamous cell carcinoma and one fibro-sarcoma was found in the DNP-$NiSO_4$ water group; one early carcinoma and one papilloma was found in the DNP-Ni gel group. However, no tumor has yet been found in rats treated with DNP or nickel alone. Liu Yi-feng et al repeated this experiment and showed that 2 NPC, 2 cancers of the nasal cavity and one cancer of palate were found in the rats treated with DNP and Ni gel, but no tumor was induced in other experimental groups. Liu Yi-feng et al showed that after feeding with 1% $NiSO_4$ solution the Ni contents of nasopharynx, esophagus, trachea, lung and some other organs of rats increased significantly. This suggests a possible affinity of Ni to nasopharynx.

Deng Cheng-zong et al reported that the sister chromatid exchange (SCE) rate of CHO cells and human lymphocytes can be increased by the addition of $NiSO_4$ to the medium. The rate of peripheral lymphocytes of workers in electroplating factory was higher than that of nickel non-contacters. After the workers have changed, their work for a few years, the SCE rate dropped significantly.

3. The genetic factor of NPC has also been proposed. Some NPC high risk families have been found. In Ye-Liang family, 11 NPC patients and one mammary cancer were found among 49 members of this family.

Ou Bao-xiang et al studied the HLA profiles of NPC patients in comparison with that of normal persons. It was shown that B_{17}, Bw_{46} and Aw_9 antigen frequencies were more prevalent in NPC patients. Furthermore, DR double blank showed higher frequency in NPC patients, whereas A_{11} and DRw_9 showed lower frequency in NPC patients than in normal subjects, but this remained to be confirmed by larger scale investigation. Yuan Hua-ye et al showed that A_2Bw_{46} haplotype had been found in NPC patients with familial history of cancer.

Ou Bao-xiang et al showed that there is a higher SCE rate of peripheral lymphocytes in NPC patients (8.96 ± 0.22 SCE/ metaphase) than in normal subjects (5.74 ± 0.42). This may indicate a higher instability of the chromosomes of NPC patients. Long Jiang-bin, Li De-rui and Huang Yuan studied also the unscheduled DNA synthesis (UDS) activity of peripheral lymphocytes of NPC patients and normal subjects, and showed that the DNA repair function expressed by UDS in NPC patients is lower than that in normal subjects, while SCE induced by some polycyclic hydrocarbons and physical factors was significantly higher than in NPC patients.

Long Jiang-bin et al had determined the glucose-6-phosphate dehydrogenase (G6PD) activities of erythrocytes and leukocytes in 137 NPC patients, 80 with other types of cancer and 116 controls. They found that the frequency of G6PD deficiency of NPC (2.9%) or other cancer patients (1.3%) was significantly lower than that in controls (9.5%) and the G6PD activities of NPC and other cancer patients, excluding G6PD deficient subjects, were higher than that of the controls.

LITERATURES

Cited mainly from "Nasopharyngeal Carcinoma - Clinical and basic researches", Ed. by Drs. Li Chen-chuan, Pan Qi-chao, Chen Jian-jing, Scientific Publisher of Guangdong, 1984 Guangzhou.

Herpes Viruses and Virus Chemotherapy, R. Kono, editor

THE MORBIDITY AND POSSIBLE CAUSE OF CERVICAL CARCINOMA IN CHINA - A REVIEW

CHEN MIN-HUI[1], SUN YU[1] and JIANG WEN-JIN[2]

Department of Cell Biology, Virus Research Institute, Hubei Medical College, Wuchang, China[1]. Department of Oncology, Second Teaching Hospital, Hubei Medical College, Wuchang, China[2].

Cervical cancer is one of common diseases with the mortality at second position of women's cancer mortality and at fourth position of all the malignancy mortality of Chinese population (1). For early detection and early treatment, a mass screening for cervical cancer has proceeded in many districts of China for many years. Now an attempt is being made in many districts of the Country to report the morbidity of cervical cancer based primarily on Pap smears of screening cervico-vaginal samples and then on biopsies.

MORBIDITY

According to Yang Da-Wang's review, based on 140 reports from different districts of 25 provinces and autonomous regions, an average morbidity rate, $138.74/10^5$, of cervical cancer in about 8 million (7,735,057) women examined during the past 15 years was estimated (2). However, due to a plan of early detection and early treatment which has been supported and encouraged by the government, the morbidity has been decreasing in number year by year. According to the reports from 16 provinces in 1974-1982 (2-11), the average morbidity of cervical cancer was $98.93/10^5$ of 645,866 women examined (Table 1). It was obviously lower than that reported by Yang. The average morbidities of carcinoma in situ and dysplasia were higher than that of cancer (Table 2).

In Table 1, it has also shown the morbidity rates of large cities such as Peking, Shanghai, Wuchang, Nanjin, Qindao and Tianjin were lower than that of the mountain area such as Jingan, Wufun, Funxan, Lioyang etc. It is most likely that there were some geographical high risk areas with a high cervical cancer incidence, such as Jingan (6), Wufun (7) and Lioyang (11). Thus an attention of some epidemiological studies has been concentrated on these areas with comparision with low incidence areas.

AETIOLOGICAL STUDIES

By use of an enzyme-labelled immune solid phase method, Chen Wen-Kai (13) reported on a prevalence rate of HSV infection in married women of Wufun. Among 77 serum samples tested, only 5 samples were negative for both HSV-1 and HSV-2 antibody, 72 samples contained antibodies either to HSV-1 or to

TABLE 1

MORBIDITY OF CERVICAL CANCER IN CHINA

Locality	Ca. per cases exam.	Morbidity(10^5)	Year reported	Reference
Beijing*	9/22,946	39.22	1980	(3)
Shanghai*	6/40,450	14.83	1977	(4)
Tianjin*	11/15,515	70.89	1974	(2)
Wuchang*	2/12,794	7.81	1978	(5)
Nanjin*	23/212,032	10.84	1982	(2)
Chendu*	47/108,988	43.12	1978	(2)
Qindao*	1/13,360	7.48	1978	(2)
Jingan	50/9,625	519.49	1982	(6)
Sangtao	34/11,784	288.55	1978	(2)
Wufun	5/3,365	148.58	1982	(7)
Shanxi	73/49.100	148.67	1976	(2)
Nanzhau	35/4,082	863.8	1980	(8)
Xinjiang	118/88,803	132.88	1978	(9)
Funxan	26/16,705	754.26	1982	(10)
Lioyang	174/19,864	875.96	1981	(11)
Baotu	25/16,453	151.95	1979	(12)
Total	639/645,866	98.93		

* Large cities

TABLE 2

MORBIDITIES OF CERVICAL CANCER IN SITU AND DYSPLASIA

Locality	Ca. in situ /No. exam.	Morbidity (10^5)	Dy./No. exam	Morbidity (10^5)	Year	Reference
Jingan	176/75,658	232.62	486/75,658	642.36	1982	(6)
Xinjiang	36/88,803	40.53	68/88.803	76.57	1978	(9)
Lioyang	92/19,864	463.21	277/19,864	1394.48	1981	(11)
Wufun	38/13,010	292.08	95/13,010	730.2	1982	(7)
Total	342/197,335	173.31	926/197,335	469.25		

HSV-2 or both. Using the same method Den Shui-Sen (14) compared the levels and geometric mean titres (GMT) of serum HSV-2 antibodies in women with cervical cancer with that in matched controls from 5 different parts of the Country. He showed that either the frequency of HSV-2 antibody or the value of GMT was significantly higher in Cases than in Controls. Additionally, according to this report, 100% of women were infected by HSV-1 as judged by occurrence of serum HSV-1 antibody. The GMT of serum antibody to HSV-2 in women with cervical cancer and controls was also detected with the ELISA method by Fen Jue-Sun et al. in 1982 (15). The value of GMT was 249.3 in Cases and 62.9 in Controls. No difference of frequency of HSV-2 antibody between Cases and Controls was stated.

A comparison of frequencies of antibody to HSV-2 among women at different ages in high incidence with that among the matched groups in low incidence areas was reported by Yang Xue-Zhi et al. (4) and Liu Zhi-Hui et al. (16). Comparing Jingan (high incidence area) with Peking (low incidence area), Yang showed that the frequency of HSV-2 antibody among the population of Jingan was lower only in the group of ages 0-9 and higher in all groups of over 10. Liu compared another high incidence area, Wufun, with the low incidence area, Wuchang. She showed that the frequency of HSV-2 antibody was higher in all age groups of Wufun than that in all the age-matching groups of Wuchang. Additionally, she also demonstrated that the GMT of HSV-2 antibody in age groups 11-20 and 21-30 of high incidence areas revealed significantly higher than that in age matching groups of low incidence areas. Like other professionals who have done similar work in other parts of the world, the above mentioned studies a tempted to relate the HSV-2 infection with cervical cancer.

M. H. Chen et al. (17) was the first in China to detect the HSV-2 specific antigen in exfoliated cells from cervico-vagina of cervical cancer patients of Wuchang with the indirect immuno-fluoresence method. He showed a positive reaction in 100% of the cases, in 9% of controls and in 45% of chronic cervico-vaginitis. Years later, Jiang Wen-Jin et al. (18) used the unlabelled anti-body PAP method to detect HSV-2 specific antigen in exfoliated cells from Cases and Controls in Wufun. According to her observation, the positive results were found in 50% of the Cases and in 31% of the Controls. The difference of percentage between the two reports might be due to the diffe-rent method used, or due to the specimens coming from different districts.

In China, M. H. Chen's group (19-21) has established animal model with the HSV-induced cancer. Most of the mice tested survived one year, which were intravaginally challenged with HSV-2 or HSV-1, once or repeatedly in the beginning period of experiment. The viruses used were living or UV-inactivated. It demonstrated that the yeilds of cancer have increased in number when a UV-inactivated HSV-1 or HSV-2 was used repeatedly. It was very interesting that the induction of the cancer could be enhanced by a promoting agent, croton oil. This establishment of animal model was very important not only because of demonstrating the oncogenic potential of HSV but also because of its availability in researching the efficacy of some drugs or vaccines against HSV-induced cancer.

As determined by both Dot and Southren DNA blot hybridization method, the fragments of HSV-2 DNA in cells of the cervical cancer were detected in 3/5 of cases by Cui Hui-Yun (22). Further studies on the viral DNA in cervical cancer cells with these methods were stated to be in progress and the results were being awaited with interest.

REFERENCES

1. Li P, Li JY (1980) Chinese J Oncol 2:1
2. Yang DW et al. (1984) In: Proceedings of the National Conference on Cervical Cancer in Jiangxi
3. Liu YF et al. (1984) Cited from 2
4. Tao N et al. (1977) Obstet and Gynecol Articles of Shanghai
5. Jiang WJ et al. (1978) In: Prodeedings of Conference on Cancer in Wuchang
6. Yang XZ et al. (1984) Cited from 2
7. Chen HZ et al. (1984) Cited from 2
8. Yi Q (1984) Cited from 2
9. Wang UZ, Lu M (1984) Cited from 2
10. Zhang H (1984) Cited from 2
11. Yuan SX et al. (1984) Cited from 2
12. Jiang Y (1984) Cited from 2
13. Chen WK (1978) In: Proceedings of the National Conference on Clinical Technology
14. Den SS (1984) Cited from 2
15. Feng JS et al. (1982) Acta Virol Sin 2:37
16. Liu ZH et al. (1984) Cited from 2
17. Chen MH et al. (1979) Chinese J Oncol 1:255
18. Jiang WJ et al. (1984) Cited from 2
19. Chen MH et al. (1981) In: Hiroshi Shiota et al. (eds) Herpesviruses. Excerpta Medica, Amsterdam-Oxford-Princeton
20. Chen MH et al. (1980) Acta Biol Exper Sin 13:273
21. Men YK, Chen MH in the press
22. Cui HY (1984) Cited from 2

HUMAN CYTOMEGALOVIRUS AND KAPOSI'S SARCOMA

ENG-SHANG HUANG AND LYNN SMILEY

Department of Medicine, Department of Microbiology and Immunology and Cancer Research Center, University of North Carolina at Chapel Hill, Chapel Hill, North Carolina 27514 (U.S.A.)

INTRODUCTION

Kaposi's sarcoma (KS) is an idiopathic, multifocal, pigmented, hemorrhagic sarcoma which has an extremely obscure nature. It was first described in 1872 by a Hungarian dermatologist, Dr. M. Kaposi (1). This tumor is characterized by the appearance of multicentric, hyperpigmented, vascular, cutaneous nodules usually localized to the lower extremities (1-4). Before 1950, KS was a rare tumor occurring in elderly white men (mean age 63 years) in Eastern Europe and North America who had an Italian or Jewish ethnic origin (3,5,6). Rare cases have been found in people of other races and ethnic background. KS in this group has been referred to as "classic Kaposi's sarcoma". It has an annual incidence of 0.02 to 0.06 per 100,000 population in the United States (3,5,7). Classic Kaposi's sarcoma is often relatively benign. Patients usually have asymptomatic violaceous plaques or nodular skin lesions. New lesions frequently occur near the original tumor site, but they may appear on any part of the body such as on the upper extremities, head and neck. Although spontaneous regression of lesions has occurred, untreated tumors may increase in size and become fungated and ulcerated. In advanced stages, disseminated disease can occur with lesions appearing in lymph nodes and visceral organs. The detailed clinical manifestations of classic Kaposi's sarcoma have been given elsewhere (1,3,4,6).

In the 1950's, it was reported that Kaposi's sarcoma also occurs in an endemic belt located in equatorial Africa (such as Zaire, Uganda, etc.) among the black population (2-4,8). Approximately 9% of all tumors reported in Uganda are Kaposi's sarcomas. African KS is not restricted to older men. It occurs in young adults between the ages of 25-45 years with a male to female ratio of 17:1 (2-4,6). Although the benign form of the disease is most common, the more aggressive disseminated Kaposi's sarcoma is also observed. The generalized lymphadenopathic form of KS which has a high mortality is also frequently seen in this endemic area in black children between the ages of 2 and 15 years (2,6).

In the early 1970's, with the advent of organ transplantation, an increased incidence of Kaposi's sarcoma was observed in transplant recipients who received immunosuppressive therapy (9-11). Also, it was observed that patients with malignancies and autoimmune diseases who received antimetabolites and corticosteroids developed Kaposi's sarcoma (9-11). These patients' ages ranged from 23-59 years (mean age 42 years) and the male to female ratio was 2.3:1. In one study, Harwood et al. (12) reported that all 12 of the renal transplant recipients who developed KS were either of Jewish or Mediteranean background. This indicates a role for genetic factors in susceptibility to this particular tumor. Widespread dissemination, with visceral involvement is often seen in this group. It is noteworthy that organ transplant recipients also have a high incidence of cytomegalovirus infection.

From 1979 to the present, more than 1,400 cases of disseminated Kaposi's sarcoma have been diagnosed in patients with the Acquired Immunodeficiency Syndrome (AIDS) in metropolitan areas such as New York City and Los Angeles (13). This type of Kaposi's sarcoma is referred to as "Epidemic Kaposi's sarcoma" to distinguish it from the classic KS seen in elderly Europeans and North Americans and the endemic KS seen in Africa. Epidemic Kaposi's sarcoma has occurred primarily among homosexual and bisexual men, hemophiliacs and drug addicts, who are much younger (mean age 38 years) than patients with classic KS. Epidemic Kaposi's sarcoma is frequently associated with opportunistic infections such as CMV and Pneumocystis carinii pneumonia. This new epidemic KS is a more widely disseminated tumor with mucocutaneous, lymph node and visceral involvement (3,6,14). The early involvement of lymph nodes and visceral organs is similar to that seen in the lymphadenopathic and rapidly fatal form of KS occurring endemically in African children. The skin lesions vary from an early patch lesion to hyperpigmented, nodular, violaceous lesions appearing later. The lesions appear anywhere on the body from the lower extremities to the trunk, face, genital organs, etc. The histopathology of early patch lesions of epidemic Kaposi's sarcoma shows an increased number of dilated, irregularly-shaped endothelial lined vascular spaces, infiltrated with lymphocytes and plasma cells (6). In the nodular stage, the lesions are infiltrated with spindle cells and atypical endothelial cells. Table 1 compares features of classic and epidemic KS; including mean age, sex ratio, geographic distribution, etc.

TABLE I

COMPARISON OF CLASSIC AND EPIDEMIC KAPOSI'S SARCOMA

	CLASSICAL K.S.	EPIDEMIC K.S.
Male:female ratio	10-15:1	Predominantly male
Mean age	63	38
Ethnic origin	Jewish and Mediterranean ancestry; rare among Anglosaxons	Mixed; homosexual and bisexual men, Haitians, drug addicts
Immune status	No obvious dysfunction	Profound depression of cellular immunity
Geographic distribution	No clustering	Predominantly in New York, Los Angeles, San Francisco and other large metropolitan areas
Clinical features	1. Skin lesions localized on lower extremities	1. Generalized skin lesions
	2. Rare lymphadenopathy and visceral involvement	2. Common lymphadenopathy and frequent visceral involvement
	3. Frequently associated with 2nd malignancy	3. High incidence of opportunistic infections; especially cytomegalovirus infection
Annual incidence in the United States	0.02-0.06 per 100,000 population	From 1979 to August 1984 over more than 14,000 cases

* After Table 1 of reference 6.

The etiology of Kaposi's sarcoma is still unclear and is expected to be multifactorial. Host characteristics, such as a genetic predisposition, an immunocompromised state, and also infectious agents and environmental factors (such as life style) perhaps all play important roles in the development of this disease.

Among the infectious agents, cytomegalovirus was found to be the most common infection in patients with Kaposi's sarcoma (14,15). Dr. G. Giraldo and Dr. E. Beth have spent a great deal of effort in searching for a viral agent associated with this tumor. In cell lines derived from KS biopsy specimens from a Zairian patient, they isolated a CMV strain, termed K9V (16,17). The CMV strain K9V was further analyzed by DNA restriction fragmentation and was found to share significant homology with the transforming CMV strain called Major (Mj) which was spontaneously released from a prostate cell line established in Dr. F. Rapp's laboratory.

In addition, Giraldo and his colleagues performed an extensive seroepidemiologic analysis of European and American KS patients which revealed a specific association with CMV, but not EBV, HSVI or HSVII. African patients with a similar clinical course also had high titers of antibody to CMV. However, since CMV infections occur commonly in healthy Africans; a biostatistical significance could not be established in these patients (15). It is difficult to determine the etiological association of CMV with Kaposi's sarcoma by means of biostatistical and molecular biological approaches at the present time. Therefore, the observations presented here from our studies, and those of others, may merely reflect an epidemiological association rather than an etiological one.

In collaboration with Dr. Giraldo and his colleagues, we have examined classic and endemic KS tumor biopsies for the existence of CMV-specific nucleic acid sequences and viral specific macromolecules by DNA reassociation kinetics analysis, <u>in situ</u> hybridization and immunofluorescence testing. In one set of studies, viral DNA and RNA could be detected in 5 out of 10 tumor biopsies and virus specific antigens could be demonstrated in 80% of specimens. In contrast, no HSV-2 or EBV DNA sequences or their viral specific macromolecules could be detected. CMV DNA levels ranged from 0.25-1 genome equivalent per cell (18,19).

In a recent study of homosexual men with KS, Dr. L. Drew et al. (14) found that CMV could be isolated from body secretions, semen, or blood in 7 out of 9 patients. CMV specific antigens could be detected by immunofluorescence in KS tissues from 6 out of 9 patients, and CMV RNA was detected in 2 out of 3 patients tested by <u>in situ</u> nucleic acid hybridization. In collaboration with McDougall and Galloway, Dr. Fenoglio (20) also demonstrated the existence of CMV RNA in KS cells derived from biopsy tissue. On the other hand, negative data has been reported by Dr. Fleckenstein's laboratory using less sensitive Southern blot hybridization with a subgenomic DNA probe (47).

As indicated above, the association of CMV with KS has been suggested by seroepidemiologic analysis and also by the identification of CMV macromolecules in KS biopsies and in cell lines derived from KS tissue. Additional indirect evidence is provided by the demonstration of the oncogenicity of CMV in tissue culture systems. Several investigators (21-27) have found that CMV is able to stimulate cellular DNA, RNA and macromolecular synthesis both in permissive and non-permissive cells. Boldogh et al. (23) demonstrated that the expression of a very early CMV gene product was necessary for the stimulation of cellular DNA synthesis and also that this function was UV-resistant. CMV also stimulates the synthesis of numerous enzymes involved in celllular proliferation (30-37) which supports the oncogenic potential of this virus (Table 2).

TABLE 2

ONCOGENIC POTENTIAL OF HUMAN CYTOMEGALOVIRUS IN VITRO

EVENTS	REFERENCES
Stimulation of host cell macromolecules synthesis	
Cellular DNA	21-27
Cellular RNA	28,29
Mitochondria DNA	22
Cellular enzymes	
DNA polymerases (α,β)	30,31
Thymidine kinase	32,33
Ornithine decarboxylase	34
Plasminogen activator	35
DNA dependent RNA polymerase	36
Exonuclease	37
Topoisomerase	37
Morphological transformation of mammalian cells	
Hamster embryonic fibroblast	38,39,43
Rodent cell	42,44
Human fibroblast	40,41

In addition to stimulating host cell macromolecular synthesis, CMV can morphologically transform mammalian cells and these transformed cells are tumorigenic in laboratory animals (38,43). To further identify the transforming region(s) of the CMV genome, DNA fragments have been studied in their ability to transform mammalian cells (41-43). Two distinct transforming DNA fragments have been identified: a 2.9 kb subfragment of the Hind III E fragment, (map unit between 0.123-0.14), of AD169 strain (42) and Towne strain Xba IE fragment (43). A CMV transforming gene has therefore been mapped near the vicinity of the immediate early gene area.

In addition to the demonstration of transforming DNA fragments in human CMV, Spector and Vacquier (45) and Gelmann _et al_ (46) found that about 5-6 regions of human CMV DNA share DNA sequence homology to the 5' half of v-myc DNA; but not to any of the other retroviral oncogenes examined. To study the possible relationship between myc sequences and the transforming ability of the human CMV genome, we used the purified 1.5 kb pst-1 myc-specific subgenomic probe derived from MC38 plasmid DNA (kindly provided by Dr. M. Bishop) to determine the location of a myc specific sequence in low passage Towne strain CMV DNA. Our results indicate that myc related sequences do exist in Towne strain CMV DNA when examined under high stringent hybridization conditions. One area with a high degree of homology has been located near the transforming area (our preliminary observation). Based on the biological characteristics of human cytomegalovirus as reported, it is very likely that CMV has oncogenic potential.

SUMMARY

The association of CMV with KS has been suggested by seroepidemiological and molecular biological studies. Additional supporting evidence for the etiological role of CMV in KS is based on the oncogenicity of CMV as demonstrated by _in vitro_ experiments. At the present time, more conclusive evidence is needed to prove its etiological role in KS.

REFERENCES

1. Kaposi M (1872) Arch Dermatol Syphilol 4:265-273

2. Taylor JF, Templeton AC, Vogel CL, et al. (1971) Int J Cancer 8:122-135

3. Safai B, Good R (1981) Ca: A Cancer Journal for Clinicians 31:2-12

4. Kungu A, Gates DG (1981) Antibiot Chemother 29:38-55

5. Giraldo G, Beth E, Buonaguro FM (1984) Antibiot Chemother 32:1-11

6. Friedman-Kien AE, Ostreicher R (1984) Overview of classical and epidemic Kaposi's sarcoma. In: Friedman-Kien, AE, Laurenstein LJ (eds.) AIDS, the Epidemic of Kaposi's Sarcoma and Opportunistic Infections. Masson Publishing Co., USA, pp 23-36

7. Taff ML, Siegal FP, Seller SA (1982) Am J Forensic Med Pathol 3:259-264

8. Kaminer B, Murray JF (1950) S Afr J Clin Sci 1:1-25

9. Klepp O, Dahl O, Stenwig JT (1978) Cancer 42:2626-2630

10. Penn I (1979) Transplantation 27:8-11

11. Stribling J, Wertzner S, Smith GR (1978) Cancer 42:442-446

12. Harwood AR, Osoba D, Hofstader SL, et al. (1979) Am J Med 67:759-769

13. Update: Acquired Immunodeficiency Syndrome (AIDS)-United States Centers for Disease Control. (1984) MMWR 33:337-339

14. Drew WL, Conant MA, Miner RC, et al. (1982) Lancet ii:125-127

15. Giraldo G, Beth E, Henle W, et al. (1978) Int J Cancer 22:126-131

16. Giraldo G, Beth E, Coeur P, Vogel CL, Dhru DS (1972) J Natl Cancer Inst 49:1495-1507

17. Giraldo G, Beth E, Haguenau F (1972) J Natl Cancer Inst 49:1509-1513

18. Boldogh I., Beth E, Huang ES, Kyalwazi KS, Giraldo G (1981) Int J Cancer 28:469-474

19. Giraldo G, Beth E, Huang ES (1980) Int J Cancer 26:23-28

20. Fenoglio CM, Oster MW, Gerfo PI, et al. (1982) Human Pathol 15:955-959

21. St Jeor S, Albrecht TB, Funk FD, Rapp F (1974) J Virol 13:353-362

22. Furukawa T, Sakuma, S, Plotkin SA (1976) Nature 262:414-416

23. Boldogh I, Gonczol E, Gartner L, Vaczi L (1978) Arch Virol 58:289-299

24. DeMarchi JM, Blankenship ML, Brown GS, Kaplan AS (1978) Virology 89:643-646

25. DeMarchi JM, Ben-Porat T, Kaplans AS (1977) Virology 97:457-463

26. DeMarchi JM, Kaplan AS (1979) Virology 82:93-99

27. DeMarchi JM (1981) Virology 114:23-38

28. Tanaka S, Furukawa T, Plotkin SA (1975) J Virol 15:297-304

29. Furukawa T, Tanaka S, Plotkin SA (1975) Proc Soc Exp Biol Med 148:211-214

30. Huang ES (1975) J Virol 16:298-310

31. Hirai K, Furukawa T, Plotkin SA (1976) Virology 70:251-255

32. Estes JE, Huang ES (1977) J Virol 24:13-21

33. Zavada V, Erban V, Rezacova D, Vonka V (1976) Arch Virol 52:333-339

34. Isom HJ (1979) J Gen Virol 42:265-278

35. Yamanishi K, Rapp F (1979) J Virol 31:415-419

36. Tanaka S, Ihara S, Watanabe Y (1978) Virology 89:179-185

37. Huang ES, Boldogh I, Baskar, JF, Mar EC (1984) The molecular biology of human cytomegalovirus and its relationship to various human cancers. In: Giraldo E and Beth E (eds.), The Role of Viruses in Human Cancer, Vol. II, pp. 169-194.

38. Albrecht T, Rapp F (1973) Virology 55:53-61

39. Boldogh I, Gonczol E, Vaczi L (1978) Acta Microbiol Acad Sci Hung 25:269-275

40. Geder L, Lausch R, O'Neill F, Rapp F (1976) Science 192:134-1137

41. Huang ES, Boldogh I, Mar EC (1983) Human cytomegaloviruses: Evidence for possible association with human cancer. In: Phillips LA (ed.): Viruses Associated With Human Cancer, New York:Marcel Dekker, pp. 161-193

42. Nelson JS, Fleckenstein B, Galloway, DA, McDougall JK (1982) J Virol 43:83-91

43. Clanton DJ, Jariwalla RJ, Kress C, Rosenthal LJ (1983) Proc Natl Acad Sci USA 80:3826-3830

44. Nelson JA, Fleckenstein B, Jahn G, Galloway DA, McDougall JK (1984) J Virol 49:109-115

45. Spector DH, Vacquier JP (1983) Proc Natl Acad Sci USA 80:3889-3893

46. Gelmann EP, Clanton DJ, Jariwalla RJ, Rosenthal LJ (1983) Proc Natl Acad Sci. USA 80:5107-5111

47. Rüger R, Colimon R, Fleckenstein B (1984) Antibiot Chemother 32:43-47

Herpes Viruses and Virus Chemotherapy, R. Kono, editor

INACTIVATED HERPES SUBUNIT VACCINE IN THE PREVENTION OF INFECTION, LATENCY AND CERVICAL CANCER IN MICE - A REVIEW

M. H. CHEN and G. R. B. SKINNER*

Department of Cell Biology, Virus Research Institute, Hubei Medical College, Wuchang, China. *Department of Medical Microbiology, the Medical School, University of Birmingham, U.K.

Since vaccine may prevent many diseases, it is natural to develop a vaccine to prevent diseases induced by herpes simplex virus (HSV). The vaccine which has to be developed is important not only because of the prevalence of clinical diseases such as herpes ophthalmicus, herpes encephalitis, herpes genitalis, neonatal and recurrent herpes infection, but also because of the close relation between the infection of herpes simplex virus type 2 (HSV-2) and cervical cancer in humans (1-3).

Lipchutz firstly showed that immunization may prevent rabbits from HSV infection (4). Years later, some reports showed that acute HSV infection and death could be prevented by immunizing animals with living or killed HSV (5). However the problem of latent infection in sensory ganglia remained to be settled. It is of interest in this regard that it was the fear of potential oncogenicity of living or inactivated HSV which has led to the development of vaccine without viral DNA. Thereafter, there were reports that compared the immune efficacy of viral glycoprotein with that of the virion (6-8).

Skinner and his coworker have developed an inactivated subunit vaccine (Ac NFU-BHK) whose preparation and designation were reported previouly (9). In brief, the vaccine was prepared by detergent and formaldehyde treatment of HSV-1 infected baby hamster kidney cells, followed by removal of virus particles by ultracentrifugation over 20% sucrose at 100,000g for 5 hr. Proteins were precipitated by acetone at -20°C. Vaccine was stored as a dried pellet in a dry enviroment. In the experiments mice received two vaccinations of test or control vaccine intraperitoneally at an interval of two weeks, each inoculation contained an equivalent of 10^7 cells. Exposure of the mouse cervix to virus was carried out by placing a sterile cotton wool pledget soaked with virus suspension against the cervix. Mice were routinely challenged with 1×10^6 pfu of HSV-2, living or inactivated. The efficacy of this vaccine will be evaluated in this review.

In the first set of experiments, the prevention of acute infection was studied. There was a significant protection of Ac NFU-BHK-immunized mice as judged by the criteria: 1. Virus yield was clearly depressed as early as 24 hr following virus challenge and remained below control levels until the last day of sampling which was 7 days following virus challenge. 2. The proportion of mice showing specific viral cytopathic effects and non-specific inflammatory changes in Pap smears was also lower in Ac NFU-BHK-immunized animals. The difference between immunized and control mice was generally more striking on the 7th day rather than immediately following virus challenge. 3. The extent of local infection, as judged by plus designations was lower in Ac NFU-BHK-immunized animals, but there was a less striking difference than with other criteria of virus infection. 4. The mortality rate was significantly reduced from 92% in control mice to 29% in NFU-BHK-vaccinated mice.

The second set of experiments was undertaken to examine the efficacy of vaccination towards prevention of HSV-2 induced cervical cancer and latency. In this part, strain 333 of HSV-2 used was inactivated with UV-light, and inoculated intravaginally once a week for 23 times. There was a significant protection of the vaccine against the HSV-2 induced cancer as judged by the incidence of precancer and cancer in the vagina or/and cervix over an experimental period of one year (Figure 1 and Table 1). These data demonstrate

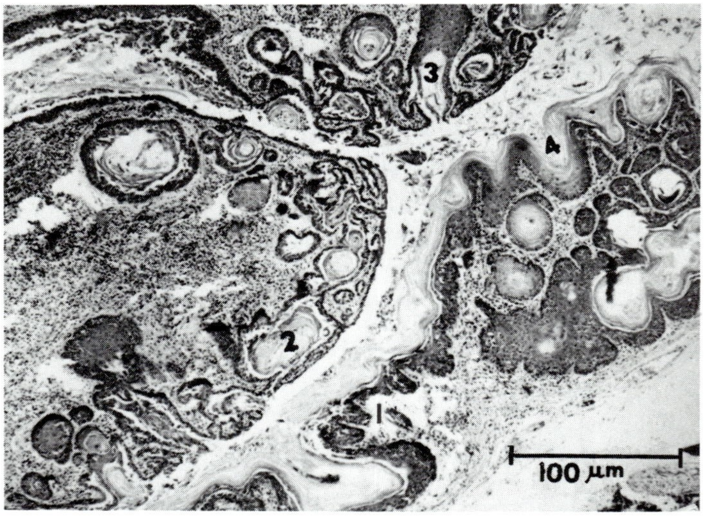

Fig. 1. Micrograph of mouse vagina and cervix. Showing precancer and cancers induced by HSV-2. 1. Precancer of vagina, 2. Cancer of cervix, 3. Cancer of vagina.

TABLE 1

EFFICACY OF VACCINATION AGAINST TYPE 2 HERPES VIRUS INDUCED CERVICAL CANCER

	Cervical Cancer			
	Survivors	Pre-invasive	Invasive	Total
(1) Vaccination with virus challenge	75	9(12%)	5(7%)	14(19%)
(2) Control vaccination with virus challenge	69	21(30%)	15(22%)	36(52%)
(3) Virus challenge alone	97	28(29%)	17(17%)	46(47%)
(4) Challenge with control uninfected cell extract	51	0(0%)	0(0%)	0(0%)

that exposure of the mouse cervix and vagina to HSV-2, induced cervical and/or vaginal cancer, including precancer, in 47% of unimmunized mice and in 52% of mice immunized with control vaccine. However, immunization of mice with vaccine Ac NFU-BHK reduced the frequency of the cancer to 19% ($P < 0.005$). None of mice receiving control uninfected cell extract developed cervical cancer. The titres of serum antibody were estimated by the enzyme linked immunoabsorbant assay (ELISA) technique with HSV-1 and HSV-2 viral antigens prepared from strain SM44 and strain 333 respectively. The geometric mean titres of serum antibody against HSV-1 and HSV-2 in mice who did or did not develop cancer is shown in Table 2. As expected, vaccinated mice (Group 1) had a significantly higher titre of type 1 antibody as judged by type 1/type 2 ratio values than unvaccinated challenged mice (Group 2 and 3) ($P < 0.05$). Mice which developed cancer (Group 6) had a significantly higher titre of type 2 antibody as judged by type 1/type 2 ratio values than did mice which did not develop cancer (Group 5). These results are in general accord with sero-epidemiological studies of preinvasive and invasive cervical carcinoma in human subjects (1-3), and suggests that a vaccination programme towards prevention or modification of herpes genitalis may reduce the prevalence of cervical carcinoma in population subgroups who are at risk.

In the second set of experiments, the efficacy of the vaccine towards prevention of the latency of HSV-2 (strain 333) in mice which survived over one year after virus challenge was also studied by the co-culture method. The percentages of animals harboring latent virus in their lumbosacral spinal ganglia and trigeminal ganglia in both immunized and non-immunized groups were not significantly different.

TABLE 2

ANTIBODY TITRES IN MICE ONE YEAR FOLLOWING THE FIRST IMMUNIZATION

	Survivors	Number of mice (%)	Geometric mean titres of antibody and their ratio HSV-1	HSV-2	HSV-1/HSV-2
(1) Vaccination with virus challenge	9	1(11)	118.5 (±7.8)	43.5 (±7.6)	2.7
(2) Control vaccination with virus challenge	9	2(22.2)	27.4 (±11.5)	87.0 (±2.2)	0.31
(3) Virus challenge alone	10	2(20)	13 (±10.4)	36.8 (±4.6)	0.35
(4) Challenge with control uninfected cell extract	23	0(0)	8 (±2.5)	6 (±2.9)	1.3
(5) Mice without cancer from Groups 1, 2 and 3	23	0(0)	58.8 (±11.9)	40.7 (±10.3)	1.4
(6) Mice with cancer from Groups 1, 2 and 3	5	5(100)	32 (±7.9)	147 (±1.8)	0.21

Although there were higher titres of HSV-1 antibody appearing in the vaccinated groups which effectively protected animals from acute HSV-2 infection and death, and also reduced the rate of HSV-2 induced cancer, the vaccine Ac NFU-BHK could not prevent the animals from latency in sensory ganglia. While elucidation of the precise mechanisma involved must await further investigation, the results obtained from clinical studies by Woodman (10) showed that a similar vaccine, Ac NFU_1 (S^-) MRC 5, can prevent recurrent episodes of herpes genitalis. Therefore, whether the vaccine has efficacy against latency or not should not interfere with its development.

REFERENCES

1. Nahmias AJ, Norrild B (1980). Oncogenic potential of herpes simplex

virus and their association with cervical neoplasia. In Rapp F (eds): "Oncogenic Herpesviruses", CRC Press, Inc., 2:25.

2. Skinner GRB. Thouless ME, Jordan JA (1971). Antibody to type 1 and type 2 herpes virus in women with abnormal cervical cytology. Br J Obstet Gynaecol 78:1031.

3. Adam K, Kaufman RH, Melnick JL, Levy AH, Rawls WE (1973). Seroepidemiologic studies of herpes virus type 2 and carcinoma of the cervix III. Am J Epidemiol 98:77.

4. Lipchutz B (1921). Untersuchungen ueber die Etiologie der Krankheiten der Herpesgruppe. Arch Dermatol Syph 136:428.

5. Anderson WA, Kilbourne EO (1961). Immunization of mice with inactivated herpes simplex virus. Proc Soc Exp Med 107:518.

6. Zweerink HJ, Martiney D (1981). Immune responses in mice against herpes simplex virus: Mechanisms of protection against facial and ganglionic infection. Infect Immun 31:267.

7. Rajcani J, Kutinova L, Vonda V (1980). Restriction of latent herpes virus infection in rabbit immunized with subvival herpes simplex virus vaccine. Acta virol 24:183.

8. Kitces EN, Payne WJ, Morahan JR, PS, Tew JG, Murray BK (1978). Herpes simplex virus vaccine: Protection from stomatitis, ganglionitis, encephalitis and latency. In de-The G, W, Rapp F (eds): "Oncogenesis and Herpesviruses III, Part 2" Lyon: IARC Scientific Publications No. 24, P 1027.

9. Skinner GRB, Williams DR, Buchan A, Whitncy J, Harding M, Bodfish K (1978). Preparation and efficacy of an inactivated subunit vaccine (NFU_1 BHK) against type 2 herpes simplex virus infection. Med Microbiol Immunol 166:119.

10. Woodman CBJ, Buchan A, Fuller A, Hartley C, Skinner GRB, Stocker D, Sugrue D, Clay JC, Wilkins G, Wiblin C, Melling J (1983). Efficacy of vaccine Ac NFU_1 (S^-) MRC5 given after an initial clinical episode in the prevention of herpes genitalis. Br J Vener Dis 59:311.

V BIOCHEMICAL, BIOLOGICAL AND CLINICAL EXPERIENCE WITH ANTIVIRAL DRUGS

Herpes Viruses and Virus Chemotherapy, R. Kono, editor

GLYCOSYLATION INHIBITORS: MODE OF ACTION AND CLINICAL EFFICACY

H.A. BLOUGH*, R. KUMARASAMY*, M. MASSARE*, R.L. GIUNTOLI[§], S. SPRECHER-GOLDBERGER[†], AND L. THIRY[†]

*Department of Ophthalmology and [§]Gynecological Oncology, University of Pennsylvania, Philadelphia, Pa. 19104 (U.S.A.) and [†]Institute Pasteur of Brussels, 1180 Brussels (Belgium)

INTRODUCTION

Eukaryotic glycoproteins and those of enveloped viruses are dependent upon the peptide sequence Asn-Xaa-Thr (X represents any amino acid except Pro or Asp[1-2]). This sequence serves an an acceptor site for *N*-linked oligosaccharides for the transfer of dolichol-linked intermediates (to the nascent polypeptide chain). Thus, any chemotherapeutic strategy targeted towards blocking the synthesis and charging of the polyprenol intermediate(s), its transfer and/or the resultant processing of the oligosaccharide, either to become "high mannose", complex or hybrid types should be effective. This inhibition will interfere with the assembly of the virion and abort other biological parameters viz. attachment, fusion (viral-cell, cell-cell) and release. When used appropriately, 2-dGlc possesses unique antiviral activity in man and has been successfully used to treat human genital herpes[3].

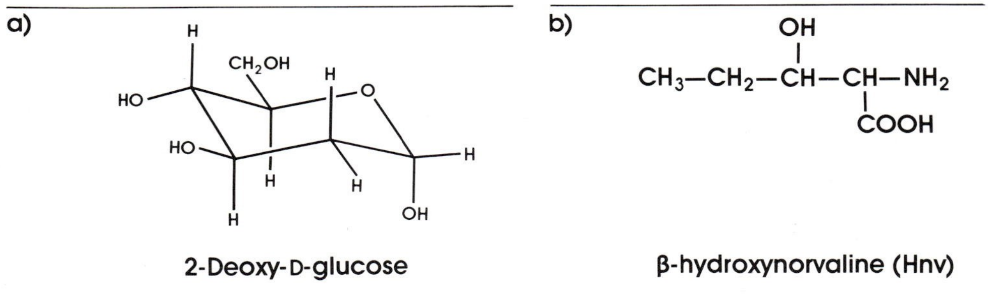

Fig. 1. Glycosylation inhibitors.

PROCEDURES AND RESULTS

2-dGlc is a simple monosaccharide (Fig. 1a) which when incorporated into dolichol intermediate(s) interferes with the elongation of the oligosaccharide(s), viz. producing short chains which are not transferred to the viral polypeptide(s)[4]; 2-dGlc is also a competitive inhibitor of glycosphingolipid biosynthesis[5]. While its effect on viral function is well known[6-7], it is anticipated that viral receptors (which are glycoproteins) would be altered. Using a retrovirus model, and monoclonal antibodies (MCA) directed against baboon endogenous virus (BaEV) in a human cell line, it is evident (Table 1) that treatment of these cells for five days inhibited viral release (syncytia forming units). With MCA plus [^{125}I] Staph A protein, it was observed that viral glycoprotein synthesis was markedly reduced although the "internal protein" of BaEV was unaffected. Treatment of the human cell line(s) with 2-dGlc reduced the viral receptor density by ∿35% using MCA D_{12} as a probe; cell viability and an enzyme marker, human alkaline phosphatase were unaffected by 10 mM 2-dGlc (Table 1).

TABLE 1

EFFECT ON BABOON ENDOGENOUS MARKERS BY A204(M7) CELLS TREATED WITH 10mM 2-dGlc

Parameter Assayed	24 h treatment		Daily treatment for 5 days	
	No drug	2-dGlc	No drug	2-dGlc
Viral syncytium forming units released into the supernatant	102±18[a]	32±7	53±9	25±1
Cell-associated antigens				
Viral gp detected with antibody A_6	304±55[b]	574±75	960±39	664±48
C_9	238±62	562±41	710±20	449±60
Viral internal protein, with F_{12}	446±86	789±55	942±164	752±47
Cell receptor to the virus detected with antibody D_{12}	5074±195	4511±216	2944±103	1820±72
Human alkaline phosphatase	308±73	337±71	474±21	529±52

[a] 200μl of supernatant medium of A204(m7) cells producing BaEV were seeded in 4 wells containing semi-confluent RSA cells; syncytia were counted after 24 h at 37°C. Results show the mean of syncytia ±S.D.

[b] A204(m7) cells were frozen, thawed and sonicated. Solid phase RSA with [^{125}I] Staph A protein were done in quadruplicate.

The substitution of Hnv in place of Thr into the peptide increases the intra-atomic distance so the hydrogen bond between GlcN (and Hnv) is not favorable; thus when BHK-21 cells were treated with 5-10 mM Hnv and challenged with HSV-1 (HF), viral yield was reduced ∿95% and endogenous fusion was completely blocked[8]. By polyacrylamide gel electrophoresis (Fig. 2) and immuno-affinity column chromatography of [^{3}H]GlcN-labeled cells, all viral glycoproteins were markedly reduced (Fig. 2). As was anticipated, these effects of Hnv could be reversed with Thr (Fig. 2). Further, Hnv appears to be incorporated into non-glycosylated viral proteins, viz. thymidine kinase and DNA polymerase, the resultant change in configuration and/or active site results in a four- to six-fold decrease in both HSV-induced enzymes (data not shown).

As a follow-up to our earlier study on 2-dGlc as an effective anti-viral agent[3], 200 women with genital herpes viral infections were evaluated in an open study. 71 were initial (mean age 23.5 years); 129 were recurrent (mean age 29.5 years). 90% of the initial cases were seen within three days; the recurrent cases within 1.1 days. Patients were selected by history, clinical evaluation and positive culture. They were treated both intra-vaginally and topically with 2-dGlc in a creme base; subjective signs of pain, dysuria, pruritis, and fever were evaluated. *84% experienced total relief within 48-72 hours,* thus confirming earlier results. Healing time following therapy was 6.3 days. Unlike acyclovir, *which appears to induce a persistent state,* the recurrence rate in patients with initial disease and treated within 5 days with 2-dGlc was <10% over a one to five year follow-up (Fig. 3). With recurrent disease, 33% were "cured" with no outbreaks after one to five years (one to three treatments with 2-dGlc). Of the remainder, 55.5% were improved (Fig. 4). Of the "improved" group, retreated with higher dosages on an intermittent basis, recurrence was reduced from 13-25 per year to two to four per year (Fig. 5). Patients (with recurrent disease) were evaluated (on an historical basis) with a one-sided paired t-test (the t-value = 11.118); this analysis allowed us to reject the null hypothesis with a confidence level of 99.5%.

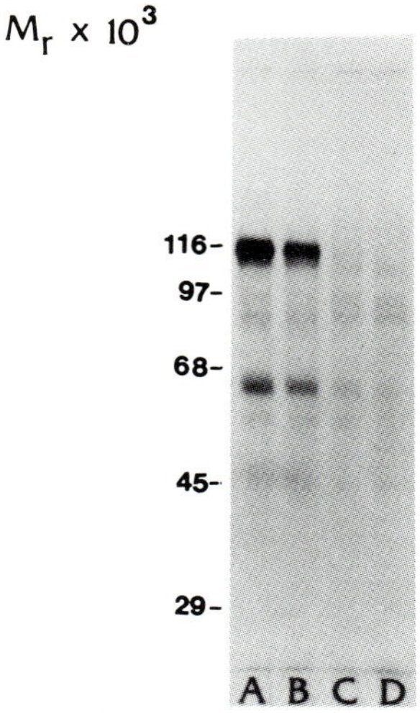

Fig. 2.Effect on HSV glycoproteins [^{3}H]GlcN label; A control; Hnv conc. B, 1 mM; C, 5 mM; D, 10 mM

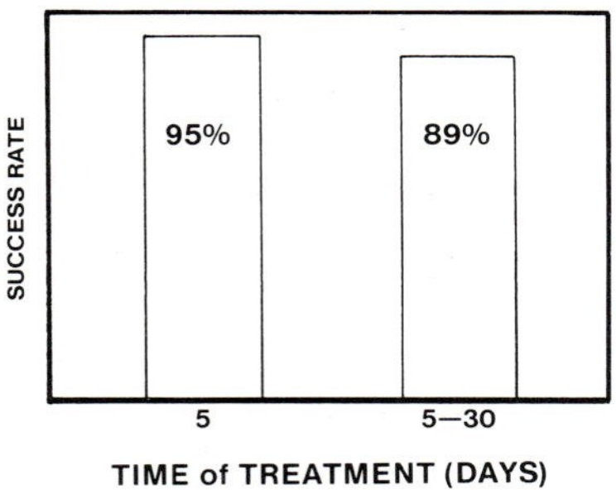

Fig. 3. Percentages of Success with initial HSV. Reinfections were excluded (Success = no recurrences 1-5 years.)

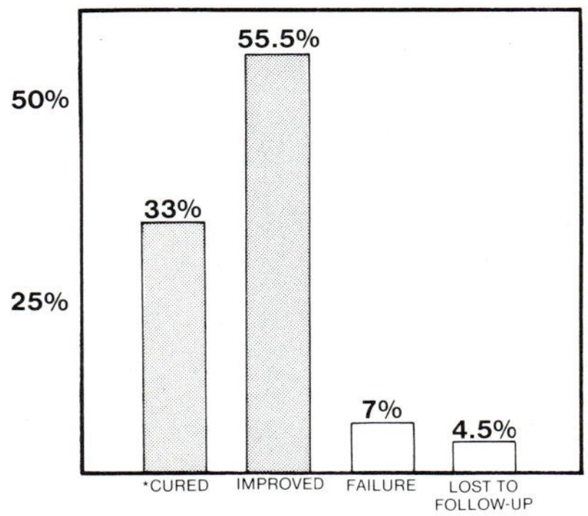

Fig. 4. The effect of 2-dGlc treatment on recurrent genital herpes in women. (Cured = no recurrences, 1-5 years.)

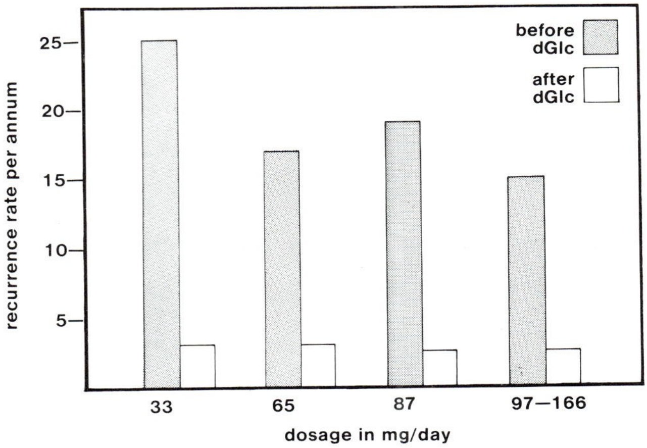

Fig. 5. The effect of 2-dGlc on the recurrence rate in females. (This refers to the 55.5% who are improved following therapy. Groups represent different dosage levels.)

In summary glycosylation inhibitors possess unique broad spectrum antiviral activity acting on the membrane level. 2-dGlc is very effective in the treatment of genital herpes virus infections in females. Because of the lack of toxicity of 2-dGlc, and its action on certain retroviruses and their receptors, it may be useful in the treatment of life-threatening diseases e.g. AIDS.

ACKNOWLEDGEMENTS

This study was supported by grants from the Rupp Foundation, and Caisse Générale d'Epargne et de Retraite and from Fonds de la Recherche Scientifique Médicale. HAB was the recipient of a special travel award from the Appel Charitable Foundation.

REFERENCES

1. Struck DK, Lennarz WJ, Brew K (1978) J Biol Chem 253: 5786-5794
2. Bause E (1979) FEBS Lett 103: 296-299
3. Blough HA, Giuntoli RL (1979) JAMA 241: 2798-2801
4. Datema R, Schwarz RT (1978) Eur J Biochem 90: 505-516
5. Suzuki Y, Blough HA (1982) Biochim Biophys Acta 810: 221-229
6. Courtney RJ, Steiner SM, Melnick MB (1973) Virology 52: 447-455
7. Blough HA, Ray EK (1980) Pharmac Ther 10: 669-681
8. Kumarasamy R, Blough HA (1984) Virology 138. In press.

© 1985 Elsevier Science Publishers B.V. (Biomedical Division)
Herpes Viruses and Virus Chemotherapy, R. Kono, editor

EFFECTS OF ACYCLOVIR ON ULTRASTRUCTURAL LOCALIZATION OF VIRAL ANTIGENS IN CULTURED SIRC CELLS INFECTED WITH HERPES SIMPLEX VIRUS

HIDETO YOSHIDA, HIROSHI SAKATA, YUJI HIRAKAWA, NOBORU HIYAMA, TOSHIYUKI IWAMOTO*

Dept. of Ophthalmology, Hiroshima Univ. School of Med., 1-2-3 Kasumi,Hiroshima
*Dept. of Pathology, Hiroshima Hospital of JNR, Futabanosato, Hiroshima, Japan

INTRODUCTION

Changes in the localization of viral antigens brought about by the presence of acyclovir(ACV) were studied using immunoelectron microscopy. We compared the results with those of IDU [1].

MATERIALS AND METHODS

Materials and methods has been described elsewhere[1]. Briefly, monolayers of SIRC cells were inoculated with herpes simplex virus type 1 (HSV) at input multiplicity of 10. After adsorption for an hour, monolayers were washed and transfered to the medium containing ACV at 10 µg/ml. The virus was susceptible to ACV (MIC=0.7 µg/ml). Cells were cultured for 3, 6, 12, 18 hours after inoculation and a direct enzyme antibody method was employed for immunoelectron microscopy.

RESULTS

At 3 hours of infection, reaction products began to appear in the cytoplasm and nuclei in both the control and ACV treated group. The amounts increased during the subsequent hours of observation. In the control group, there was diffuse intense immuno-reaction in the cytoplasm and nuclei and dense accumulations of reaction products were seen on the cell surfaces. In ACV treated cells the reaction was much decreased. Intranuclear antigens were present as focal accumulations of granular deposits, and cytoplasmic stainings were very much reduced in degree; deposit on the cell surface was a rare finding. The focal appearance of the intranuclear antigenic deposits gave characteristic "speckled pattern" **(Fig. 1-A).**

In standard electron microscopy, progeny virus particles were markedly reduced in number. In addition, the nucleocapsids had diminished electron density and the cores appeared hollow and empty. No enveloped particles were found. In immunoelectron microscopy the particles in the control group were stained as dense black dots, while in the presence of ACV viral particles were not detectable with immunostaining alone. After counterstaining by uranyl acetate, viral particles were detectable but no immune deposits were found in them **(Fig. 1-B).**

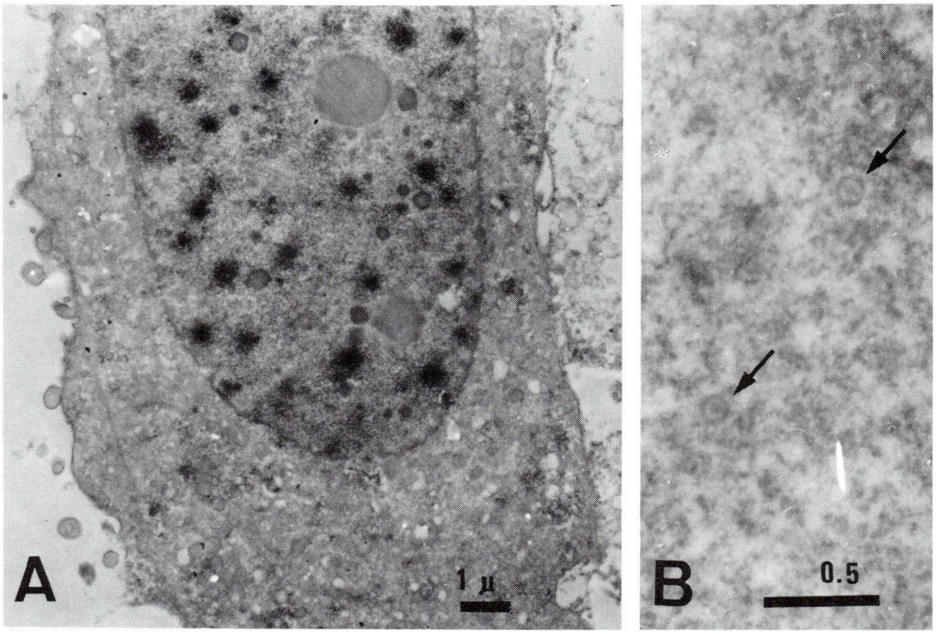

Fig. 1. Immunoelectron micrographs of HSV infected cells in the presence of ACV at 12 hours of infection.

A. (No counterstaining) Nucleus is stained in a "speckled pattern" and cytoplasm is stained slightly. Virus particles are not detectable with immunostaining alone. **B.** (with counterstaining by uranyl acetate) Viral particles are seen but no immune deposits are seen on them.

DISCUSSION

In our previous study[1], we reported reduction of immune deposits and viral particles by treatment with IDU. The effects were more pronounced in cytoplasm than in nucleus and viral particles were not significantly altered morphologically.

In the presence of ACV, immune deposits and progeny particles were decreased in much higher degree and intranuclear antigen preserved its focal pattern of distribution until later hours of infection giving the characteristic pattern of the deposits. Viral particles were not reactive with the antibody we used. In addition in ACV treated cells, cores appeared hollow or empty suggesting deficient DNA synthesis[2]. These results may give a morphological evidence that ACV does not interfere with early phase of protein synthesis but it is followed by inadequate protein synthesis probably because of impaired DNA synthesis.

REFERENCES

1. Yoshida H, Sakata H, Hiyama N, Iwamoto T (1983): Jpn. J. Ophthalmol., 27, 321.
2. Nii S, Rosenkranz HS, Morgan C, Rose HM (1968): J. Virol., 3, 1163.

STRAINS OF VARICELLA-ZOSTER VIRUS (VZV) RESISTANT TO 1-β-D-ARABINOFURANOSYL-E-5-(2-BROMOVINYL)URACIL (BV-araU)

TAKASHI SAKUMA, TATSUO SUZUTANI, HIDEKI KAWAI and MASANOBU AZUMA
Department of Microbiology, Asahikawa Medical College, Asahikawa 078-11, Japan

INTRODUCTION

BV-araU is a potent inhibitor of the replication of herpes simplex virus type 1 and VZV in human embryonic lung (HEL) cells (1,2). We have reported that strains of VZV resistant to BV-araU were isolated from VZV-infected Vero cells which were pulse-treated with IUdR and/or BUdR and then treated with BV-araU, while they could not be isolated from VZV-infected cells treated with BV-araU alone. These BV-araU resistant strains (BV-araU^r) were classified into two classes according to drug susceptibility and thymidine kinase (TK) activity. YSR and 018 strains showed high resistance to IUdR and BUdR and the same TK activity level as that in mock-infected cells. Meanwhile, 03 and 07 strains had low resistance to IUdR and BUdR, and had two to three times the TK activity of mock-infected cells (3).

In order to clarify the relation between resistance and TK activity, neutralization tests of viral TK activity were performed by using several anti-VZV guinea pig sera immunized with various VZV strains.

MATERIAL AND METHODS

Compounds. BV-araU was kindly supplied by Dr. H. Machida, Research Laboratories, Yamasa Shoyu Co. Ltd., Choshi, Japan. IUdR and BUdR were purchased from Wako Chemical, Ltd., Osaka, Japan. (methyl-^{3}H)thymidine (41 Ci/mmol) was purchased from Amersham International plc., England.

Viruses. The Oka strain of VZV was kindly supplied by Dr. M. Takahashi, Research Institute for Microbial Diseases, Osaka University, Osaka, Japan. The YS strain was isolated in our laboratory on HEL cells from the vesicular fluid of a patient with varicella. BV-araU^r strains were obtained as described previously (3). Briefly, YS strain-infected Vero cells were treated with 10 to 20 μg of IUdR or BUdR or both per ml for 24 h, and then replenished with fresh maintenance medium. After 48 h incubation, 0.1 to 1.0 μg of BV-araU per ml was added and cultivated until a cytopathogenic effect was apparent. Cloning from the resistant strain was carried out by the plaquing method with free virus of VZV in a medium containing 1 μg of BV-araU per ml on HEL cells (Fig.1).

TK activities and drug susceptibilities of these strains are summarized in Table 1.

Antisera. Antisera were prepared from guinea pigs immunized four times with various VZV strains passaged more than 15 times through guinea pig embryo cells.

Fig. 1. Isolation process of BV-araU^r strains

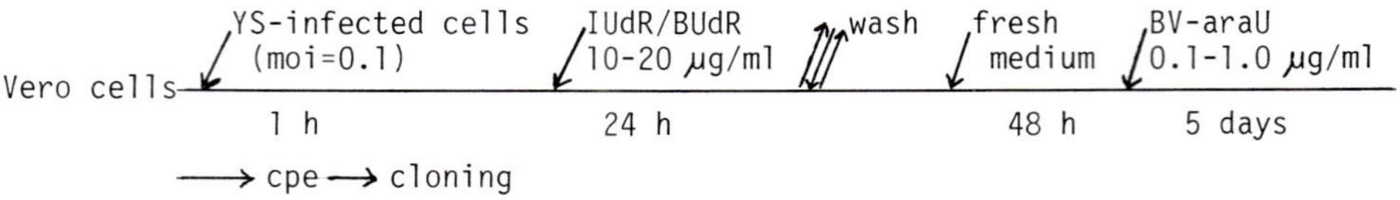

Table 1. Thymidine kinase activity in cells infected with VZV strains and their susceptibilities to drugs

Cells infected with	Relative thymidine kinase activity in infected cells	MIC (μg/ml) for 50 % PFU reduction for		
		BV-araU	IUdR	BUdR
Mock	1.0			
Oka	67.2	0.0006	0.4	0.5
YS	64.6	0.0005	0.3	0.5
YSR	1.2	5.8	1.9	8.0
03	2.2	5.2	0.78	1.5
07	3.0	4.7	0.39	3.0
018	1.0	7.4	1.6	7.6

Data from Sakuma, 1984 (3).

Immune adherence hemagglutination (IAHA) titers of these sera to VZV are shown in Fig. 2.

Assay of TK activity and neutralization test. TK assay was performed as described previously (3). 25 μl of crude enzyme material was mixed with 25 μl of serially diluted anti-VZV serum, incubated for 15 min at 37 °C, and then 50 μl of reaction mixture (13 mM ATP, 13 mM $MgCl_2$, 0.26 M Tris-hydrochloride [PH 8.0], and 1 μCi of [^{3}H]thymidine [0.2 μM]) was added. After incubation for 15 min at 37 °C, the reaction was terminated by adding 25 μl of cold 50 % trichloroacetic acid. Reaction products were separated by spotting 20 μl of the terminated mixture onto Whatman DE-81 disks. The radioactivity retained on the disks was measured.

RESULTS

Neutralization patterns of viral TK activity in YS strain- infected cells by various antisera. Anti-YS sera at the 32 IAHA titer neutralized 50 % of YS strain induced viral TK activity. However, anti-07-1 and anti-03-5 sera required higher titers than 512 or 4,096 IAHA titers to neutralize the YS strain-induced viral TK activity. On the other hand, anti-018-2 and anti-YSR sera could not neutralize the viral TK activity (Fig. 2). The neutralization pattern of the Oka strain-induced TK activity was almost the same as that of YS strain (data not shown).

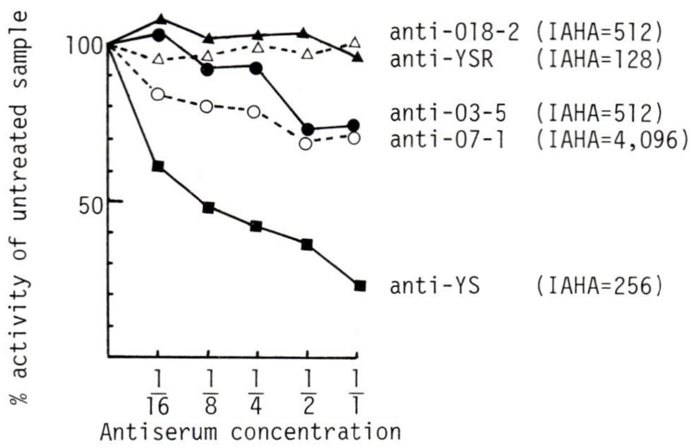

Fig. 2. Effect of various antisera on thymidine kinase activity of YS strain-infected HEL cells.

These results suggest that a small amount of viral TK is produced in 03-5 and 07-1 strain-infected cells, meanwhile, 018-2 and YSR strain-infected cells may produce no viral TK.

Effect of anti-YS and anti-07-1 sera on comparable TK activities of YS and 07-1 strain-infected cells. The above results do not eliminate the possibility that the 03-5 and 07-1 strains produce a regular amount of viral TK with a slight change in the conformation of the active site of the TK molecule, and for that reason, the anti-03-5 and anti-07-1 sera show a reduced neutralization titer to YS strain-induced TK activity. If so, then it might be possible to demonstrate experimentally that neutralization patterns of the YS and 07-1 strain-induced TK activities, which were adjusted to the same activity level relative to that of mock-infected cells, by anti-YS and anti-07-1 sera are different from each other.

In this experiment, relative TK activities of original YS-enzyme and 07-1-enzyme materials to that of mock-infected cells were 23.8 and 3.2, respectively. So, YS strain-induced TK activity diluted to 1:8 is comparable to the activity of undiluted 07-1 strain-induced TK. As shown in Fig. 3, no difference was detected in the neutralization patterns of the diluted YS strain- and 07-1 strain-induced TK by anti-YS and anti-07-1 sera. In contrast to the high IAHA titer of anti-07-1 serum, low neutralization titers of this antiserum to diluted YS strain- and 07-1 strain-induced TK were observed (Fig. 3, b).

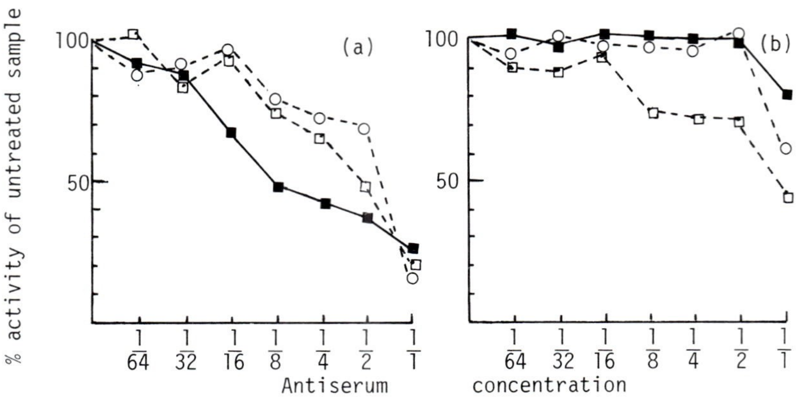

Fig. 3. Effect of antiserum on thymidine kinase activity. Anti-YS antiserum (a) or anti-07-1 antiserum (b) was added to YS- and 07-1-enzyme materials. Symbols;(■—■) original YS-TK, (□---□) 1:8 diluted YS-TK, (○---○) original 07-1-TK

DISCUSSION

The results reported here show that the BV-araU^r strains contain at least two kinds of mutant. TK-gene expression of YSR and 018-2 strains may be completely suppressed or deleted. On the other hand, TK-gene expression of 07-1 and 03-5 strains was reduced as compared with that of the YS strain, suggesting that the efficiency of TK-mRNA synthesis in 07-1 strain-infected cells may be reduced for some reason, such as a modulation of the TK promotor gene. Susceptibility of 07-1 and 03-5 strains to BV-araU was comparable to that of YSR and 018-2 strains, but the susceptibility of 07-1 and 03-5 strains to IUdR and BUdR was high compared with YSR and 018-2 strains. These results suggest that an altered substrate affinity of TK also occurred in 07-1 and 03-5 strains. Darby et al. have reported a similar phenomena with HSV type 1 (4). Further biochemical and molecular studies are needed to settle these problems.

REFERENCES

1. Machida H, Kuninaka A & Yoshino H (1982) Antimicrob. Agents Chemother. 21: 358-361
2. Machida H & Sakata S (1984) Antiviral Res. 4: 135-141
3. Sakuma T (1984) Antimicrob. Agents Chemother. 25: 742-746
4. Darby G, Field H. G. & Salisbury S. A. (1981) Nature (London) 289: 81-83

THE EFFECT OF TUNICAMYCIN ON CELL SURFACE ALTERATIONS INDUCED BY A STRAIN OF HERPES SIMPLEX VIRUS TYPE 2.

EHUD KATZ and HAIM GAMLIEL

Department of Virology, Hebrew University-Hadassah Medical School and
Department of Hematology, Hadassah University Hospital, Israel.

INTRODUCTION

Herpes simplex virus type 2 (HSV-2) assembles by budding from the cell membranes during its maturation. Several strains of HSV cause cell fusion, a process which depends on both the virus strain and the type of cell being infected. A mutant of HSV-2 that induces extensive fusion of BSC1 and vero cells, but which fails to do so in human fibroblasts, was isolated in our laboratory (1). This virus, in addition to induction of fusion, grows in the presence of acycloguanosine (ACG), because of inducing low levels of thymidine kinase and therefore was named HSV-2-ACG.

Tunicamycin is an antibiotic which inhibits glycosylation of proteins and has previously been shown to significantly reduce the infectious yield of HSV (2, 3). In the present study we studied, using scanning electron microscopy, the effects of tunicamycin on the fusion of BSC1 caused by HSV-2-ACG and on the accumulation of virus-like particles on the surface of the cells.

RESULTS

First, the growth of HSV-2 and HSV-2-ACG, in the presence of ACG and tunicamycin, was followed. BSC1 cells were infected with HSV-2 and HSV-2-ACG. Following adsorption, M199 medium containing ACG (50 μM) or tunicamycin (50 μg/ml), was added. The cells were harvested at 22 hours after infection and the infectivity of the virus was determined by plaque assay. The two viruses grow very efficiently in untreated BSC1 cells, however, in the presence of ACG, the infectious titer of HSV-2 is significantly reduced, while the mutant HSV-2-ACG grows normally. The growth of the two virus strains is significantly inhibited by tunicamycin.

HSV-2 infected cultures are less uniform, as compared to uninfected cells, showing a large proportion of rounded-up cells. Multiple elongated microvilli, sometimes arranged in clusters covering these cells, are seen, using scanning electron microscopy. Infection of BSC1 cells by the mutant HSV-2-ACG, in the absence or presence of ACG leads to fusion of cells. The cells are polygonal and flattened, showing very active surfaces characterized by an increase in the number of microvilli. The microvilli appear with extensive bud-like swellings beside aggregates of virus-like particles.

Examination of HSV-2-ACG infected cultures in the presence of tunicamycin reveals a complete inhibition of both cell-fusion and the accumulation of virus-like particles on the cell surface. Although some cells are rounded-up, they usually display a reduced number of microvilli, while a few cells are extremely smooth in nature, showing undulated surfaces or exaggerated blebs.

DISCUSSION AND CONCLUSIONS

In contrast to wild-type infection, HSV-2-ACG induces extensive cell fusion and the gigantic cells formed display very active surfaces, characterized under scanning electron microscopy by an increase in the number of microvilli, as compared to uninfected BSC1 cells, and by accumulation of budding of virus-like particles on the cell surface. In these cells virus particles seem to massively bud even through the membrane of the microvilli. Tunicamycin prevents the fusion induced by HSV-2-ACG and also the egression of virus particles through the surface of the cells. The present study supports previous reports (4, 5, 6, 7), which have indicated that a fusion-promoting viral factor may be a membrane glycoprotein. Tunicamycin, by inhibiting glycosylation of this factor, may prevent it from functioning in the fusion process.

REFERENCES

1. Katz E, Margalith E (1982) Arch Virol 74:111-123
2. Katz E, Margalith E, Duksin D (1980) Antimicrob Agents Chemother 17:1014-1022
3. Pizer LI, Cohen GH, Eisenberg RJ (1980) J Virol 34:142-153
4. Gallaher WR, Levitan DB, Blough HA (1973) Virology 55:193-201
5. Keller JM (1976) Virology 72:402-409
6. Knowles RW, Person S (1976) J Virol 18:644-651
7. Levitan DB, Blough HA (1976) J Virol 18:1081-1087

A detailed description of this study, which includes photographs of scanning electron microscopy, has recently been published by us in Scanning Electron Microscopy Vol. 1983 IV pp. 2037-2045.

Herpes Viruses and Virus Chemotherapy, R. Kono, editor

STUDIES ON ANTIVIRAL ACTIVITY OF SEVERAL HYDROLYSABLE TANNINS

MANABU TAKEHARA, MASAYUKI TAKECHI AND YASUO TANAKA

Department of Microbiology, Kobe University School of Medicine, Kobe; and Department of Pharmacognosy, Faculty of Pharmaceutical Science, Kinki University, Higashi-Osaka (Japan)

INTRODUCTION

Several antiherpetic tannins have been purified from buds of Syzygium aromatica and roots of Paeonia species (1). Among these hydrolysable tannins tested antiviral activity, the most active substances against herpes simplex virus type 1 (HSV-1) were eugeniin and 1,2,3,4,6-penta-O-galloyl-D-glucose (PGG) (2).

In this report, antiviral effects of PGG on HSV growth in several mammalian cell cultures and also on the infectivity of cell-free viruses were studied.

MATERIALS AND METHODS

Hydrolysable tannin

1,2,3,4,6-pentagalloylglucose (PGG) shown in Fig. 1 was purified by the column chromatography through Sephadex LH-20 and Lichroprep RP-18 after methanol extraction from Gallae chinensis.

Cell cultures

The cell lines used in these experiments were FL, MA-104, Vero and BHK-21 cells. These cells were grown in Eagle's minimum essential medium containing 0.03 % L-glutamine and 5 to 10 % inactivated calf serum, and incubated at 37°C.

Viruses

Herpes simplex virus type 1 (HSV-1, HF strain) and vesicular stomatitis virus (VSV, N.J. strain) were prepared in FL cell cultures.

Interferon and double-stranded RNA

Human interferon (HuIFN)-α was kindly supplied from Nippon Chemical Research, Kobe, and Green Cross Co., Osaka, Japan. A double-stranded (ds) RNA preparation was obtained by the cold phenol method from purifi-

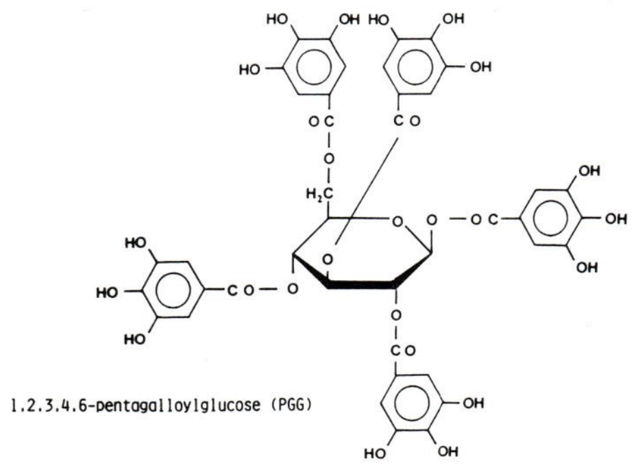

Fig. 1. Chemical structure of PGG

ed rice dwarf virus (RDV) (3).

RESULTS

Effect of PGG on HSV-infected MA-104 cells

Different concentrations of PGG were added 1hr post-infection (p.i.) to MA-104 cells. Treatment of HSV-infected cells with 3 to 50 μg/ml of PGG caused significant reduction of virus yields. However, inhibitory effects on the virus growth by treatment with PGG before infection were lower. A long incubation for 10 to 20 hr after addition of PGG p.i. prevented profoundly the virus growth. The inhibitory rate of virus production in HSV-infected BHK-21 cells was apparently lower than those in FL, MA-104 or Vero cells.

Effect of PGG on cell-free HSV

Different concentrations of PGG were incubated for 1 hr at 37°C with HSV diluted with phosphate buffer saline. Each sample was titrated for residual infectivity by plaque assay using MA-104 cell. The infectivity was neutralized strongly by 10 to 100 μg/ml of PGG.

A combined effect with PGG, HuIFN-α and dsRNA on HSV or VSV growth

The FL cell cultures were exposed to HuIFN (200 to 1,000 IU/ml) or RDV-RNA (30 μg/ml), and incubated at 37°C for 18 to 24 hr. The cells were infected with the viruses and PGG (25 μg/ml) was then added at 1 hr p.i. to the medium. These combined treatment caused a marked enhancement of inhibition on the virus growth in comparison with treatment of PGG alone. No influences were shown in the inhibition by PGG or IFN against HSV production in FL cells, even when PGG and IFN were added simultaneously after mixing both samples before or after virus infection.

From our results, it was suggested that the antiviral activity is based on a binding of galloyl groups in tannin molecule to cell membrane or viral surface proteins. It seems also likely that these activities are dependent on the number of galloyl or hexahydroxydiphenoyl group in the tannins.

REFERENCES

1. Takechi M, Tanaka Y (1981) Planta medica 42 : 69-74
2. Takechi M, Tanaka Y (1982) Planta medica 45 : 252-253
3. Takehara M, Suzuki N (1973) Arch Ges Virusforsch 40 : 291-299

EFFECTS OF NUCLEOSIDE ANALOGS IN INHIBITION OF EPSTEIN-BARR VIRUS

J.-C. LIN, D.J. NELSON, C.U. LAMBE, E.I. CHOI AND J.S. PAGANO

Lineberger Cancer Research Center, University of North Carolina, Chapel Hill, N.C. 27514 and the Wellcome Research Laboratories, Research Triangle Park, N.C. 27709

INTRODUCTION

We recently reported that several nucleoside analogs, E-5-(2-bromovinyl)-2'-deoxyuridine (BVDU), 1-(2-deoxy-2-fluoro-β-D-arabinofuranosyl)-5-iodocytosine (FIAC), 1-(2-deoxy-2-fluoro-β-D-arabinofuranosyl)-5-methyluracil (FMAU), and BW B759U or 9-(1,3-dihydroxy-2-propoxymethyl)guanine (DHPG), have prolonged effects in suppressing Epstein-Barr virus replication, even after the drugs are removed from persistently infected cell cultures (1,2). In the present studies we have characterized the efficacy of each drug in parallel with ACV, and compared the extent of phosphorylation of BW B759U and ACV.

MATERIALS AND METHODS

Treatment of cells with drugs. Exponentially growing P3HR-1 cells were spun down and suspended in fresh medium containing different concentrations of drugs (0, 0.01, 0.1, 1, 10 and 100 μM) for 14 days (2). The number of EBV genome copies per cell was determined (3).

Determination of viral ED_{50} and ED_{90}. The number of EBV genome copies per cell after drug treatment was plotted against drug concentrations, and viral ED_{50} and ED_{90} were determined from the plots.

Determination of ID_{50} for cell growth. During drug treatment, cells were counted daily. The number of cells after 4 days of growth was plotted against drug concentration, and cell ID_{50} was determined from the plot.

Nucleotide analysis by high-pressure liquid chromatography. Raji cells were superinfected or mock-infected with EBV. ^{14}C-BW B759U (50 μCi/μmole) or ^{14}C-ACV (53.8 μCi/μmole) were added 8 hrs or 24 hrs after infection and pulsed for 4 hr. Perchloric acid cell extracts were prepared and assayed by high-pressure liquid chromatography (4).

RESULTS

Relative efficacy of drugs. A dose-dependent inhibitory effect was observed for each drug tested. The number of EBV genome copies per cell was plotted against drug concentrations. From the plots we determined the viral ED_{50} value for each drug. The same graphical method was used to determine the cell growth ID_{50} in P3HR-1 cells. On the basis of these data, we calculated the therapeutic index (ID_{50}/ED_{50}) for each drug.

TABLE I

INHIBITORY ACTION OF NUCLEOSIDE ANALOGS

DRUG	ED_{50}	ID_{50}	THERAPEUTIC INDEX ID_{50}/ED_{50}
ACV	0.3	250	833
BW B759U	0.05	200	4000
BVDU	0.06	390	6500
FIAC	0.005	5	1000
FIAU	0.005	1	200
FMAU	0.0065	1	154

The relative potencies of these drugs on the basis of anti-EBV activities are: FIAC=FIAU>FMAU>BW B759U>BVDU>ACV; and on the basis of the therapeutic index: BVDU>BW B759U>FIAC>ACV>FIAU>FMAU.

Anabolism of BW B759U and ACV in superinfected Raji cells. To assess the molecular mechanisms of the greater activity of BW B759U and as a first step in understanding the more prolonged inhibitory effect of BW B759U over ACV (2), the kinetics of phosphorylation of the drugs in superinfected Raji cells were analyzed. EBV infection produced a rapid and marked increase in BW B759U phosphorylating activity, and this activity was 100-fold greater than that of ACV (Table 2).

TABLE 2

PHOSPHORYLATION OF BW B759 AND ACV IN SUPERINFECTED RAJI CELLS

DRUG	P MOLES TRI-P/10^6 CELLS	
	8 hr	24 hr
^{14}C-BW B759U	10.7	10.8
^{14}C-ACV	0.03	0.13

DISCUSSION

The studies presented herein clearly demonstrated that BW B759U, BVDU, FIAC, FMAU and FIAU are potent inhibitors of EBV replication in culture. The anti-EBV activity of these compounds appear to be more or less selective in that they inhibit viral replication at concentrations of drug which are to varying degrees not cytotoxic or cytostatic.

Like other nucleoside analogs, both BW B759U and ACV could be preferentially phosphorylated in infected cells (Table 2) in contrast to the low level of phosphorylation in uninfected cells (data not shown). Whether the prolonged anti-EBV activity of BW759, FIAC, FMAU and BVDU previously observed (1,2) are related to the accumulation of a stable pool of drug triphosphates remains to be determined.

In contrast the ACV which is a chain terminator, a large amount of incorporation of BW B759U internally into viral DNA strands was observed in HSV-infected cells (5). The formation of larger quantities of BW B759U-triphosphate than ACV-triphosphate in superinfected Raji cells may facilitate the incorporation of BW B759U into the internucleotide chain of EBV DNA. Thus, the viral DNA-containing BW B759U moieties internally may interfere with the rate of DNA chain elongation relative to unmodified primer (6). It has been documented that HSV-induced DNA polymerase has integrally associated exonuclease activity (7). There is some indication that EBV-induced DNA polymerase also has exonuclease activity (8). Exonuclease may play a role in affecting drug action due to excision of the terminally incorporated drug moieties, allowing at least temporary recovery of primer-template capability. Under these circumstances, the antiviral activity of a nucleoside analog such as ACV with a potential of chain-terminating would be expected to be more reversible than the analog such as BW B759U that incorporates into the internucleotide chain of viral DNA. Therefore, the apparent difficulty of the excision of BW B759U moieties incorporated internally may account for the more prolonged inhibitory effect of BW B759U over ACV.

ACKNOWLEDGEMENTS

We thank Barbara Leonard for typing the manuscript, Drs. T. Krenitsky of Burroughs Wellcome Company for ^{14}C-ACV and ^{14}C-BW B759U, C. McLaren of Bristol-Myers Company for FIAC, FMAU and FIAU, and E. DeClercq for BVDU.

This work was supported by Public Health Service grants 5-P01-CA-19014 and AI-17205 from the National Cancer Institute.

REFERENCES

1. Lin JC, Smith MC, Cheng YC, Pagano JS (1983) Science 221:578-579
2. Lin JC, Smith MC, Pagano JS (1984) J Virol 50:50-55
3. Lin JC, Smith MC, Pagano JS (1982) Virology 117: 186-194
4. Furman PA, Lambe CU, Nelson DJ (1982) Am J Med 73(1A): 14-17
5. Cheng YC, Grill SP, Dutschman GE, Nakayama K, Bastow KF (1983) J Biol Chem 258:12460-12464
6. Frank KB, Chiou JF, Cheng YC (1984) J Biol Chem 259:1566-1569
7. Ostrander M, Cheng YC (1980) Biochim Biophys Acta 609:232-245
8. Clough W (1979) Biochemistry 18:4517-4521

SELECTIVE INHIBITION OF HUMAN CYTOMEGALOVIRUS REPLICATION BY 1-β-D-ARABINOFURANOSYL-5-FLUOROURACIL: A POSSIBLE BI-FUNCTIONAL ANTIVIRAL AGENT.

SATORU SUZUKI,* MINEO SANEYOSHI,* CHIKAO NAKAYAMA* and YUKIHIRO NISHIYAMA**

* Faculty of Pharmaceutical Sciences, Hokkaido University, Sapporo 060,
** Nagoya University School of Medicine, Nagoya 464, Japan.

INTRODUCTION

It has been shown that a number of compounds exhibit highly selective inhibitory effects against herpes simplex viruses (HSV). However, only few selective inhibitors for human cytomegalovirus (HCMV) are known. We found that 1-β-D-arabinofuranosyl-5-fluorouracil (ara-FU) exhibited antiviral activity at low concentration against HCMV. We describe here the presumed mechanism of action of ara-FU on the replication of HCMV with regard to the dTTP pool size in infected cells and the viral DNA polymerase system.

MATERIALS AND METHODS

Cells and virus. Human embryonic fibroblasts (HEF) cells and AD169 strain of HCMV were used.

Compounds. Ara-FU was synthesized in our laboratory[1] and its 5'-triphosphate (ara-FUTP) was synthesized from ara-FU according to the method as described previously[2]. Other related compounds were also synthesized in our laboratory[3,4].

Virus plaque assay. Monolayers of HEF cells in 24 well plates (Linbro) were infected with 120 pfu of the virus. After 1 hr adsorption period at 37°C, the cultures were overlaid with 2 ml of 0.5% agarose in Eagle's MEM containing appropriate concentrations of inhibitors. After the incubation period of 7 days, the plaques were counted using a dissecting microscope at x20 magnification after fixation and staining.

Assay for DNA polymerase. Viral DNA polymerase was partially purified from HEF cells infected with HCMV. Purification of the polymerase was carried out according to the methods as described previously[5]. The standard mixture for the polymerase (25 µl) contained 50 mM tris-HCl (pH 7.8), 4 mM $MgCl_2$, 0.5 mM dithiothreitol (DTT), 100 mM ammonium sulfate, 75 µM concentrations of dATP, dGTP, dCTP and [^{3}H]dTTP (0.3 µCi/nmol), 2.5 µg activated salmon sperm DNA and enzyme. The reaction mixture was incubated at 37°C for 15 min. After incubation, 20 µl aliquots were transferred to DEAE cellulose paper disc (Whatman DE-81). The discs were washed with 5% Na_2HPO_4 six times, twice with 95% ethanol and dried. Remaining radioactivity was measured in a Packerd liquid scintillation counter with toluene scintillator.

Determination of dTTP pool size. The quantitative analysis of dTTP pool size was performed by the enzymatic procedure[6] with some modifications. Monolayers of HEF cells in 10 cm dish were infected with HCMV at a moi of 3. After adsorption at 37°C for 1 hr, fresh media containing nucleoside analogues were added. Cells were collected after incubation at 37°C for 72 hr. Extracts of cells were prepared as described previously[7]. The reaction mixture for determination of dTTP (50 µl) contained 50 mM tris-HCl (pH 7.8), 4 mM $MgCl_2$, 0.5 mM DTT, 25 µg native salmon sperm DNA, 35 µM concentrations of dATP, dCTP and [^{3}H]dGTP (0.6 µCi/nmol). Samples or dTTP standards and 0.063 units of DNA polymerase I Klenow fragment (P-L) were added to the mixture. The reaction mixture was incubated at 37°C for 30 min. After incubation, 40 µl aliquots were transferred to DE-81 paper disc. Remaining radioactivity was measured according to the same method described above.

RESULTS AND DISCUSSION

Drug concentrations which reduced plaque numbers to 50% (ID_{50}) against HCMV are shown in Table I. Ara-FU was found to be the most effective against HCMV among the 5-halo-ara-Us tested and its ID_{50} value was 3.8 µM. 5-Halo-ara-UTPs exhibited competitive inhibition with dTTP for HCMV-DNA polymerase (data not shown), and their apparent Ki values are summarized in Table II. The Ki value of ara-FUTP for the polymerase was larger than the other 5-halo-ara-UTPs.

TABLE I

ANTIVIRAL ACTIVITY OF 5-HALO-ARA-Us AND THE RELATED COMPOUNDS AGAINST HCMV.

Compounds	ID_{50} (µM)
Ara-FU	3.8
-ClU	115
-BrU	35.6
-IU	111
-T	119
-U	40

TABLE II

Ki VALUES OF 5-HALO-ARA-UTPs FOR HCMV-DNA POLYMERASE.

Compounds	Ki (µM)
dTTP	3.4 (Km)
Ara-FUTP	10
-ClUTP	1.5
-BrUTP	2.5
-IUTP	2.0
-TTP	1.0
-UTP	2.4

The dTTP pool size in HEF cells was stimulated approximately 33 fold by the virus infection. In contrast, treatment with ara-FU decreased the size of dTTP pool about 50% (Table III).

TABLE III

EFFECTS OF ARA-FU ON THE dTTP POOL SIZE.

Samples	dTTP (pmol/7x10^6cells)
Mock	2.38
Mock + ara-FU*	2.02
HCMV infected	78.8
HCMV infected + ara-FU*	44.9

*In the presence of 74 μM ara-FU for 72 hr.

From these findings, it seems reasonable to assume that ara-FU acts as a bi-functional inhibitor (self-potentiator) of HCMV replication. Ara-FU is phosphorylated by cellular thymidine kinase of which activity is enhanced by HCMV infection[8]. The resulting ara-FUMP inhibits cellular thymidylate synthetase[9], which in turn decreases the dTTP concentration. The viral DNA polymerase is inhibited by ara-FUTP. The dTTP competes with ara-FUTP for the DNA polymerase. As the dTTP pool size is reduced, the inhibitory effect of ara-FUTP becomes more efficient. On the other hand, other 5-halo-ara-UMPs except ara-FUMP do not inhibit thymidylate synthetase. Therefore, their inhibitory effects on HCMV are considered to be weaker than those of ara-FU. The scheme of action presented below will explain why ara-FU is effective against HCMV at low concentration.

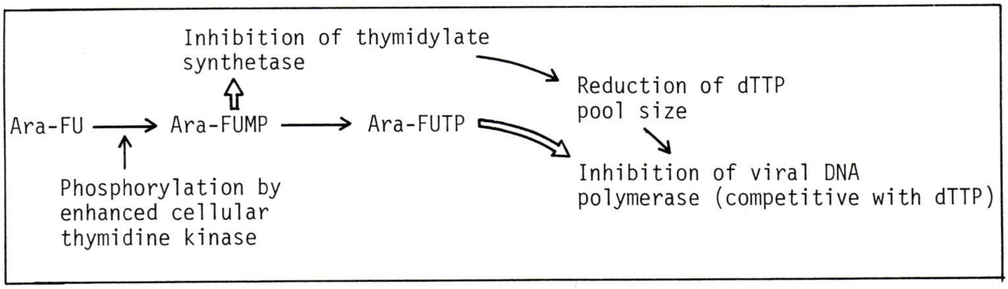

Fig.1. Proposed inhibition scheme of ara-FU against HCMV.
⇨ ; inhibition site.

ACKNOWLEDGEMENT

This work was supported in part by Grant-in-Aid for Cancer Research from the Ministry of Education, Science and Culture of Japan.

REFERENCES

1. Saneyoshi M, Inomata M, Fukuoka F (1978) Chem. Pharm. Bull. 26: 2990
2. Yamaguchi T, Saneyoshi M (1984) Chem. Pharm. Bull. 32: 1441
3. Ono K, Ogasawara M, Ohashi A, Matsukage A, Takahashi T, Nakayama C, Saneyoshi M (1982) Biochemistry 21: 1019
4. Nakayama C, Machida H, Saneyoshi M (1979) J. Carbohydr. Nucleosides Nucleotides 6: 295

5. Nishiyama Y, Suzuki S, Yamauchi M, Maeno K, Yoshida S (1984) Virology 135: 87
6. North T, Bestwick R, Mathews K (1980) J. Biol. Chem. 255: 6640
7. Tanaka K, Yoshioka A, Tanaka S, Wataya Y (1984) Anal. Biochem. 139: 35
8. Zavada V, Erban V, Rezacova D, Vonka V (1976) Arch. Virol. 52:333
9. Nakayama C, Wataya Y, Santi D, Saneyoshi M, Ueda T (1981) J. Med. Chem. 24: 1161

THERAPEUTIC EFFICACY OF INTERFERON ON HSV-1 OCULAR INFECTION IN MICE

YOSHIKAZU SHIMOMURA, YUICHI OHASHI, HITOSHI WATANABE, HISASHI HOSOTANI, SHIGERU KINOSHITA, REIZO MANABE, KOSABURO SATO*, AND TORU WADA

Department of Ophthalmology, Osaka University Medical School, Osaka (Japan)
Shionogi Research Laboratories, Shionogi & Co.,Ltd., Osaka (Japan)*

INTRODUCTION

Several investigators have studied the therapeutic efficacy of topically applied human interferon (IFN) on herpetic keratitis. (1-3) These results have suggested that the antiviral action of IFN is mainly prophylactic. To the best of our knowledge, instillation of IFN has been mostly used for the treatment of herpetic keratitis. Iontophoresis is a well-documented method ensuring the delivery of higher drug concentrations in ocualr tissues when compared with simple instillation. (4)

In the present study, we utilized iontophoresis of IFN in the treatment of murine herpetic keratitis and compared its efficacy with that of instillation or systemic administration.

MATERIALS AND METHODS

Virus inoculation Scarified corneas of C57BL/6 male mice (6 weeks old) were inoculated with 10 ul suspension of HSV-1 Fukuda strain (2×10^4 pfu/eye).

Systemic IFN-treatment Murine IFN-α/β (either 10^5 or 10^3 IU/mouse) was administered intraperitoneally for 5 consecutive days beginning 2 hours after the virus inoculation.

Topical IFN-treatment Murine IFN-α/β (10^3 IU/eye) was administered topically in two different ways (instillation or iontophoresis) for the treatment of herpetic eye infection. The topical treatment was done for 3 consecutive days beginning 2 hours after the virus inoculation.

Instillation. Ten ul of murine IFN-α/β solution were instilled twice a day.

Iontophoresis. A sterile cup was centered on the cornea with its edge placed at the inside of the limbus. Murine IFN-α/β solution was added to the eye cup. The anode made contact with IFN solution and the cathode was attached to the ear. A direct current (0.6 mAmps) was applied for 6 minutes. (5) Iontophoresis was performed once a day.

Clinical evaluation of HSV ocular infection in mice We examined the corneal and periocular lesions of infected mice with the aid of a slit lamp and fluorescein staining. The eye whose clinical scores were zero at 8 days post-inoculation was regarded as a cured eye.

Assay for the latent infection At 28 days post-inoculation, infected mice were killed to take out the trigeminal ganglia. Each ganglion was placed in the culture medium and incubated for 5 days at 37 C. The supernatent of each culture was assayed for the infectivity using CV-1 cell monolayers.

RESULTS AND DISCUSSION

The results are shown in this table.

	Systemic Treatment		Topical Treatment		Non-Treatment
	10^3IU	10^5IU	Instillation	Iontophoresis	
Tested Eyes	24	32	12	9	24
Cured Eyes	9(38%)	26(81%)*'	3(25%)*	5(56%)	5(21%)'
Latency	24(100%)	28(88%)*	10(83%)	3(33%)*'	23(96%)'

*' In the column of Cured Eyes;there was a significant difference ($p<0.005$).
*' In the column of Latency;there was a significant difference ($p<0.005$).

The efficacy of intraperitoneal administration of IFN-α/β (10^5 IU/mouse) on acute ocular HSV infection was superior to that of the other treatments. In spite of more efficient delivery of the drug, the clinical scores were worse in the eyes treated with iontophoresis. This may be that the iontophoretic treatment was cytotoxic to the cornea. (6) In fact, the incidence of latent infection in the trigeminal ganglia was significantly less in the animals treated with iontophoresis than those treated systemically. We suppose that the iontophoretic treatment with IFN inhibited the multiplication of the virus in the cornea effectively to block the establishment of the latent infection, whereas intraperitoneal administration could not provide enough IFN with the cornea to do so. However, this would be the case only if the iontophoresis with IFN is started from the early course of the infection.

REFERENCES

1. Sundmacher R, Neuman-Haefelin D (1976) J Infect Dis 133 (suppl.):A160-164
2. Kaufman HE, Meyer RF, Laibson PR, Waltman SR, Nesburn AB, Shuster JJ (1976) J Infect Dis (suppl.):A165-168
3. Jones BR, Coster DJ, Falcon MG, Cantell K (1976) J Infect Dis 133 (suppl.): A169-172
4. Hill JM, Park N-H, Gangarosa LP, Hull BS, Tuggle CL, Bowman K, Green K (1978) Invest Ophthalmol Vis Sci 17:473-476
5. Willey DE, Trousdale MD, Nesburn AB (1984) Invest Ophthalmol Vis Sci 25: 945-950
6. Shimomura Y, Gangarosa LP, Kataoka M, Hill JM (1983) Invest Ophthalmol Vis Sci 24:1588-1594

NUCLEOSIDE POOLS OF ACYCLOVIR TREATED HERPES SIMPLEX TYPE 1 INFECTED CELLS

JOHAN HARMENBERG, GUNNAR ABELE AND BRITTA WAHREN

Department of Virology, National Bacteriological Laboratory, S-105 21 Stockholm, (Sweden)

INTRODUCTION

A number of modern antitumor and antiviral substances utilize viral or cellular deoxythymidine kinases (dTKs) for activation of the drugs. Examples of these compounds are acyclovir (ACV), bromovinyldeoxyuridine, jododeoxyuridine, 5-fluorouracil and 5-fluorodeoxyuridine. Addition of the natural substrate of dTK which is deoxythymidine (dThd) may therefore decrease the activity of these substances (1, 2).

ACV was found to exert less antiviral activity in African green monkey kidney (GMK) cells than in other cells tested (3). It was necessary to use a 20-100 times higher concentration of ACV in GMK cells as compared to human fetal lung fibroblast (HL) cells to achieve a similar antiviral activity (3). It has been shown that uninfected GMK cells contain higher levels of dThd than uninfected HL cells (1). Herpes simplex virus (HSV) infection and ACV treatment may alter the cellular metabolism of nucleosides. To clarify the importance of naturally occurring nucleosides, we studied the nucleoside pools of HSV infected and uninfected GMK and HL cells with and without antiviral substances.

MATERIAL AND METHODS

Chromatographic conditions

High performance liquid chromatography (HPLC) analysis was performed on a liquid chromatograph (Waters Assoc., Milford, Mass., USA). Conditions as previously described (4).

Sample preparation

Stationary GMK and HL cells were infected with HSV-1 (moi = 4), mock infected or HSV-1 infected with the addition of ACV, for 9 h. Subsequently the cells were extracted in 0.5 M $HClO_4$ (perchloric acid, PCA). After centrifugation the supernatant was neutralized with 4 M KOH and 0.4 M KH_2PO_4. After another centrifugation the supernatant was loaded onto a Sep-Pak C_{18} cartridge. Sep-Pak procedure as previously described (4).

RESULTS AND DISCUSSION

Nucleoside pools of herpes simplex type 1 (HSV-1) infected and uninfected GMK and HL cells have been analysed with high performance liquid chromatography (HPLC). Deoxythymidine and adenosine were the only nucleosides found in measurable amounts. The dThd pool seemed to be selectively increased in uninfected and infected GMK cells, but not in HL cells. dThd was also the only nucleoside excreted to the medium. HSV-1 infection reduced the dThd concentration of GMK cells. Addition of ACV to HSV-1 infected GMK cells induces an abortive infection. This resulted in a dThd concentration similar to that of uninfected GMK cells. dThd added to HSV-1 infected GMK and HL cells reduced the antiviral action of ACV as measured by a plaque reduction assay. ACV is known to be activated mainly by HSV induced deoxythymidine kinase (dTK), an enzyme which utilizes dThd as a substrate. The poor antiviral activity of ACV in GMK cells as compared to HL cells may be explained by the presence of dThd in GMK cells.

REFERENCES

1. Harmenberg J (1983) Intervirol 20:48-51
2. Larsson A, Brännström G, Öberg B (1983) Antimicrob Agents Chemother 24:819-822
3. Harmenberg J, Wahren B, Öberg B (1980) Intervirol 14:239-244
4. Harmenberg J, Larsson A, Hagberg C-E (1983) J Liq Chromatogr 6:655-666

INCORPORATION OF (E)-5-(2-BROMOVINYL)-2'-DEOXYURIDINE INTO DEOXYRIBONUCLEIC ACID OF VARICELLA-ZOSTER VIRUS (TK^+- AND TK^--STRAINS)-INFECTED CELLS

T. YOKOTA[1], K. KONNO[1], S. SHIGETA[1] and E. DE CLERCQ[2]
[1]Department of Bacteriology, Fukushima Medical College, Fukushima 960, Japan and
[2]Rega Institute for Medical Research, Katholieke Universiteit Leuven, B-3000 Leuven, Belgium

Recently we isolated a mutant varicella-zoster virus strain (TK^--VZV) which is resistant to (E)-5-(2-bromovinyl)-2'-deoxyuridine (BVDU) and (E)-5-(2-iodovinyl)-2'-deoxyuridine (IVDU) and does not induce viral thymidine kinase (TK) activity in infected cells (1,2). The TK^--VZV strain and the parent (TK^+-VZV) strain induce comparable levels of viral DNA polymerase activity (3). The 5'-triphosphate of BVDU (BVDUTP) has been evaluated for its inhibitory effects on the activity of TK^+-VZV DNA polymerase, TK^--VZV DNA polymerase and cellular DNA polymerase (3). From the results obtained it is clear that the selective inhibitory action of BVDU on VZV replication primarily depends on a specific phosphorylation by the viral TK. However, this does not exclude the possibility that a differential inhibitory effect of BVDUTP at the DNA polymerase level further contributes to the selective inhibition of VZV replication by BVDU. In this study, we investigated the incorporation of IVDU into viral and cellular DNA of TK^+-VZV-, TK^--VZV- and mock-infected cells.

(^{125}I)-IVDU was synthesized at the Rega Institute (Katholieke Universiteit Leuven) essentially as described previously (4). Human embryo fibroblast (HEF) cells were infected with TK^+-VZV or TK^--VZV. After 24 hours of incubation, the cells were pulse-labeled with (^{125}I)-IVDU or (^{3}H)-deoxythymidine (dT) at a final concentration of 20 µM (IVDU) or 0.05 µM (dT). VZV- or mock-infected flasks were harvested at the indicated times (Fig. 1). Acid-precipitated radioactivity was determined. The results for the time-response curve of cellular uptake of (^{125}I)-IVDU are shown in Fig. 1. The uptake of (^{125}I)-IVDU was confined to cells infected with TK^+-VZV; no uptake of (^{125}I)-IVDU could be demonstrated with either TK^--VZV- or mock-infected cells. (^{3}H)-dT was taken up by either TK^+-VZV- or mock-infected but not TK^--VZV-infected cells.

Viral and cellular DNAs from VZV-infected cells were separated by isopycnic centrifugation in CsCl gradients and the extent of incorporation of IVDU into DNA was estimated by determining the differences in the DNA densities (5,6). The DNAs isolated from TK^+-VZV-infected cells grown in the presence of (^{125}I)-IVDU exhibited a significant shift in the buoyant density of viral DNA (density increase from 1.71 to 1.747 g/ml) and a slight shift in the buoyant density of host DNA (density increase from 1.70 to 1.717 g/ml). In marked contrast with the DNAs isolated from TK^+-VZV-infected cells, the DNAs isolated from TK^--VZV- or mock-infec-

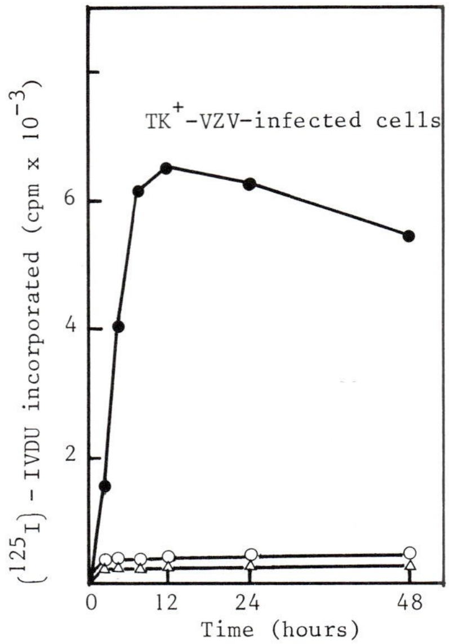

Fig. 1. Time-response curve of cellular uptake of $[^{125}I]$-IVDU.

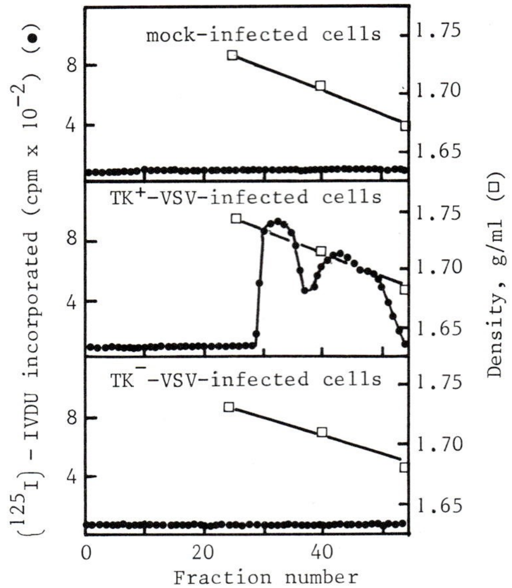

Fig. 2. Isopycnic CsCl centrifugation of DNA from VZV-infected cells.

ted cells did not exhibit a detectable incorporation of $[^{125}I]$-IVDU (Fig. 2). The failure to find any incorporation of $[^{125}I]$-IVDU into DNA of mock- or TK^--VZV-infected cells can be explained by the unability of IVDU to serve as substrate for the cellular TK. Vice versa, the incorporation of $[^{125}I]$-IVDU into DNA of TK^+-VZV-infected cells can be regarded as a direct consequence of its specific phosphorylation by the viral TK. Whether the incorporation of IVDU into viral DNA is proportional to, and/or responsible for, the anti-VZV action of the compound is an interesting hypothesis that is worth pursuing.

REFERENCES

1. Shigeta S, Yokota T, Iwabuchi T, Baba M, Konno K, Ogata M, De Clercq E (1983) J Infect Dis 147:576-584

2. Yokota T, Ogata M, Shigeta S (1983) Fukushima J Med Sci 29:101-111

3. Yokota T, Konno K, Shigeta S, De Clercq E (1984) Mol Pharmacol, in press

4. De Clercq E, Heremans H, Descamps J, Verhelst G, De Ley M, Billiau A (1981) Mol Pharmacol 19:122-129

5. Allaudeen HS, Chen MS, Lee JJ, De Clercq E, Prusoff WH (1982) J Biol Chem 257: 603-606

6. Mancini WR, De Clercq E, Prusoff WH (1983) J Biol Chem 258:792-795

EFFECTS OF AN EXTRACT OF HYPERICUM ERECTUM ON HERPES SIMPLEX VIRUS

JUNKO RENARD - NOZAKI AND TAIJEONG KIM
Department of Microbiology, Tokyo Medical College,
6-1-1, Shinjuku, Shinjuku-ku, Tokyo, 160 (Japan)

INTRODUCTION

Despite the development of vaccins against pathogenic viruses there is a dire need for antiviral agents in case of immunodeficiency or infection with low response to vaccination. It is under those circumstances that we discovered that a substance contained in Hypericum erectum had antiviral effects on a broad spectrum with comparatively low cytotoxicity[1].

In this paper we present our experiments on this substance in a system of herpes simplex virus(HSV) and Vero cells as well as our investigation into its participation in the activation of macrophages(Mø)[2] and natural killer (NK)[3] cells considered, like interferon, to play an important role in the defense reaction of the organism in case of viral infection.

MATERIALS AND METHODS

Antiviral agents

Extraction of the antiviral substance(AVS) from Hypericum erectum. The crude material was extracted from the plant with 50% methanol and treated as follows: Chromatography with XAD-7 column, adjustment to pH3, distribution with ethyl acetate, readjustment to pH6 and chromatography with Cellulofine GH-25 column.

Acyclovir(ACV). Sumitomo Kagaku Co., Japan.

Virocidal action of AVS

A mixture of two equal volumes of HSV(HF strain, 10^7 $TCID_{50}$/ml) and AVS(100, 200, 400 µg/ml) was stored at 37°C or room temperature. The quantity of infectious virus was examined by micro-assay method based on CPE.

Virostatic action of AVS

Vero cells were grown as monolayer in 6-well plates(ø35mm) and the HF strain (5 x 10^3 $TCID_{50}$) was used to infect the Vero cells. The remaining virus was removed and, after addition of 2 ml of maintenance solution(MS), AVS was added at various concentrations. The virus, intra and extracellular, was harvested after incubation for 24h. The titration was carried out by micro-assay method.

Relation between virus yield and duration of treatment

AVS was added to the MS for treatment of the infected cells during 6 or 12 h. Then fresh MS, without AVS, was substituted and virus yields were examined.

Activating effect of Mø

Adherente cells(Mø>95%) were obtained from the peritoneal cavity of AVS injected(100 µg, s.c.) mice(ICR,5W,♂) and the activity of Mø was examined with as marker the consumption of glucose in the culture medium(RPMI1640 + 10% FBS).

Activating effect of NK cells

Spleen cells, used as effector cells, were taken from AVS injected mice while target cells were Vero cells alone, HSV infected(12 h) Vero cells ans YAC-1 cells. NK cells activity was examined by ^{51}Chromium release assay.

RESULTS

Judging from the action of the *Hypericum erectum* extract(Fig.1) on non-cell associated virus, inactivation increased with AVS concentration and incubation time but was not dependent on the temperature(Tab.1).

Dried plant
← extracted with 50% MeOH
Extract
← concentrated by rotary evaporator
Centrifugation
Supernatant
XAD-7 c.c.
← eluted with 80% MeOH
Eluate
← adjusted with HCl to pH 3
Centrifugation
Supernatant
← distributed with EtOAc
Aqueous layer
← adjusted with NaOH to pH 6
Cellulofine GH-25 c.c.
← eluted with DW
Peak II
AVS

Molecular weight : approx. 1000
pH stability : 2, 4, 7, 9
Heat resistance : 10 min at 100°C
UV absorbance(λ max. in DW) : 280
Biuret reaction : -
Ninhydrin reaction : -
Anthrone reaction : +
Iron(III) chloride reaction : +

Fig.1. Extraction, purification and properties of AVS

		Infectious virus ($TCID_{50}$/0.05ml)		
		0'	30'	60'
AVS	50 µg/ml	1×10^7	1×10^5	1×10^2
	100 µg/ml	1×10^7	1×10^1	0
	200 µg/ml	1×10^6	0	0
Control(DW)		1×10^7	1×10^7	1×10^7

Tab.1. Virocidal action of AVS on HSV(HF/Vero, 37°C or room temp.)

As for virus multiplication in host cells, inhibition was observed with the addition of 10 μg/ml of AVS, and with 25 μg/ml the yields of virus, intra and extracellular, decreased significantly. This virostatic effect was about the same as that of ACV used for control(Tab.2).

Concentration		Virus yield($TCID_{50}$/0.05ml)		
		AVS	ACV	Cont.
10 μg/ml	Intracellular	10^3	10^2	10^4
	Extracellular	10^2	10^0	10^3
25 μg/ml	Intracellular	10^2	10^1	
	Extracellular	0	0	
50 μg/ml	Intracellular	0	0	
	Extracellular	0	0	

Tab.2. Dose response of AVS to virus yield(HF/Vero, 24 h incubation)

Table 3 shows the virus yields in the cultures incubated for an additional time of 18 or 12 h after treatment with AVS respectively for 6 or 12 h. When the treatment was conducted for 12 h, the difference in yield became evident.

			Virus yield($TCID_{50}$/0.05ml) Duration of treatment		
			0-6 h	0-12 h	0-24 h
AVS	10 μg/ml	Intracellular	1×10^4	1×10^3	1×10^3
		Extracellular	1×10^2	1×10^2	1×10^2
	50 μg/ml	Intracellular	5×10^3	1×10^3	0
		Extracellular	1×10^2	1×10^1	0
ACV	10 μg/ml	Intracellular	1×10^4	1×10^3	1×10^2
		Extracellular	1×10^3	1×10^1	1×10^0
	50 μg/ml	Intracellular	1×10^3	1×10^3	0
		Extracellular	1×10^2	1×10^0	0
Control(DW)		Intracellular			1×10^4
		Extracellular			1×10^3

Tab.3. Relation between yield and duration of treatment(HF/Vero, 24 h incubation)

DISCUSSION

In vitro, as stated above, AVS showed both virocidal and virostatic effects on HSV. Its mechanism is being investigated.

Results *in vivo* indicated that AVS activated Mø and NK cells(Tab.4), suggesting that it could induce interferon.[4)5)] However the experiments performed along this line were negative. It seems therefore to activate Mø and NK cells, not through interferon, but directly.

Mø activity*

		After injection of AVS	
		1 day	3 days
Source of Mø	AVS injected	26.5	39.7
	DW injected	4.1	3.9

NK cells activity**

Source of spleen cells	Target cells	Incubation time	
		5 h	10 h
AVS injected	Non infected Vero	10.1	8.2
DW injected	"	7.3	8.9
AVS injected	HSV infected Vero	19.4	32.7
DW injected	"	4.4	6.5
AVS injected	YAC - 1	71.6	57.8
DW injected	"	19.0	10.3

* % of glucose consumption in the medium after 48 h incubation of Mø(1×10^6)
** % of ^{51}Cr release using spleen cells as effector cells(E/T = 40/1)

Tab.4. Effects of AVS on Mø and NK cells

The chemical composition of AVS has yet to be established. Pending that, as only one spot was detected in a TLC analysis using 2 systems of solvents, it is believed that the substance is comparatively pure. Judging from its chemical properties(Fig.1) it could be a Flavone glycoside[6] and analysies by NMR, Mass spectrography, etc., are scheduled to clarify this point.

REFERENCES

1. Renard-Nozaki J, Kim T, Atanasiu P (1984) Antiviral Action of an Extract of Hypericum erectum on Enveloped Viruses. Sixth International Congress of Virology. September 1-7, Sendai,Japan
2. Allison A C (1974) On the Role of Mononuclear Phagocytes in Immunity against Viruses. Progr. Med. Virol. 18: 15
3. Santoli D, Koprowski H (1979) Mechanism of Activation of Human Natural Killer Cells against Tumor and Virus Infected Cells. Immunological Rev. 44: 125-163
4. Santoli D, Trinchieri G, Koprowski H (1978) Cell Mediated Cytotoxicity against Virus-infected Target Cells in Human. II Interferon Induction and activation of Natural Killer Cells. J. Immunol. 121: 532-538
5. Gidlund M, Orn A, Wigzell H, Senik A, Gresser I (1978) Enhanced NK Activity in Mice Injected with Interferon and Interferon Inducers. Nature 273: 759
6. Hayashi K (1980) Plant Pigments - An Introduction to Research and Experiments Yokendo Ltd, Tokyo, pp174-201

CAN 9-ANILINOACRIDINES ELIMINATE LATENT HERPES?

PAUL N. GOLDWATER*, CAROL GUNN*, KAREN E. FLYNN*, BRUCE C. BAGULEY+

* Department of Immunobiology and + Cancer Research Laboratory, University of Auckland School of Medicine, Private Bag, Auckland, New Zealand.

INTRODUCTION

Amsacrine, a 9-aminoacridine (4), has clinically useful activity in the treatment of acute leukaemia (1) and has been shown to have antiviral activity against vaccinia and other viruses (3). Anilinoacridines bind to ds DNA by intercalation of the acridine chromophore (5). The anilino portion projects into the minor groove of the DNA double helix (2) and substituents para to the attachment point of the anilino ring project away from the DNA and might interact with a second macromolecular species. Substitution of the anilino ring results in significant changes in biological activity of the molecule. We have identified a number of compounds with marked in vitro anti-herpesvirus activity. Some compounds have been tested in an in vitro system to demonstrate inhibition of reactivation of mouse latent ganglionic infection. Freshly explanted dorsal root ganglia from previously infected mice were exposed to drug for 24 hours. No compound, so far tested, prevented reactivation of latent infection.

MATERIALS AND METHODS

Compounds. All anilinoacridine compounds were synthesised in the Cancer Research Laboratory, School of Medicine, University of Auckland (6,7).

Virus Strain. ATCC Herpes simplex (HSV) type 1 (Strain F), type 2 (Strain G) and clinical isolates were used in antiviral assays and Strain G was used in latency studies.

In vitro antiviral assays: Inhibition of cytopathic effect in HSV-infected BHK-21 microcultures was satisfactory for assessing antiviral activity (expressed as ED_{50}). Drug cytotoxicity was assessed in uninfected cultures and expressed as CTD_{50}.

Inhibition of reactivation of latently infected ganglia. Freshly explanted dorsal root ganglia (from mice previously infected by intradermal inoculation of Strain G into the pinna) were exposed to $2ED_{50}$ of drug in growth medium (GM) for 24 hours. Ganglia were further incubated for 5 days in GM, freeze/thawed and a suspension of BHK-21 cells added. The monolayer was examined for cytopathic evidence of reactivated virus.

RESULTS

The ED_{50} and CTD_{50} of 46 derivatives of 9-anilinoacridine were determined. Cytosine arabinoside and acycloguanosine were used for comparison. The values in the table represent the mean of at least 2 separate assays against herpes simplex type 2 (clinical isolate 6177). Cell doubling times after exposure to subcytotoxic levels of all compounds tested did not differ significantly from control cultures.

Anilino ring substitution. A wide range in activity was seen for anilinoacridines substituted para to the attachment point to the acridine ring (the 1'-position). ED_{50} concentrations varied from 1.5 μg/ml to >25 μg/ml. The most effective substituents were the 1'-$NHCOOCH_3$, the 1'-$NHSO_2CH_3$, and the 1'-NH_2. Small changes in the substituents, such as the substitution of an ethyl or phenyl group, resulted in a significant diminution of activity. The $NHCOOCH_3$ group, when placed in either of the other two possible positions (2' or 3') on the anilino ring, was ineffective (compounds 11, 12). The addition of a 3'-methoxy group to compound 4 increased antiherpes activity and decreased cytotoxicity. However, similar substitution to compound 7 reduced antiviral activity.

Acridine ring substitution. Derivatives of the most active compound, 13, were not available. However, using parent compound 7, we were unable to increase antiherpes activity by substituting the acridine portion of the molecule.

Effect of anilinoacridines on reactivation of latent ganglionic infection. 10 anilinoacridine compounds with high antiherpes activity failed to prevent reactivation of latent ganglionic infection.

TABLE

ANTI-HERPESVIRUS ACTIVITY OF MONO-SUBSTITUTED AND DISUBSTITUTED ANILINOACRIDINES

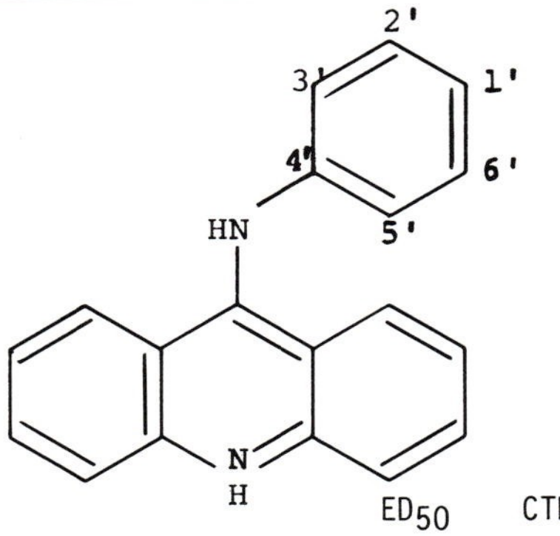

No.	Substituent	ED_{50}	CTD_{50}
1	1'-NH_2	2.4[a]	>25[b]
2	1'-$NHCOCH_3$	9.4	12.5
3	1'-$NHCONHCH_3$	6.3	12.5
4	1'-$NHCOOCH_3$	1.5	25
5	1'-$NHCOOCH_2CH_3$	6.3	>25
6	1'-$NHPO(OCH_3)_2$	6.8	<25
7	1'-$NHSO_2CH_3$	1.9	>25
8	1'-$NHSO_2C_6H_5$	3.2	>25
9	1'-OH	4.6	12.5
10	1'-$COCH_3$	5.5	12.5
11	2'-$NHCOOCH_3$	>25	>25
12	3'-$NHCOOCH_3$	12.5	25
13	1'-$NHCOOCH_3$, 3'-OCH_3	0.8	3.1
14	1'-$NHSO_2CH_3$, 3'-OCH_3	2.7	25
	Cytosine arabinoside	0.8	>25
	Acycloguanosine	0.5	>25

[a] Concentration (μg/ml) inhibiting virus induced cytopathic effect in 50% of microcultures.

[b] Concentration (μg/ml) causing visible cytotoxic changes in 50% of microcultures of non-infected cells.

ACKNOWLEDGEMENTS

This work is supported by a grant from the Auckland Medical Research Foundation.

REFERENCES

1. Arlin ZA, Sklaroff RB, Gee TS, Kempin SJ, Howard J, Clarkson BD, Young CW (1980) Cancer Res 40:3304-3306

2. Baguley BC, Nash R (1981) Eur J Cancer 17:671-679

3. Byrd DM (1977) Ann NY Acad Sci 284: 462-471

4. Cain BF, Attwell GJ (1974) Eur J Cancer 10: 539-549

5. Waring MJ (1976) Eur J Cancer 12: 995-1001

6. Denny WA, Cain BF, Attwell GJ, Hansch C, Panthananickal A, Leo A (1982) J Med Chem 25: 276-315

7. Rewcastle GW, Baguley BC, Cain BF (1982) J Med Chem 25: 1231-1235

EVALUATION OF ANTIVIRALS IN PREVENTING HERPES SIMPLEX VIRUS-INDUCED CATARACTS IN A MURINE MODEL

RAYMOND F. SCHINAZI*, R. TAYLOR SCOTT, J. ALLEN GAMMON, R. DOYLE STULTING, JOHN F.R. KUCK, JOHN D. WRIGHT AND ANDRE J. NAHMIAS.

Veterans Administration Medical Center/Emory University School of Medicine, Atlanta, Georgia 30033, U.S.A.

INTRODUCTION

Cataracts are a prominent cause of decreased vision in humans (1). Numerous cataractogenic factors have been detected including physical, chemical, predisposing metabolic and genetic conditions, associated eye disease, aging and virus infection during embryonic life (2). A surge of interest in virus-induced cataracts followed the 1964-1965 epidemic of rubella virus in the United States. In that instance cataracts in the newborn were determined to be a consequence of the mother contracting rubella during the first trimester of pregnancy. Rubella virus has been isolated from cataractous lenses of neonates (3) and the virus has been shown to persist in the lens for up to 1 year after birth. In one case virus was found after 2 years (4). More recently, Cibis and Burde (5) recovered herpes simplex virus (HSV) from the lens of a newborn with an obvious cataract, suggesting that other viruses may also cause direct pathogenic effects on the lens. A better understanding of the pathological mechanisms involved in rubella-induced cataract formation as well as other cataracts has been derived from animal studies (2,6-8) and studies of congenital rubella cases (3,4). Theories have evolved that satisfactorily explain the responsible biological and morphological changes in some experimental cataracts. These observations have been helpful in predicting similar mechanisms in humans (e.g. human galactosemia, diabetic cataract, or hypocalcemia). It is usually difficult to ascertain the exact cause or locus of the primary disturbance in the complex lens metabolism system which precipitates the opacities. The final common denominator from various insults to the lens leads ultimately to a disturbance of lens protein. However, it is conceivable that genetic mechanisms which control lens protein synthesis are the target of the primary assault. Certainly the etiology of most congenital, juvenile and senile cataracts remains ill-defined. A portion of these opacities may be caused by a viral infection or possibly by reactivation of latent virus.

The current intense interest in the myriad of diseases caused by herpes simplex viruses has made possible the discovery in this laboratory that young mice inoculated intracerebrally with HSV exhibit a high incidence of cataracts along with other pathology. To moderate or overcome the pathogenic effect of the viruses, potent selective antivirals were used; thus, depending on the antiviral drug and dose scheduling, larger numbers of treated than untreated mice survived the primary infections.

MATERIAL AND METHODS

<u>Cell culture techniques.</u> The techniques used in our virology laboratory to prepare virus stocks and titrate them by plaque assays have been described (9).

Animals and virus inoculation. Swiss outbred ICR female mice were ordered from Harlan-Sprague Dawley (Indianapolis, Ind.). The mice were housed no more than 6 to a cage and allowed to acclimatize to their new environment for 2 weeks before each experiment. They were provided water and rat chow (Ralston Purina Co., St. Louis, MO.) *ad libitum* and kept on 12 hour cycles of light and dark, under constant conditions of temperature (22° C) and humidity. The mice were grouped when 6-7 weeks old, anesthesized with Metofane (Pitman-Moore Co., Washington Crossing, N.J.), examined ophthalmologically, and carefully numbered by earmarking prior to inoculation of 0.05 ml of stock HSV at appropriate dilution in sterile phosphate-buffered saline (PBS , pH 7.4) into the right cerebral hemisphere.

Drugs and Drug Treatment. The 2'-fluoroarabinopyrimidine nucleosides were obtained from Drs. J. Fox and K. Watanabe (Sloan-Kettering Institute for Cancer Research, N.Y.). Acyclovir (ACV) and vidarabine (ara-A) were obtained from Burroughs-Wellcome (Research Triangle, N.C.) and Sigma Chemical Co. (St. Louis, Mo.), respectively. 9-(1,3-Dihydroxy-2-propoxymethyl)guanine (DHPG, 2'NDG, BIOLF-62, or BW759) was obtained from Syntex Inc. (Palo Alto, CA). Intraperitoneal treatments were begun 5 hours after virus inoculation and continued twice a day for 4 days for a total of 8 doses. The animals were examined ophthalmologically every other week for 3 months.

RESULTS

Incidence of cataracts.

Of a total of 716 mice inoculated with strains of HSV-1 (KOS) or HSV-2 (G), 407 survived; 78 (19.2%) developed unilateral or bilateral cataracts 8 weeks after virus inocuation. Eleven of 15 surviving untreated animals (73.3%) and 67 of 392 surviving drug-treated mice (17.1%) developed lens opacities. In contrast, none of 135 control mice inoculated intracerebrally with PBS developed opacities or other ocular changes (Table I). In order to confirm that the cataracts were induced by the virus and not by the drugs (10-12), high doses of the antivirals (200, 400, and 800 mg/kg intraperitoneally per day) were given to uninfected mice twice a day for 4 days. No uveitis or lens opacities were noted at 3 months after treatment in any of the mice treated with antivirals alone (data not shown).

In a prospective pilot study, 80 mice were inoculated intracerebrally with HSV-2 (60 LD_{50}) and treated with FMAU at a relatively high dose of 0.5 and 5 mg/kg (24 mice) and FMAU or FIAC at a dose of 0.1 and 15 mg/kg, respectively (56 mice). Slit lamp examination was performed on the two populations at 4, 8, and 12 weeks after brain inoculation, without the use of anesthetic.

By 4 weeks, 2 of the 56 mice treated with the relatively less effective doses of antivirals had obvious unilateral cataracts and 16 mice had died. At eight weeks, 6 additional mice developed unilateral cataracts, 1 mouse had a unilateral cataract and unilateral uveitis, and 2 mice had unilateral uveitis. At 12 weeks post-infection one mouse developed a unilateral cataract and 3 mice died (1 mouse that had developed unilateral cataracts 8 weeks after infection, one with unilateral uveitis, and a mouse with the cataract and uveitis). However, one of the mice that had developed unilateral uveitis at 8 weeks, developed 4 weeks later a unilateral cataract in the same eye. These *in vivo* observations document changes from uveitis to cataract as well as progression of disease from ocular abnormality to death. Significantly, none of the 24 mice treated with effective doses of FMAU died or developed uveitis or cataracts.

TABLE I.

FREQUENCY OF VIRAL-INDUCED CATARACTS AFTER INTRACEREBRAL INOCULATION WITH HERPES SIMPLEX VIRUSES IN OUTBRED FEMALE MICE

Dose of Virus (Strain)[a]	No. of Mice Surviving: Alive/ Total(%)[b]			No. of Surviving Mice with Opacities (%)[b]								
	Untreated	Treated[c]	Total	Untreated			Treated[c]			Total		
				OD	OS	OU	OD	OS	OU	OD	OS	OU
HSV-2 (Strain G)	10/211	373/465	383/676	3	3	1	15	15	34	18	18	35
50-600 LD_{50}	(4.7)	(80.2)	(56.7)									
				7/10			64/373			71/383		
				(70)			(17.2)			(18.4)[e]		
HSV-1 (Strain KOS)	5/10	19/30	24/40	-	-	4	-	1	2	-	1	6
1 LD_{50}	(50)	(63.3)	(60)									
				4/5			3/19			7/24		
				(80)			(15.8)			(29.2)[e]		
PBS-inoculated[d]	135/135	-	135/135	0	0	0	-	-	-	0	0	0
	(100)		(100)									
				0/135						0/135		
				(0)						(0)		

[a] Mice inoculated intracerebrally when 6-7 week old. Mice dying within 24 h of inoculation are not included.
[b] At 8 weeks after inoculation.
[c] Treated with antivirals 5 h after virus inoculation.
[d] Phosphate buffered saline.
[e] Fischer exact test for 2 x 2 tables - $p < 10^{-5}$.

We have also determined the incidence of cataracts in mice treated with different doses of experimental and licensed antivirals (Table II). In general, the most effective antiviral prevented the formation of cataracts. The two more effective drugs were FMAU and FMAC, which completely prevented cataract formation at relatively low doses. Interestingly, although ACV, ara-A, FIAC and the other drugs were effective in significantly reducing mortality at some of the doses tested, they were unable to prevent the development of cataracts in a substantial number of surviving mice. These results suggests that this mouse model could be useful in evaluating the effectiveness of new antivirals in preventing ocular sequelae of HSV encephalitis. The dose scheduling of the drugs also appears to be an important variable for controlling progression of disease.

TABLE II

INCIDENCE OF CATARACTS IN SWISS ICR FEMALE MICE AFTER INTRACEREBRAL INOCULATION WITH HSV-2 (STRAIN G, $10LD_{50}$) AND TREATMENT WITH DIFFERENT ANTIVIRALS

Drug and Dosage mg/kg[a]		Day of Examination	Mortality: No. Dead/ No. Inoc. (%)[b]	No. Surviving Mice with Opacities			% of Survivors Developing Opacities
				OD	OS	OU	
ACV	15	30	13/15 (87)	-	-	2	100
	20	60	8/12 (67)	2	1	-	75
	60	31	5/12 (42)	-	-	1	14
Ara-A	10	30	9/12 (75)	1	-	1	67
	15	30	14/15 (93)	-	-	1	100
	60	31	6/12 (50)	1	-	-	17
DHPG	2.5	59	8/17 (47)	-	-	4	44
	5.0	59	8/15 (53)	1	1	3	71
	10.0	30	14/27 (52)	1	3	5	64
FIAC	15	35	4/12 (33)	2	-	-	25
	20	35	1/12 (8)	2	-	-	18
	40	35	2/12 (17)	2	1	1	40
	80	35	0/15 (0)	-	-	-	0
FMAU	0.5	30	0/12 (0)	-	1	2	25
	5	35	0/12 (0)	-	1	-	8
	15	35	0/15 (0)	-	-	-	0
	30	35	0/15 (0)	-	-	-	0
FMAC	0.5	30	8/15 (53)	-	-	2	29
	1	30	8/15 (53)	-	-	-	0
	5	30	0/15 (0)	-	-	-	0
FEAU	50	30	9/12 (75)	1	-	-	33
	100	30	1/15 (7)	1	-	-	7

[a] Given 5h after virus inoculation. Dose schedule, twice a day for 4 days

[b] Calculated on day 30

Optimization of cataract formation

We have also carried out a long-term prospective pilot study to determine the optimum conditions necessary to induce cataracts i.e. maximum number of mice developing cataracts and minimum attrition rate among virus inoculated mice. The results are summarized in Table III.

TABLE III

PILOT EXPERIMENT TO DETERMINE THE INCIDENCE OF CATARACTS IN SWISS FEMALE MICE AFTER INTRACEREBRAL INOCULATION WITH HSV-2 (STRAIN G)

Group	Brain Inoculation	Treatment[a]	Dose of Drug[b]	No. of mice dead/ Total (%)[c]		No. Surviving
A	PBS (control group)	PBS	-	0/30	(0)	30
B	PBS (drug-control group)	FIAC	60	0/27	(0)	27
C	HSV-2 (500 LD_{50})	PBS	-	10/10	(100)	0
D	HSV-2 (500 LD_{50})	FIAC	60	20/60	(33)	40

INCIDENCE OF CATARACTS IN GROUP D[d]

Day of examination after virus inoculation	No. animals examined	No. of Surviving Mice with Opacities OD	OS	OU	Total No.	(%)
29	40	4	5	8	17	(42.5)
59	40	7	5	9	21	(52.5)
126	39	5	4	12	21	(53.8)

[a] Intraperitoneally, twice a day for 4 days.
[b] Mg/kg per day.
[c] On day 29.
[d] None of the animals in group A or B developed cataracts or other ocular changes by day 126 after intracerebral inoculation with PBS.

The experimental design was similar to that described in the Materials and Methods Section. Briefly, the mice were earmarked and grouped. At 6 weeks of age, the mice were anesthetized and inoculated with virus (strain G of HSV-2; about 500 LD_{50}). By day 29 after infection, all the virus control group had died (mean day of death, MDD = 3.40 ± 1.07). However, only 33% (20/60) of the virus-inoculated mice in the FIAC-treated group died (MDD = 10.21 ± 4.20) and no mice died in either the uninfected control group or uninfected drug control group. The incidence of cataract among the virus-infected treated mice by day 29 was 43% (17/40). Four, 5 and 8 animals had obvious OD, OS and OU cataracts, respectively. The progressive changes were monitored for an additional 3 months. By day 126 after virus inoculation, 5, 4 and 12 animals had OD, OS and OU cataracts respectively. The incidence of bilateral cataract had increased from 20% to 31%

had OD, OS and OU cataracts respectively. The incidence of bilateral cataract had increased from 20% to 31% and the percent of animals with cataracts increased from 43% to 54%. None of the control mice inoculated with PBS or FIAC (60 mg/kg/day; bid x 4d) developed cataracts or other ocular changes.

Virological, immunological and pathological findings.

Infectious virus could not be recovered at 3 months after inoculation from homogenized extracts of the eyes and brain. However, latent virus (defined as negative isolation of virus from tissue homogenates and positive explant culture) was isolated from two-thirds of the trigeminal ganglia explants homogenized on day 14 after sacrifice. The HSV-antibody titer in the serum of mice inoculated with virus that developed opacities and those that did not was compared to uninfected mice. Serum titers three months after inoculation of randomly selected groups of infected mice (including mice with cataracts) was > 1:256 by virus plaque neutralization assay (by enzyme-linked immunosorbent assay the titer of most mice was > 1:12,800), whereas PBS-inoculated mice had titers of < 1:4.

Documentation of the gross morphology of cataracts was carried out by photography under a stereo microscope. Low power magnification of the cataract as compared to clear lens is shown in Figure I and II. One of the unusual features of the advanced stage of this HSV-induced cataract is a thick white opaque cap over the posterior pole of the lens. This appears to be extracapsular, but it is strongly adherent to the capsule, making it sometimes difficult to remove the lens intact. This part of the lens capsule is known to be the thinnest and most porous part, and it could well be that it is the route of penetration of virus into the lens, if, indeed, there is penetration. Obviously, virus penetration is of great interest to us, and we plan to investigate the morphological and virological changes of the lens capsule.

Pathological ocular changes in mice inoculated with virus or phosphate-buffered saline were studied by light microscopy. The histopathological findings included necrotizing retinitis, granulomatous reaction, posterior migration of lens epithelium, liquefaction of lens fibers, lens shrinkage, fibrous metaphasia of lens epithelium and focally calcified glial scar. A selection of histopathologic sections of normal and cataractous mouse eyes is shown in Figures III-VI.

It should be stressed that the virus infected animals developing unilateral or bilateral cataracts are not debilitated. They continue to gain weight and lead "normal" lives, except for the blindness. They maintain all the reflexes found in apparently normal littermates (infected and uninfected), including blinking reflexes.

DISCUSSION

During studies of new potent antivirals on the development of herpes encephalitis in mice, cataracts and other ocular lesions formed in a significant proportion of the surviving animals. Three other independent reports on the development of lens opacities in mice following intracerebral inoculation with HSV support our findings. While studying the turnover of brain catecholamines in outbred Swiss mice after HSV intracerebral infection, Lycke and Roos (13) noted opacities in one-third of the survivors. No attempt to characterize the opacities was made. More recently, Field *et al* (14) noted the same phenomenon in inbred Balb/c mice inoculated intracerebrally with acyclovir-resistant HSV variants [28% (14 mice) incidence of opacities at 3 months after infection]. These studies have been expanded in an attempt to explain this phenomenon in terms of virus spread from the brain to the eye and antigen distribution in the CNS (15-17). In an abstract by Siegel

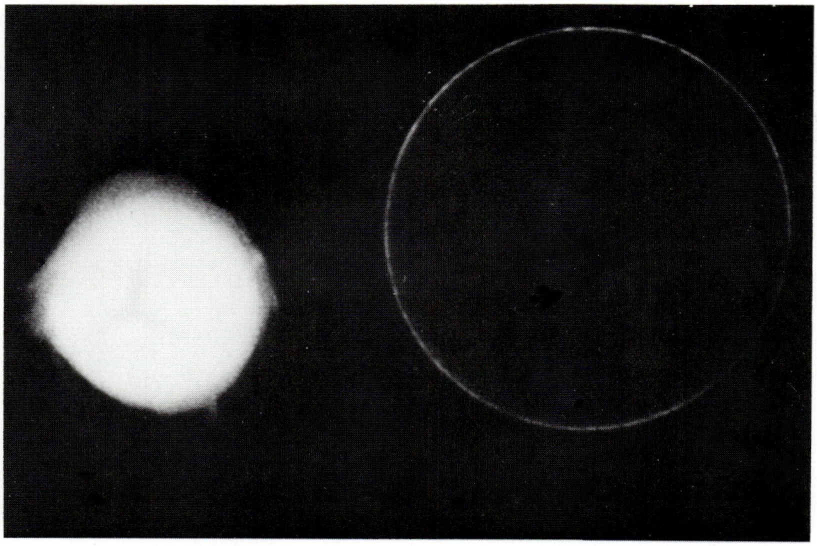

FIGURE I. Gross morphology of lenses from herpes-infected mouse, showing one clear lens (right) and one cataract of which only nucleus remains from the dissection.

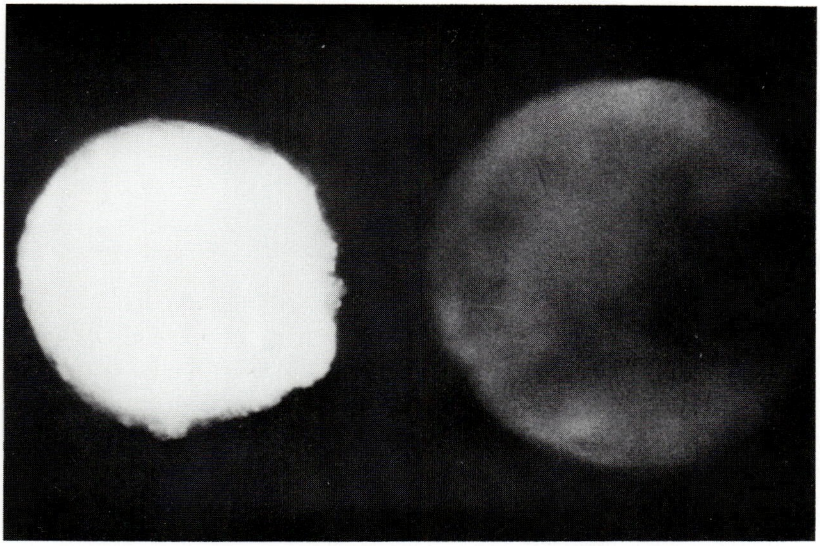

FIGURE II. Lenses from herpes-infected mouse, showing one immature cataract and one resorbing mature cataract.

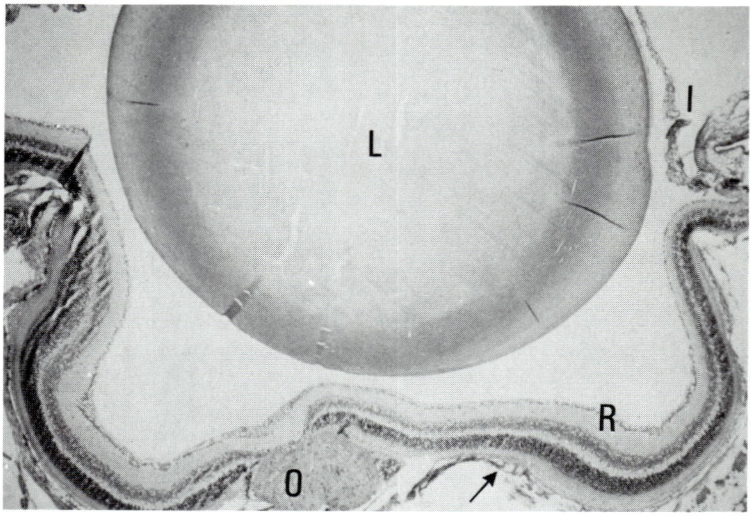

FIGURE III. Uninvolved eye. The lens (L), iris (I), retina (R), choroid (arrow) and optic nerve (O) are intact. H & E, X30

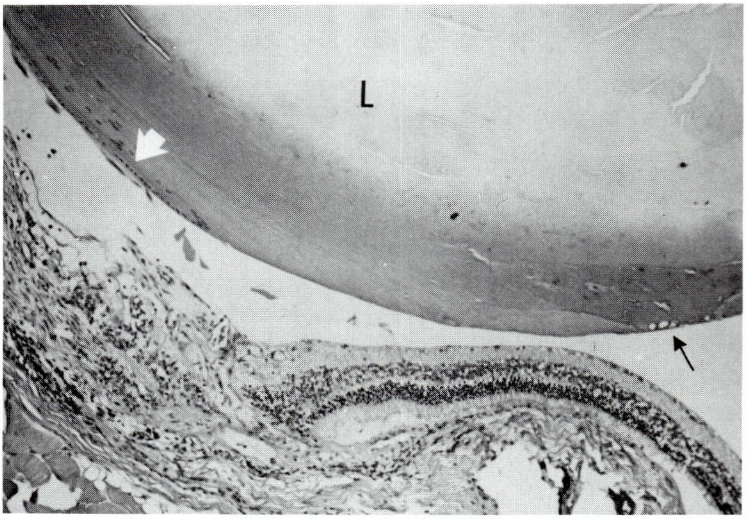

FIGURE IV. Left eye of mouse sacrificed 2 months after virus infection. Focal retinal involvement takes the form of thickening and disruption of retinal tissue; reactive proliferation of retinal pigment epithelium and choroidal inflammatory infiltration (lower left field in photomicrograph); early posterior migration of lens epithelium (white arrow); and mild liquefaction of lens cortex (black arrow). H & E, X75

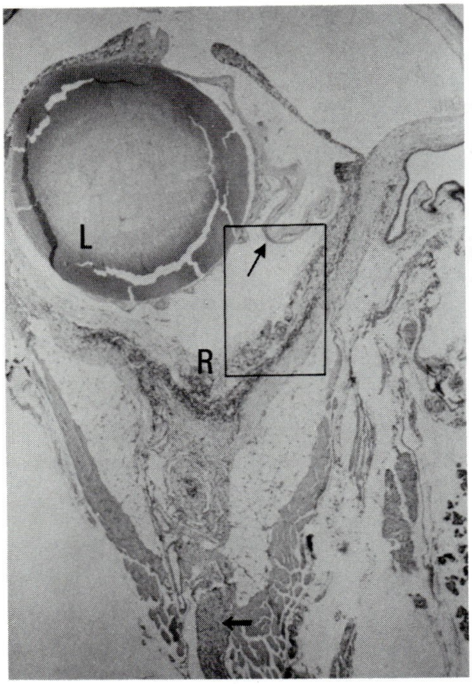

FIGURE V. Severely affected cataractous eye, with marked loss of lens cortex (L); wrinkling of lens capsule and proliferation with fibrous metaplasia of lens epithelium (arrow), replacement of retina by focally calcified glial scar with persistent, chronic granulomatous inflammatory reaction (R); and adjacent choroidal atrophy. The optic nerve (heavy arrow) is markedly atrophic. H & E, X30.

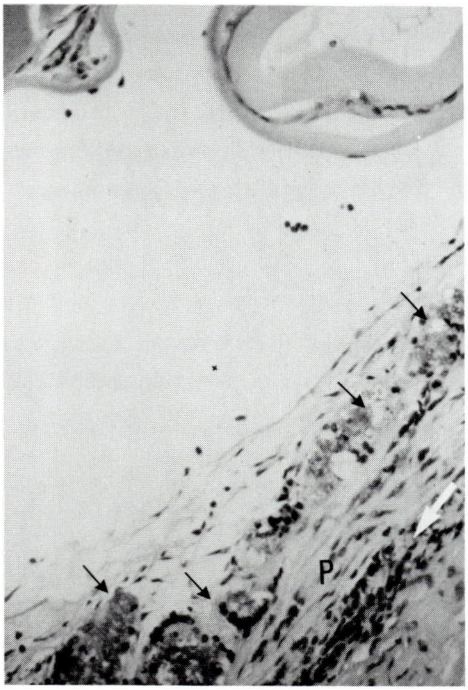

FIGURE VI. Same eye (inset). The wrinkled lens capsule and proliferated lens epithelium appear in the upper field. The atrophic, gliotic retina is focally calcified (arrows), and associated epithelial and foreign-body giant cells characterize the persistent granulomatous infiltration. There is proliferation with fibrous metaplasia of the retinal pigment epithelium (P), and the atrophic choroid contains a round cell inflammatory infiltrate (white arrow). H & E, X132.

et al (18) and in a more recent publication (19) [9.4% (6 mice) incidence of opacities at 11 days after infection], the pathological ocular changes following intracerebral inoculation of mice with HSV-1 were reported. HSV particles were found on the retina by electron microscopy during early virus spread. Of significance is that Field *et al* developed their model using only drug-resistant variants, while we have developed what we believe to be a more clinically relevant model which uses wild-type viruses, which are drug sensitive. It should be stressed that the retinal tropism of HSV is not limited to ACV-resistant HSV strains; wild-type virus will also produce retinitis and cataracts provided the dose of virus is non-lethal or antiviral drugs are used to moderate the pathogenic effect of the virus.

In our mouse model, the onset of cataract formation and ocular changes can be precisely monitored. By careful observations during the early stages of the experimental protocol, it is possible to detect early *in vivo* changes in the eye.

This model is particularly relevant clinically for the following reason. Significant reduction in mortality has been documented in well controlled clinical trials which have established the efficacy of vidarabine therapy for patients with herpes encephalitis or neonatal herpes (20, 21). However, survivors of these infections are frequently left with severe disability (20-22). For example, patients may sustain visual loss due to cataract formation and other lesions of the visual system. There are several well documented cases of patients with herpes encephalitis and/or neonatal herpes who, subsequent to the primary involvement, developed eye lesions (see references cited in 14 and 19). These lesions are similar to those found in our animal model. It is also likely that the incidence of morbidity will increase in patients recovering from HSV encephalitis and neonatal herpes parallel to the development of newer, more effective antivirals (23). Indeed, there is a precedent for this phenomenon in antibacterial therapy (24). For example, following the introduction of effective drugs for bacterial meningitis, chronic disabilities in meningitis survivors became increasingly apparent. By learning with this model the mechanism(s) by which the virus spreads from the brain or other sites to the eye causing these lesions, we may discover how to prevent or better treat these visual handicaps associated with severe herpetic infections. This mouse model may also be useful in predicting the effectiveness of new antivirals in preventing ocular lesions induced by HSV in humans.

ACKNOWLEDGEMENTS

This investigation was supported in part by funds from the National Institutes of Health (AI 18600 and AG 04214) and by a Merit Award from the Veterans Administration. Part of this work was also presented at ARVO 1984 [see Invest. Ophthalmol Vis Sci (1984) 25 S:23].

REFERENCES

1. Hammond EC, Spalter HF (1973) Am J Ophthalmol 76:389

2. Van Heyningen R (1969) In: Davson H (ed), The Eye (ed 2, Vol 1). Academic Press, New York

3. Cotlier E, Fox J (1966) In: Dardenne MU, Nordmann J (eds) Biochemistry of the eye. S.Karger, Basel, pp 467-477 and references cited therein

4. Merser MA, Harley JD, Hertzberg R, Dorman DC, Murphy MA (1967) Lancet ii, pp 387-388 and references cited therein

5. Cibis A, Burde RM (1971) Arch Ophthalmol 85:220-223

6. Kuck JFR (1970) In: Graymore CN (ed) Biochemistry of the Eye. Academic Press, New York

7. Kinoshita JH (1975) Invest Ophthalmol 4:786-799

8. Van Heyningen R, Pirie A (1967) Biochem J 102:842-852

9. Schinazi R, Peters J, Williams CC, Chance D, Nahmias AJ (1982) Antimicrob Agents Chemother 22:499-507

10. Hollwich F, Boateng A, Kolck B (1975) In: Bellows JG (ed) Cataract and Abnormalities of the Lens. Grune and Stratton Inc, New York

11. Pavan-Langston D, Park NH, Lass J, Papale J, Albert DM, Lin TS, Prusoff WH, Percy DH (1982) Proc Soc Exp Biol Med 170:1-7

12. Kuck JFR (1977) In: Dikstein S (ed) Drugs and Ocular Tissues. S Karger, Basel

13. Lycke E, Roos B-E (1975) J Neurol Sci 26:49-60

14. Field HJ, Anderson JR, Wildy P (1982) J Gen Virol 59:91-99

15. Anderson JR, Field HJ (1982) Neuropathol Applied Neurobiol 8:277-287

16. Anderson JR, Field HJ (1983) J Neurol Sciences 60:181-195

17. Anderson JR, Field HJ (1984) Brit J Exp Path (in press)

18. Siegel FL, Sibrack CD, Peiffer RL (1982) Federation Proceedings Abstract 2495, New Orleans, p 697

19. Peiffer RL, Dekker Jr, CD, Siegel FL (1983) Assoc Res Vis Ophthalmol 24:1070-1078

20. Whitley RJ and Alford CA (1981) In: Nahmias AJ, Dowdle W.R., Schinazi RF (eds) The Human Herpesviruses - an interdisciplinary perspective. Elsevier North-Holland, New York, pp 478-495

21. Whitley RJ, Soong S-J, Linneman C, Liu C, Pazin G, Alford CA and the NIAID Collaborative Antiviral Study Group (1982) J Am Med Assoc 242:317-320; and Whitley *et al* (1983) Pediat 72:778-785

22. Chin D, Edis R (1982) Lancet, ii, 870

23. Schinazi RF, Prusoff WH (1983) Pediat Clin N Am 30:77-92

24. Feldman WE, Ginsburg CM, McCracken GH, Jr, Allen D, Ahmann P, Graham J, Graham L (1982) J Pediat 100:209-212 and references therein.

VI CLINICAL EXPERIENCES WITH ANTIVIRAL DRUGS AND INTERFERON

ACYCLOVIR TREATMENT FOR HERPES SIMPLEX VIRUS ENCEPHALITIS

H.SHOJI, M.ARAMAKI, M.KAJI, Y.KITAHARA[1], Y.KURODA[2], S.OHTANI[3]

1st Dept of Internal Medicine, Kurume University School of Medicine,
1 Dept of Internal Medicine, Kyushu Rosai Hospital, 2 Dept of Neurology, Saga Medical School, 3 Tokyo Seninhoken Hospital, Japan.

Herpes simplex virus (HSV) encephalitis is now one of the most common causes of nonepidemic encephalitis in Japan. Antiviral drugs have been administered because of the high mortality of this disease (1,2). We present here the results of acyclovir (ACV) treatment for HSV encephalitis.

PATIENTS AND ACV TREATMENT

Seven patients had HSV encephalitis including one with meningitis. The diagnosis was made from a combination of the clinical findings, CT, EEG and antibody response (CF and ELISA) to HSV in serum and CSF, though these antibodies' response was apt to be proved retrospectively. ACV 10 mg/kg was given intravenously by infusion three times daily for 10 days. In principle, ACV treatment was applied at the acute stage, except for the two patients to whom it was alternately with Ara-A aministration.

RESULTS

The outcome of ACV tretment in the 7 cases is shown in Table 1. One patient died of an accidental complication, and the mortality of our series was 14 %. Two patients who received the alternative therapy with Ara-A had severe sequelae - tetraplegia and apallic state respectively. The remaining four had good recoveries. The only side effects were slight elevations of the serum GOT, GPT and

TABLE 1
SUMMARY OF ACV TREATMENT

Cases	CF	ELISA*	Drugs	Neurol. status**	Outcome
1 38/M	+	+	Ara-A→ACV	lethargy	tetraplegia
2 27/F	+	+	ACV	lethargy	no sequelae
3 64/F	+	+	ACV	coma	death
4 4m/F	+	-	ACV	lethargy	no sequelae
5 50/M	+	+	Ara-A→ACV	coma	apallic state
6 18/M	+	n.d.	ACV	lethargy	no sequelae
7 36/F	-	-	ACV	stupor	no sequelae

*CF>64 in serum or >1 in CSF ** on the beggining of ACV
ELISA>1.5 in CSF (by Dr.Mizutani)

LDH in two patients.

Next, we would like to present the ACV treatment for two cases: a severe form of HSV encephalitis and a meningitis type.

Case 3, a 64 year-old female, was admitted to our hospital on the 7th day after the appearence of neurological symptoms. On admission, her state was comatose. CSF examination revealed moderate pleocytosis. CT and EEG exhibited localized abnormalities in the right temporal and frontal lobes. Immediately ACV treatment was begun. She responded to pain stimulation on the 10th day of the treatment. But she acutely died of gastrointestinal bleeding 1 month after admission. An autopsy was not performed. Significant increases of CF and ELISA were confirmed retrospectively. Case 4, a 4 month-old girl, was admitted to our hospital on the 4th day after the appearence of meningeal signs. On admission, severe herpetic eruptions were observed periorally. Moderate pleocytosis was present, but CT and EEG showed no abnormalities. This case was reparded as HSV meningitis, and ACV treatment was begun. The skin eruptions and neurological signs improved rapidly within a few days after treatment began.

DISCUSSION

ACV is an antiviral drug with selective activity against the herpes groups. Results of ACV double blind studies to HSV encephalitis have now been published. Recently Skölderberg et al reported ACV reduced the mortality rate (19%) compared to Ara-A treatment (50%). Although our study was uncontrolled trial, ACV treatment showed efficacy in the evaluation of the neurological findings, sequelae etc.. In the one case of death, delayed start of ACV administration might be related to the bad prognosis. On the other hand, severe brain swelling often occurs in this encephalitis. Infusion is restricted during the acute stage. It may be pointed out that ACV could be given with small infusions because of good solubility.

REFERENCES

1. Whitley J R, Soong S-J et al. (1977) Adenine arabinoside therapy of biopsy-proved herpes simplex encephalitis. N Engl J Med 299:289-294.
2. Ohtani S, Aoyama Y et al. (1982) Therapeutic effect of Ara-A on herpes simplex virus encephalitis. J Jpn Ass Infect Dis 56:799-824.
3. Sköldenberg B, Forgren M et al. (1984) Acyclovir versus vidarabine in herpes encephalitis. Lancet II:707-711.

Herpes Viruses and Virus Chemotherapy, R. Kono, editor

CLINICAL EVALUATION OF ACICLOVIR FOR THE TREATMENT OF HERPES VIRUS INFECTION IN THE IMMUNOCOMPROMISED HOSTS

T. MASAOKA

Department of Internal Medicine, Center for Adult disease, Osaka

INTRODUCTION

Herpes infection is often complicated in immunocompromised patients. For its treatment, however, no reliable drug has been available.

Aciclovir developed by Wellcome Foundation was reported to be very effective for such diseases.

In order to clarify the efficacy and toxicity of Aciclovir in immunocompromised patients, a phase II study and a randomised controlled study were conducted by the Aciclovir study group in Japan.

PATIENTS AND METHODS

In the phase II study, 144 patients with VZV, HSV or CMV infections were treated with Aciclovir 5mg/kg 3times/day × 5days (Table 1).

The underlying diseases were mainly leukemia, lymphoma and solid tumors.

Table 1.

Phase II Study of Aciclovir in Immunocompromised Patients
—patients' background—

background \ causative virus		VZV	HSV	CMV	not determined	total
No. of cases		92	25	4	23	144
Sex	Male	45	8	2	16	71
	Female	47	17	2	7	73
Age (mean 41.5 y/o)	−20	24	6	2	6	38
	21−50	26	8	2	14	50
	51−	42	11	0	3	56
Start of Aciclovir* (mean 5.84th day)	1− 3	36	12	0	8	56
	4− 6	34	6	0	6	46
	7−	22	7	4	7	40
Daily dosage* (mg/kg/day)	<15	11	2	0	4	17
	15	73	21	3	14	111
	>15	8	2	1	3	14
Days of administration	mean 8.0days (range 3 − 56days)					

* 2 patients were excluded due to prophylactic use after BMT

Table 2. Criteria of response

Excellent	3 days
Good	5 days
Fair	7 days
No response	later than 7 days

In the double blind (DB) controlled study, 20 patients were treated with Aciclovir 5mg/kg 3times/day × 7days and 18 patients with manitol as placebo. In this study no significant differences in background factors were observed between the groups. Criteria of response was shown in Table 2.

RESULTS

In the phase II study, Aciclovir gave a very high response rate (Table 3) which was observed by the rapid improvement in pain, erythema, vesicle formation and crusting.

There was a tendency for the response to be better when Aciclovir administration was started earlier (Fig 1).

Side effects were mild and reversible and were seen in only five of 144 patients (Hepatic injury and skin rash occured in the same patient). (Table 4)

Table 3. Response to Aciclovir in Phase II Study

Causative virus	Disease	No. of Cases	Clinical Efficacy				not evaluated
			excellent	good	fair	no response	
VZV	Herpes Zoster	83	33 (40.7)	42 (51.8)	6 (7.4)	0	2
	Varicella	9	1	8	0	0	0
HSV	Herpes Simplex local	24	11 (45.8)	10 (41.7)	3 (12.5)		
	Herpes Simplex generalized	1	0	1	0	0	0
CMV		4	1	1	1	1	0
not determined		23	2	7	6	2	6
Total		144	48 (33.3)	69 (47.9)	16 (11.1)	3 (2.1)	8 (5.6)

( ) : %

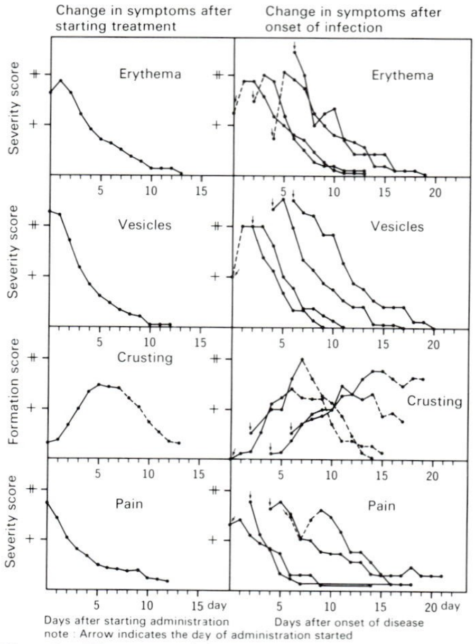

Fig. 1. (Phase II study)

Table 4. Side Effects (144 cases)

Side effects	Relation to Aciclovir		
	Sure	Probable	Uncertain
Hepatic injury	1	2*	5
Skin rash	0	2*	1
Albuminuria	0	1	0
Nausea	0	0	1
Vasopressin demand increased	0	0	1
Total	1	5	8

* in the same patient

In the DB study, statistically significant differences ($p < 0.05$) were observed in effective rate, general improvement and the grade of erythema on the 6th and 7th days after starting administration (Fig 2, Table 5).

Table 5.

Randomised Controlled Study of Aciclovir

Aciclovir : 5 mg/kg × 3 times/day × 7 days

Placebo : mannitol

Drug		Aciclovir	Placebo
Total No. of cases		20	18
Cases used for analysis		17	10
Effective rate*		82.4%	30.0%
Grade of erythema*	(on day 6)	1.29±1.16	2.40±1.08
	(on day 7)	1.18±1.13	2.20±1.32
Grade of general improvement*	(on day 6)	2.35±1.06	1.30±1.42

* significant at $p < 0.05$

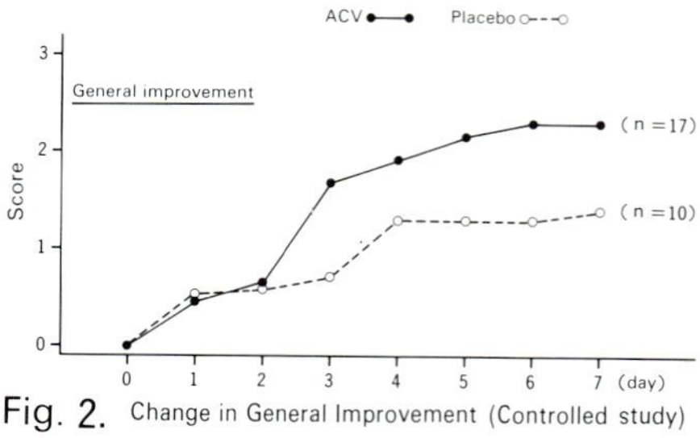

Fig. 2. Change in General Improvement (Controlled study)

CONCLUSION

In the phase II and DB study Aciclovir was highly effective against VZV and HSV infections. The response was better when treatment was started earlier. There were no serious side effects.

Aciclovir is considered very promising for the treatment of such viral disesase because it is very effective and shows few side effects.

LOW DOSE ORAL ACYCLOVIR PROPHYLAXIS AGAINST HERPESVIRUS INFECTIONS IN RENAL ALLOGRAFT RECIPIENTS *

LINDA SEALE, CAROL JONES, SHASHI KATHPALIA, GEORGE GEE JACKSON, MARTIN MOSES and DONALD PACKHAM

The Section of Infectious Diseases, Department of Medicine and Transplant Surgical Unit, Department of Surgery, University of Illinois Hospital, University of Illinois College of Medicine at Chicago, USA

In a double-blind, randomized controlled study, low dose oral acyclovir given prophylactically was compared to placebo in 39 patients receiving renal transplants. Prophylaxis was begun prior to transplantation with a single 400 mg dose, and was continued post-operatively for thirty days, at a dose of 200 mg every eight hours if renal function was adequate. Acyclovir prophylaxis prevented viral shedding in all but 1 of 18 (6%) drug treated patients, while 14 of 21 (67%) of placebo recipients shed virus during the 30 day period of prophylaxis. At the completion of the 90 day trial period, overall 9 of 17 (54%) acyclovir recipients had no positive cultures, compared to only 2 of 19 (11%) placebo recipients. Both trends were statistically significant, the first at a level of less than 1/1000 and the latter less than 5% chance. Clinically apparent disease was present in 13 of 17 (76%) culture positive, placebo treated patients at the end of 90 days, whereas lesions due to HSV developed in only 3 of 8 (13%) culture positive patients previously treated with acyclovir. The exacerbation of HSV infection was significantly more frequent in persons of the black race and in those above 40 years, the median age of the group. Male patients and those given an allograft from a living related donor had fewer episodes of infection than females and persons with a cadaver allograft. Immunosuppression with azathioprine and antilymphocyte globulin or cyclosporine had no difference on the frequence of infection. All patients received prednisone. Prophylactic acyclovir reduced the frequency, delayed the appearance and ameliorated the severity of recurrent HSV infection in these patients. No toxicity or adverse responses were observed.

* The investigation was supported by a grant fund from the Burroughs Wellcome Company, Research Triangle Park, North Carolina

EXPERIENCE WITH ACYCLOVIR AFTER HERPES VIRUS INFECTION IN RENAL TRANSPLANTED PATIENTS

DENNIN, R.H., SCHULZ, E., DAHLHOFF, K., SACK, K.
Institut für Medizinische Mikrobiologie und Klinik für Innere Medizin; Medizinische Hochschule Lübeck, Ratzeburger Allee 160, 2400 Lübeck 1, Fed. Rep. Germany

Introduction

Mucocutaneous herpes simplex virus (HSV) infections are frequent events in patients after immunosuppressive therapy; after kidney transplantation morbidity rates in the range of 50% have been reported (1); mostly with good prognosis - but sporadic disseminated infections occur including the central nervous system.
Acyclovir represents a drug for effective therapy of HSV caused diseases with only rare side effects; furthermore with ciclosporine a new immunosuppressive drug is available which enhances the transplant survival and further is supposed to reduce the risks for infections compared to previous immunosuppressive regimen (2).
From this point of view the present study should demonstrate the incidence of HSV-infections/diseases, the usefulnes of diagnostic parameters as well as the virus chemotherapy with kidney transplanted patients under modern regimes of immunosuppressive therapy.

Patients and Methods

54 patients - kidney transplanted between 6/1982 and 2/1984-were studied; immunosuppressive therapy was with ciclosporine and prednisolone (exceptions: 2 patients were treated with azathioprine/prednisolone); ciclosporine therapy: initial dosage 14 mg/kg/d reduced to 6 to 8 mg/kg/d in the course of 3 to 6 month; ciclosporine concentration was controlled by blood level determinations.
Specimens for HSV isolations were throat gargles and vaginal smears resp. conjunctival smears collected in physiological NaCl-solution; HeLa cell cultures were incubated with the specimens; culture medium: MEM, hepes buffered + 2.5% calf serum; antigen-typing of the HSV-isolates was done with a monoclonal antibody test system.

Results

Herpes simplex virus could be isolated from 22 of the 54 patients; 11 of the 22 showed clinical signs of HSV infections: stomatitis, vulvovaginitis and conjunctivitis.

All HSV isolates were of serotype 1.
2/11 patients with clinical signs were treated by reduction of ciclosporin dosage only; this was at the time when acyclovir wasn't yet available. The other 9/11 patients with clinical signs were treated with acyclovir (5 mg/kg/d for 5 to 8 days). Patients treated with acyclovir showed reduction of symptoms very quickly; all patients treated with acyclovir even with severe course of the disease reported they were free of pains 1 to 2 days after acyclovir treatment began. in 10 of the 11 patients the infectious process remained locally; the one case with disseminated HSV-retinitis could only be stopped by acyclovir but the defect remained at the stage the treatment began.
With one exception it failed to isolate HSV after acyclovir treatment began: the days and weeks thereafter. The one exception is one patient who developed a second HSV caused disease: conjunctivitis.

Herpes Viruses and Virus Chemotherapy, R. Kono, editor

VIRAL RESISTANCE IN CLINICAL PRACTICE: SUMMARY OF FIVE YEARS EXPERIENCE WITH ACYCLOVIR

DAVID W. BARRY, M.D. AND SANDRA NUSINOFF LEHRMAN, M.D.

Departments of Clinical Investigation and Virology, Burroughs Wellcome Co., 3030 Cornwallis Road, Research Triangle Park, N.C.

Changes in the sensitivity of microorganisms to chemotherapeutic agents during the course of therapy is a universal phenomenon. "Resistance", defined as a change to markedly decreased sensitivity, has been induced in vitro by virtually all antibacterial, antifungal, antiparasitic and antiviral agents. Our studies with acyclovir, therefore, were undertaken to determine the frequency, circumstances, and clinical implications of the development of resistance in patients receiving antiviral therapy.

The quantitative relationship between the in vitro susceptibility of herpes simplex virus to acyclovir (ACV) and the clinical response to therapy has not been established in man. Sensitivity results, expressed as the concentration of drug required to inhibit by 50% the growth of virus in tissue culture ("the ID_{50} value"), vary greatly depending upon the particular assay used (1), the cell type employed (2) and the laboratory performing the test. Using a dye-uptake method in Vero cells (3) which gives ID_{50} values approximately 10-fold higher than plaque reduction assays, 1417 isolates from approximately 500 patients were examined over a 5-year period. The isolates were not randomly selected, and emphasis was given to examining in detail those virus isolates from patients where there was some suspicion that resistance might be present.

The results of dye-uptake sensitivity testing on these clinical isolates is summarized below.

CUMULATIVE DISTRIBUTION OF ACV ID_{50} BY DYE UPTAKE ASSAY
1417 ISOLATES

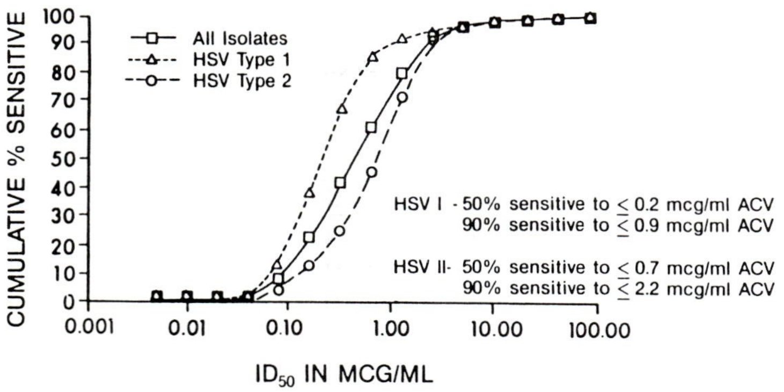

Isolates with significantly diminished sensitivity were found in some patients. They may be divided as follows:

1. Twenty patients were found to have pretherapy isolates which were significantly less sensitive to ACV than normal isolates. While the origin of this diminished sensitivity is unclear, none of the patients had received prior ACV therapy and the response to therapy with ACV could not be distinguished from that of patients whose pretherapy isolates were sensitive to ACV.

2. Viruses of significantly diminished sensitivity to ACV were isolated from nine immunocompetent patients while they were receiving ACV. Similar isolates were obtained from an additional nine patients who received only placebo. The patient's clinical course and response to therapy could not be distinguished from those patients from whom sensitive virus or no virus was obtained during the course of therapy.

3. Twelve severely immunocompromised patients shed viruses with significantly reduced sensitivity to ACV. In some, isolation of these viruses was associated with a diminished clinical response allowing the virus to be termed "resistant" (4). In all cases, the patient was severely immunocompromised (after bone marrow transplantation or because of severe combined immunodeficiency disease) and all had received prolonged or repeated courses of ACV. In some instances these viruses were shed asymptomatically and disappeared spontaneously, whereas in others, they were obtained from chronic indolent ulcers which neither worsened nor improved dramatically with further therapy. None of these viruses caused life-threatening disease in any of the patients.

4. Markedly less sensitive viruses were obtained from three patients with breakthrough recurrences during one four-month study of suppressive oral ACV (5). No such isolates were obtained from patients in a similar but larger study (6). In two of the three patients acyclovir was continued, the lesions healed rapidly, and further lesions were not observed on subsequent suppressive therapy. When ACV was discontinued the patients returned to their normal pattern of recurrence and only sensitive virus could be isolated from their lesions.

Ongoing studies are being performed in an attempt to determine the relationship of *in vitro* sensitivity, achievable serum drug concentrations and clinical response to therapy.

REFERENCES

1. Barry DW, Blum MR (1983) In: Turner P, Shand DG (eds) Recent Advances in Clinical Pharmacology. Churchill Livingstone, Edinburgh pp 57-80

2. DeClerq E (1982) Antimicrob Agents Chemother 21:661-3

3. McLaren C, Ellis MN, Hunter GA (1983) Antiviral Res 3:223-34

4. Dekker C, Ellis MN, McLaren C, Hunter G, Rogers J, Barry DW (1983) J Antimicrob Chemother 12(B):137-152

5. Straus SE, Takiff HE, Seidlin M, Bachrach S, Lininger L, DiGiovanna JJ, Western KA, Smith HA, Nusinoff Lehrman S, Creagh Kirk T (1983) N Engl J Med 310:1545-50

6. Nusinoff Lehrman S, Hunter G, Rogers J, Corey L, Davis G, Barry D (1984) Abstracts of the 24th Interscience Conference on Antimicrobial Agents and Chemotherapy

Herpes Viruses and Virus Chemotherapy, R. Kono, editor

TREATMENT OF RECURRENT GENITAL HERPES WITH PS-K

TAKASHI KAWANA
Department of Obstetrics & Gynecology, Faculty of Medicine, University of Tokyo.
7-3-1, Bunkyo-ku, Hongo, Tokyo, Japan 113

INTRODUCTION

Treatment of recurrent genital herpes is one of the biggest matter of concern. Many studies indicated that recurrence of genital herpes is not related to humoral immunity but to cell mediated immunity. Therefore some attempts have been made to prevent recurrence of genital herpes using biological responce modifiers (BRM) such as BCG[1)], Levamisol with successful result to some extent. PS-K, a proteinbound polysaccharide, is a kind of BRM developed in Japan and being used for immunotherapy of cancer. Effect of administration of PS-K on recurrent genital herpes was investigated.

PATIENTS

19 female and 5 male patients, aged 20-61 years, with recurrent genital herpes were studied. All of these patients were diagnosed by virus isolation. Two female cases were caused by HSV-1 and remaining 22 by HSV-2.

PS-K

PS-K was given at the daily dose of 3.0-5.0 gr per os.

RESULTS

1) Duration of illness

Duration of illness prior to and during administration of PS-K was compared. In all but three cases, duration of illness shortened after taking this drug. In 15 cases, it became less than half.

2) Frequency of recurrence

Frequency of recurrence per three months were compared. Nineteen out of 24 recurrent cases experienced a decrease in the frequency of recurrent infections. In three cases, recurrent episode has not occured more than 1 year.

3) Side effect

No side effect was observed at all.

EFFECT OF PSK ON RECURRENT GENITAL HERPES

Patient		Age	Sex	Type of HSV	Duration of illness (day)		Frequencies per three months	
					before	during	before	during
31	M.H.	36	F	2	10.0	3.4	2.0	1.3
100	K.N.	28	F	1	6.0	0	3.0	0*
92	M.S.	61	F	2	14.8	3.0	2.0	1.0
112	A.H.	35	F	2	10.3	2.8	2.0	2.0
122	H.H.	43	F	2	7.0	3.2	3.0	1.7
106	A.Y.	53	F	1	10.2	6.0	3.0	3.4
111	S.T.	30	F	2	10.0	4.5	3.0	1.9
142	Y.H.	32	F	2	7.0	3.0	6.0	1.5
155	K.T.	31	F	2	12.0	6.0	3.0	0.6
162	O.H.	66	F	2	5.0	3.0	3.0	0.9
168	K.U.	31	F	2	5.0	3.5	4.0	3.0
175	Y.E.	25	F	2	9.8	6.5	2.3	0.5*
200	O.K.	22	F	2	6.3	3.0	3.0	1.2
240	H.M.	23	F	2	6.6	6.3	3.0	1.0
244	K.Y.	35	F	2	10.0	5.1	6.0	3.0
251	K.S.	32	F	2	7.0	5.0	1.5	1.0
265	O.H.	20	F	2	5.6	8.1	6.0	1.6
272	A.Y.	49	F	2	10.0	4.2	3.0	4.0
285	M.Y.	23	F	2	6.8	7.5	3.0	0.8
M-4	S.T.	28	M	2	13.0	4.0	4.2	3.2
M-19	K.K.	28	M	2	14.8	3.8	1.0	1.0
M-2	I.Y.	31	M	2	14.0	7.2	2.0	0.5
M-18	N.S.	35	M	2	7.0	3.0	1.5	0.5
M-11	S.T.	36	M	2	10.0	3.0	6.0	1.5*

* No recurrence for more than 1 year

COMMENTS

Though the mechanisms, which may be involved in the efficacy of this drug, has not yet been elucidated, it seems that the activity of this drug to enhance cellular immunity observed when administered in animal and man led to this favorable effect.

If further investigation confirms these findings, PS-K may well become a useful agent in the treatment of recurrent genital herpes.

REFERENCES

1) Anderson FD, et.al (1974), obstat gynecal 43:797,

2) Kint A, et.al (1974), N. Engl. J. Med. 291:308

3) Akiyama J. et. al (1977) Can. Research 37:3042

THE MANAGEMENT OF HERPES SIMPLEX ENCEPHALITIS IN JAPAN AND SOME OF ITS RELATED PROBLEMS

T. TAKASU, S. KAMEI, E. TAMURA, S. OTANI*, H. MIZUTANI**

Department of Neurology, Nihon University School of Medicine, 30-1, Ohyaguchi-kamimachi, Itabashi-ku, Tokyo (Japan 173), Tokyo Sen-in Hospital, Tokyo (Japan)*, Virus Laboratory, Kanto Teishin Hospital, Tokyo (Japan)**

INTRODUCTION

In Japan, a research group organized in 1980 (headed by S. Ohtani) conducted a clinical trial of Adenine arabinoside (Ara-A) in herpes simplex encephalitis during the one-and-a half-year period from that year.

MATERIAL, METHODS AND RESULTS

(1) One hundred and six patients with Herpes simplex encephalitis (HSE) were collected. The year, month, place, age of onset and sex were analysed.

(2) The antibody against Herpes simplex virus (HSV) in cerebrospinal fluid (CSF) was estimated both with complement fixation (CF) and with enzyme-linked immunoadsorbent assay (ELISA). Brain biopsy was not done.

(3) ELISA was proved to be more sensitive than CF, but because of this sensitivity, even minute quantities of antibody could be detected in CSF of non-HSE patients with cerebrovascular disorder or with polyclonal stimulation.

(4) Ninety-two patients were treated with Adenine arabinoside (Ara-A ; Vidarabine) during the one-and-a half-year period from 1981 to 1982.

Of these, only 55 were diagnosed as Herpes simplex encephalitis (HSE) retrospectively.

(5) The side effects of Ara-A treatment were non-serious and transitory so far as a certain regimen was maintained.

(6) Ara-A treatment was effective in improving prognosis.

(7) However, the start of Ara-A treatment was delayed in almost three fourths of the patients.

DISCUSSION

In addition to the re-confirmation of the effect of Ara-A and its usefulness for the treatment of this encephalitis, this study revealed that actually in 74% (34/46) of the cases the treatment was started only after the third week of the illness.

For good therapecutic results, early treatment is required and for early treatment early diagnosis is required. However, unfortunately early diagnosis is not always possible. The appearance of symptoms and signs of encephalopathy makes us suspect the possibility of this encephalitis.

With more features specific for this encephalitis manifested, the validity of our diagnosis becomes more probable. Establishment of the herpes simplex etiology awaits the demonstration either of virus antigen in the brain biopsy specimen or, although less definite, of a significant rise of antibodies against the virus in serum or cerebrospinal fluid. For various reasons it takes not rarely too much time to avoid the delay in starting the treatment and in Japan brain biopsy is not feasible for social reasons.

What about the outcome that would be expected if the treatment with Ara-A were started sometime before the etiology has been established? Delay in starting the treatment and the chance of undertreatment, i.e. the chance of not treating true herpes simplex encephalitis could be avoided. On the other hand the chance of overtreatment, i.e. the chance of treating non-herpes simplex cases with Ara-A would be substantial. As a matter of fact our experience in Japan showed that the 37 out of 92 Ara-A treated cases, i.e. 40%, were not herpes simplex encephalitis if retrospectively scrutinized. Overtreatment should not be allowed if the side effect of the treatment is not tolerable. Fortunately the side effects observed in our cases were all non-serious and transitory.

CONCLUSION

The authors would like to stress the importance of intensive clinical examination of all cases of encephalopathy with all feasible means in the initial days of the illness, and to speak for starting Ara-A treatment without delay even if the etiology has not been established for some reasons. Future development of reliable and harmless measure for early diagnosis is awaited.

REFERENCES

1. Otani S, Aoyama Y et al: A clinical trial of Ara-A in the treatment of herpes simplex virus encephalitis. J Jpn Soc Infect Dis 56:799, 1982 (In Japanese with English abstract)
2. Mizutani H, Mizutani H et al: Serological diagnosis of herpes simplex encephalitis — an evaluation of ELISA for its diagnosis —. J Jpn Soc Infect Dis 57: , 1983 (In Japanese with English abstract)
3. Takasu T, Kamei S, Tamura E et al: Clinical features of herpes simplex encephalitis in Japan and some therapeutic problems. J. Jpn Soc Intern Med (in preparation in Japanese with English abstract)
4. Kamei S, Takasu T, Tamura E et al: Enzyme-linked immunoadsorbent assay (ELISA) the diagnosis of herpes simplex encephalitis. Clinical Neurology (in preparation in Japanese with English abstract)

EVALUATION OF ANTIVIRAL ACTIVITY AND THERAPEUTIC EFFICACY OF ARA-A ON CHRONIC HBV INFECTION

SHIRO SUZUKI, SHOZO WATANABE, TETSUO ITO, and TAKESHI TANAKA

Third Department of Internal Medicine, Mie University School of Medicine, Tsu, Mie, 514 (JAPAN)

INTRODUCTION

Adenine arabinoside (Ara-a) was reported to have antiviral effect to Hepatitis B Virus (HBV) and resulted in continuous depression of HBV replication in some persistent HBV infected patients, indicating therapeutic effect to chronic type B hepatitis. However the therapeutic efficacy of Ara-a treatment to chronic type B hepatitis was reportedly not so high; persistent depression of HBV replication in 30% of treated cases at most. In order to increase efficacious rate of Ara-a, many trials are now going to perform concering a schedule of Ara-a treatment or a combination with other agents.

In this paper results of our trials of 2 courses Ara-a treatment were described.

PATIENTS AND SCHEDULES OF ARA-A TREATMENT

Chronic type B hepatitis cases with positive HBeAg were treated with Ara-a of 10mg/kg/day for 4 weeks (1st course). After 2 weeks of pause, if possible, another 4 weeks of Ara-a treatment was performed (2nd course). Patients given only 1st course were called 1 course group (25 cases) and those who completed 2nd course, 2 courses group (34 cases). Diagnosis of all patients were biopsy proven. During and after the Ara-a treatment HBV markers (HBsAg, HBeAg, AntiHBs, AntiHBe, and DNA-P) were estimated using appropriate methods, and routine liver function tests and ordinary clinical observations were carried out. Only the cases with positive HBeAg at the start of Ara-a treatment were included into our study. Number of cases in each group and several other characteristics such as age, sex, etc. were summarized in Table I. There was no conspicuous difference between both groups in usual clinical backgrounds.

TABLE I

CLINICAL BACKGROUNDS OF ARA-A TREATED CASES

	1 course group	2 courses group
No. of Cases	25	34
Mean age ± S.E.	31.0 ± 1.84	32.1 ± 1.88
Sex Male	20	25
Female	5	9
Liver Histology CAH	20	27
CIH	5	7

RESULTS

DNA-P activity was significantly decreased after 1 course of Ara-a treatment comparing with pretreatment level. In 2 courses group, another Ara-a treatment resulted in more conspicuous reduction of DNA-P after the 2 courses of Ara-a. Changes of HBeAg titers expressed in cut off indices were illustrated in Fig.1. Ara-a treatment resulted in more conspicuous and significant reduction of HBeAg in 2 courses group even 6 months after the end of Ara-a treatment. As to HBsAg titers no significant change by Ara-a treatment was observed in both groups.

Decrease or normalization of serum GPT was observed and it coincided with HBeAg decrease or disappearance. No prominent adverse effect was observed except for slight bone marrow inhibition and gastrointestinal disorders.

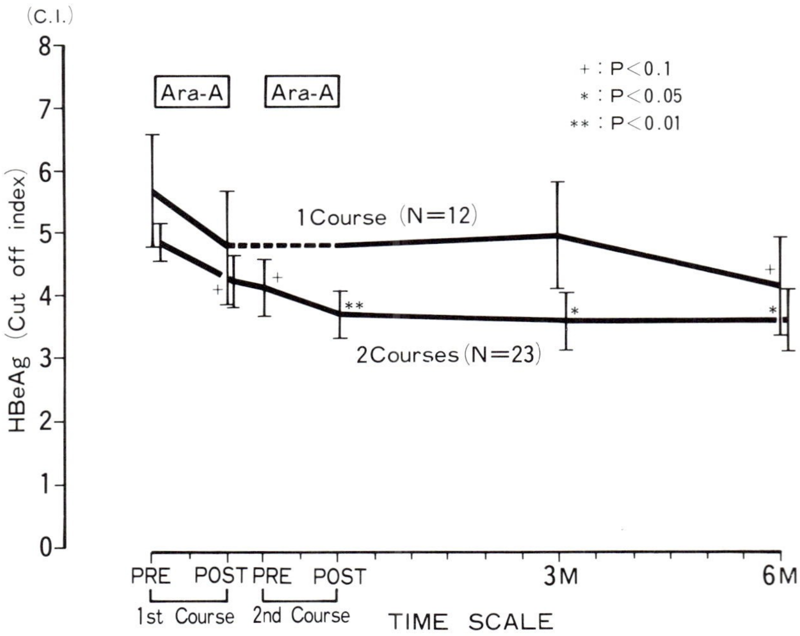

Fig. 1. Changes of HBeAg titers during and after Ara-a treatment.

CONCLUSION

Ara-a had a potent antiviral activity to chronic HBV infections. It significantly lowered DNA-P levels and HBeAg titers not only just after Ara-a treatment but 6 months later. Inhibition of HBV replication was more conspicuously observed in cases given 2 courses of Ara-a treatment. Inhibition of HBV replication coincided with lowering of transaminase levels.

INTERFERON THERAPY OF RECURRENCES OF GENITAL HERPES

LAWRENCE J. ERON, CINDY TOY, AND DONNA SANTOMAURO

Division of Infectious Diseases, The Fairfax Hospital, Fairfax, Virginia, and Medical Research, The Schering Corporation, Kenilworth, New Jersey (USA)

INTRODUCTION

Genital herpes simplex type 2 infections are most troublesome because of their tendency to recur. Trials demonstrating the efficacy of orally administered acyclovir in the treatment (1) and suppression (2) of recurrences have been successfully conducted. However, on discontinuation of the drug, no effect has been demonstrable on the frequency or severity of subsequent recurrences. Therefore, alternative strategies employing recombinant leukocyte α interferon have been designed to assay its therapeutic effect on recurrences of genital herpes (3).

MATERIALS AND METHODS

Cloned interferon α_2 or placebo was administered subcutaneously to 45 patients with frequent recurrences (eight or more in a year's time) of genital herpes. The diagnosis was confirmed by cultures of herpes simplex virus. They were randomized to receive either five million units of interferon or placebo daily during the first three days of a recurrence, beginning during the prodrome or within 12 hours of the onset of visible lesions. They were evaluated in a double-blinded fashion as to the time to symptom resolution, time to healing, and time to the next recurrence. During the next recurrence they were again randomized to receive either interferon or placebo, and evaluated as above.

RESULTS

Forty-five patients were enrolled in the study, of which 25 were males and 19 were females. During the first recurrence (Table 1), there were no differences between interferon and placebo recipients as to the time to healing (6.4 vs 5.8 days, respectively), the time to symptom resolution (4.7 vs 3.7 days, respectively), or the time to the next recurrence (41.2 vs 58.3 days, respectively).

For their next recurrence, 35 of the original 45 agreed to be randomized once again to receive either interferon or placebo. Again there were no significant differences for any of the clinically evaluable outcomes between the four groups (Table II). Differences in numbers of patients between the different parameters within a single group reflects the lack of evaluability of certain parameters within the group.

TABLE I

CLINICAL RESULTS OF THE FIRST RECURRENCE

Days to	Interferon						Placebo					
	Female		Male		Overall		Female		Male		Overall	
	N	Mean	N	Mean	N	Mean	N	Mean	N	Mean	N	Mean
healing	8	6.1	11	6.5	19	6.4	10	5.4	14	6.1	24	5.8
symptoms end	8	4.4	10	4.9	18	4.7	10	3.3	11	4.0	21	3.7
next recurrence	8	40.3	8	42.1	16	41.2	9	48.6	10	67.0	19	58.3

TABLE II

CLINICAL RESULTS OF THE SECOND RECURRENCE

Days to	Interferon-Interferon						Placebo-Placebo					
	Female		Male		Overall		Female		Male		Overall	
	N	Mean	N	Mean	N	Mean	N	Mean	N	Mean	N	Mean
healing	3	5.0	3	5.7	6	5.3	5	4.2	4	5.8	9	4.9
symptoms end	4	6.8	3	3.3	7	5.3	5	3.8	4	3.3	9	3.6
next recurrence	4	18.8	1	14.0	5	17.8	4	25.8	2	19.0	6	23.5

Days to	Interferon-Placebo						Placebo-Interferon					
	Female		Male		Overall		Female		Male		Overall	
	N	Mean	N	Mean	N	Mean	N	Mean	N	Mean	N	Mean
healing	4	5.5	5	6.0	9	5.8	4	5.5	6	4.5	10	4.9
symptoms end	4	6.0	4	4.3	8	5.1	4	4.8	6	4.0	10	4.3
next recurrence	3	29.7	3	18.0	6	23.8	2	32.0	3	26.7	5	28.8

In summary, there was no effect of interferon on the time to healing, time to symptom resolution, and time to the next recurrence. Longer time to symptom resolution was observed in female patients when compared to males ($p=0.05$). Fever, chills, fatigue, and myalgias were seen more frequently in the interferon group compared to placebo ($p<0.01$). New methods of interferon administration, other types of interferons, or combination with other antivirals (4) may yet be efficacious in the therapy and suppression of recurrences of genital herpes.

REFERENCES

1. Reichman RC, Badger GJ, Mertz GJ, et al (1984) J Am Med Assoc 251:2103-2107.
2. Straus SE, Takiff HE, Seidlin M, et al (1984) N Engl J Med 310:1545-1550.
3. Gutterman JU, Fine S, Quesada J, et al (1982) Ann Intern Med 96:549-556.
4. Fraser-Smith EB, Eppstein DA, Marsh YV, et al (1984) Antimicrob Agents Chemother 25:563-565.

© 1985 Elsevier Science Publishers B.V. (Biomedical Division)
Herpes Viruses and Virus Chemotherapy, R. Kono, editor

TREATMENT OF HEPATITIS B VIRUS INFECTED CHILDREN WITH HUMAN LEUKOCYTE INTERFERON

YASUO CHIBA, TATSURU YAMANAKA AND TOORU NAKAO

Department of Pediatrics, Sapporo Medical College, chuo-ku S.1, W.16 Sapporo, JAPAN 060

MAKOTO KURODA

Japan Red Cross Hokkaido Blood Center, Chuo-ku S.9, W.14, Sapporo, Japan 064

INTRODUCTION

Chronic infection with hepatitis B virus (HBV) is one of the important causes of liver disease in Japanese children. Recently, interferon (IFN) has been employed for the treatment of HBV chronic hepatitis in adults and some promising results have been reported. Therefore, we also initiated treatment of HBV infected children with human leukocyte IFN.

MATERIALS AND METHOD

Patients and IFN

Fifteen patients were treated with IFN. They ranged in age from 5 months to 12 years old and all of these subjects were positive for HBe antigen. Histologic examinations revealed that 7 cases had chronic active hepatitis (CAH) and 5 cases had chronic persistent hepatitis (CPH). The remaining 3 cases had minimal histologic changes which rather suggested acute hepatitis. Human leukocyte IFN was administered for 11 to 52 days per course by intramuscle inoculation, with a daily dose being ranged from 1 to $3x10^6$ units.

RESULTS

Details of the patients treated with IFN and summary of the results are presented in Table 1 and 2, respectively. In five subjects, HBe antigen disappeared shortly after the initiation of IFN treatment, while in 3 subjects HBe antigen became undetectable 1 to 4 months after termination of treatment. Although two cases appeared to respond to the treatment initially as indicated either by the significant decrease of HBe antigen titers (case M.Y.) or by the transient disappearance of HBe antigen (case T.S.), they required 3 and 2 courses of IFN treatment until HBe antigen became consistently negative. Six of the 8 subjects who lost HBe antigen had histologic diagnosis of CAH and liver tissues obtained after treatment revealed improved findings. In contrast, six of the 7 subjects who did not respond to the treatment were those with acute hepatitis or CPH.

TABLE 1.

HBe Ag Positive Patients Treated With Human Leukocyte IFN

Name	Age (Sex)	Weight	Histologic type[a]	Dose(10^6)x Days	Result[b]
S.K.	6M (F)	7Kg		1.2 x 11	-
Y.F.	6Y (F)	18Kg		2.0 x 18	+
T.O.	5M (F)	7Kg		2.0 x 21	-
K.M.	6Y (M)	23Kg	CAH	1.2 x 20	++
M.Y.	3Y (F)	15Kg	CPH	2.0 x 15	-
				2.2 x 52	-
				2.2 x 10	+
A.M.	5Y (F)	20Kg	CAH	3.0 x 28	+
M.K.	5Y (F)	25Kg	CPH	2.0 x 20	-
J.U.	2Y (M)	12Kg	CPH	2.0 x 20	-
Y.S.	9Y (M)	26Kg	CAH	2.0 x 32	++
T.T.	12Y (M)	43Kg	CAH	2.0 x 40	++
N.K.	1Y (M)	10Kg	CPH	2.2 x 28	-
Y.K.	6Y (M)	25Kg	CAH	2.2 x 48	-
T.T.	1Y (M)	10Kg	CAH	2.2 x 16	++
H.S.	10Y (M)	28Kg	CPH	3.0 x 30	+
T.S.	9Y (M)	35Kg	CAH	2.2 x 28	++[c]
				3.0 x 37	+

a) CAH, chronic active hepatitis ; CPH, chronic persistent hepatitis
b) ++, disapperance of HBe Ag within a period of IFN treatment ; + later disapperance of HBe Ag. c) HBe Ag reappeared 2 months later

TABLE 2.

Summary of IFN Treatment of HBe Ag Positive Patients[a]

Histologic type[b]	Number of Patients	Disappearance of HBe Ag			Detection of HBe Ag		
		immediate	late	no	within 6 months	after 6 months	no
CAH	7	5[c]	1	1	3	2	2
CPH	5	0	1	4	0	0	5
Others	3	0	1	2	1	0	2

a) Results confined to initial treatment
b) CAH, chronic active hepatitis ; CPH, chronic persistent hepatitis.
c) Include a patient in whom HBe Ag reappeared

Herpes Viruses and Virus Chemotherapy, R. Kono, editor

TREATMENT OF SUBACUTE SCLEROSING PANENCEPHALITIS WITH HUMAN ALPHA-INTERFERON

NAOKI MIZUTANI*, MITSUNOBU MIYAZU*, SHIN ISOMURA*, KAZUYOSHI WATANABE*, JIRO IMANISHI**,
* Department of Pediatrics, Nagoya University School of Medicine, Nagoya,
** Department of Microbiology, Kyoto Prefectual University of Medicine, Kyoto,

INTRODUCTION

Subacute sclerosing panencephalitis (SSPE) is a rare progressive disease of the central nervous system associated with persistent slow measles-like virus infection. Up to the present, there have been some attempts to treat the patient with SSPE with the progress of the research on its pathogenesis. But there is no radical treatment as yet. The aim of this study is to report the results of human alpha-interferon (IFN) therapy in five patients with SSPE, and to investigate the permeability of IFN at blood-brain barrier (BBB) after intramuscular or intravenous IFN administration.

CASES AND METHODS

Clinical features and labolatory findings of five patients with SSPE was summarized in Table 1. Used human alpha IFN was produced by the method of Cantell et al (1). As a rule, IFN was administered intramuscularly at a dose of 100-150 x 10^4 unit per day, 30-150 x 10^4 unit per day intravenously, and 1-12 x 10^4 unit per day intrathecally. The assessment of the effect was based on the changes of clinical symptoms, EEG findings, cranial CT scan findings, and measles antibody titers in serum and CSF before and after the IFN administration. Furthermore, to investigate the permeability of IFN at BBB after intramuscular or intravenous administration, serial changes of IFN titers were studied in serum and CSF simultaneously. IFN assay was performed according to the method of Havell et al (2).

RESULTS

<u>Therapeutic effect of IFN on patients with SSPE (Table 2)</u>

From October 2, 1978 through June 29, 1982, a total dose of 1300-11692 x 10^4 unit of IFN was given to each patients. The observation of clinical course was made for 26-60 months. There were no severe side effects except for temporary high fever and vomiting. No clinical improvement was observed in all cases. EEG revealed a progressive disorganization and slowing of the basic rhythm. Furthermore, sleep stage differenciation became unclear. Cranial CT scan demonstrated progressive cortical atrophy and severe dilatation of all ventricles. Measles antibody titers in both serum and CSF also unchanged (Table 2).

<u>IFN titers and permeability of IFN at BBB</u>

Table 1 Summary of clinical and labolatory findings of five patients.

Case	1. Y.T.	2. Y.H.	3. O.M.	4. N.M.	5. N.A.
Age of onset	13 y	5 y	9 y	7 y	5 y
Sex	male	male	male	male	male
Past history of measles	11 m moderate	10 m moderate	12 m moderate	12 m moderate	6 m moderate
Between measles and SSPE	12 y	4 y	8 y	6 y	4 y
Stage of Jabbour's classification	I	II	II	II	II
First chief complaint	generalized convulsion mental deterioration	changes of character gait disturbance	gait disturbance mental deterioration	mental deterioration myoclonus	delayed speech myoclonus
Initial diagnosis	epilepsy	brain tumor	degenerative disease	epilepsy	SSPE
Initial EEG findings	periodic burst & suppression	periodic burst & suppression	periodic burst & suppression	periodic burst & suppression	periodic burst & suppression
Initial cranial CT scan findings	normal	normal	low density in basal ganglia ventricular enlargement	normal	normal
Measles titer (HI)					
serum	x 512	x 512	x 512	x 128	x 128
C.S.F.	x 32	x 32	x 16	x 16	x 16
CSF findings					
IgG (mg/dl)	23	8	21	25	ND
protein (mg/dl)	80	40	75	ND	109
cell count	5/3	1/3	2/3	3/3	0/3

ND: not done

Table 2 Summary of IFN treatment.

Case	1. Y.T.	2. Y.H.	3. O.M.	4. N.M.	5. N.A.
The start of the treatment	1979. 1. 22.	1978. 10. 2.	1980. 8. 19.	1981. 4. 30.	1982. 3. 30.
Stage at the start of the treatment (Jabbour's classification)	I — II	II	II	II	II
Doses of IFN (x 10^4 IU)	5870	11692	2382	2305	1300
I.M.	5870	10300	800	1250	1300
I.V.		1350	1550	1050	
I.T.		42	32	5	
Period of observation (1984. 8. 31.)	2 y. 2 m. lost to follow up	5 y. 10 m.	4 y.	3 y. 4 m.	2 y. 5 m.
Clinical course	very slowly progressive	progressive	progressive	progressive	progressive
Measles titer (HI)					
serum pre/post	x 512 / x 512	x 512 / x 512	x 512 / x 512	x 128 / x 128	x 128 / x 128
C.S.F. pre/post	x 32 / x 32	x 32 / x 64	x 16 / x 32	x 16 / x 16	x 16 / x 16
EEG finding	progressive	progressive	progressive	progressive	progressive
Cranial CT scan finding	normal → brain atrophy ventricular enlargement	normal → brain atrophy ventricular enlargement	low density of basal ganglia ventricular enlargement	normal → brain atrophy ventricular enlargement	normal → brain atrophy ventricular enlargement

I.M.: intramuscular administration

I.V.: intravenous administration

I.T.: intrathecal administration

Intramuscular and intravenous administration of IFN elevated its serum levels with the peak level one and a half hour after administration respectively. IFN titers in CSF raised about a quarter to an eighth of that of serum, but rapidly diminished. On the other hand, serum IFN titers diminished gradually. These results indicate that the permeability of intramuscularly or intravenously administered IFN at BBB is relatively good.

REFERENCES

1. Cantell K, et al (1977) Pharmac Ther C 1: 369
2. Havell EA, et al (1972) Antimicrob Agents Chemother 2: 476

TOPICAL TREATMENT OF RECURRENT FACIAL AND GENITAL HERPES WITH HUMAN INTERFERON BETA CREAM

M. MOVSHOVITZ, M. SCHEWACH-MILLET, S. KRISS-LEVENTON, J. SHOHAM*, T. DOERNER*, AND M. REVEL**

Sheba Medical Center, Tel Hashomer, *InterYeda Ltd, Ness Ziona, **Department of Virology, Weizmann Institute of Science, Rehovot (Israel)

INTRODUCTION

The treatment of herpes simplex virus dermal infections is complicated by the recurrent nature of the disease, resulting from the poorly understood latency state of the virus in the sensory nervous ganglions afferent to facial and genital areas (1-3). The increasing number of new cases of genital herpes (4), the severe objective and subjective discomfort caused by the eruptions, the danger of infection spreading to sexual partners and to newborns, and the associated cancer risk factor (5) emphasize the need for treatment. The virus is widespread in the human population, and it is possible that patients with recurrent eruptions suffer from some temporary or cyclic cellular immunity impairment which allows the virus to multiply (6). Complete elimination of the virus seems unrealistic, and the treatment should first aim at reducing the virus load and at enhancing the immune resistance, thereby decreasing the chances of new eruptions. Interferons (IFNs) having both antiviral and immunoregulatory effects (7) and being possibly part of the natural defence mechanism deficient in the patients (8), we have experimented the use of human IFN-β in the treatment of recurrent herpes dermal infections.

To avoid side effects often caused by systemic IFN administration (9), we have used the IFN-β (Frone^R)-cream (InterYeda) for topical application on the area affected by the herpes lesions. The absence of any side effect, together with the fact that IFN does not lead to the appearance of IFN-resistant virus strains, allowed to continue this simple treatment for prolonged periods of time. We report here on a group of 31 patients with labial or genital herpes, who showed a 10-fold decrease in the number of days with recurrent herpes eruptions over a period of 2 years, as well as a clear reduction in subjective and objective symptoms.

MATERIALS AND METHODS

Patients were followed at the outpatient dermatological clinic of the Sheba Medical Center, Tel Hashomer, Israel. Patients suffering from facial (12 cases) or genital herpes (19 cases) with recurrences every 0.5-3 months entered the study. All had been followed for several months, some from 1 to 18 years prior

TABLE 1

EFFECT OF TOPICAL APPLICATION OF IFN-β (FRONE) CREAM ON RECURRENT HERPES

Case Nbr.	Months before Frone	Months of Frone treatment	Sex	Age	Locali-zation	Time between* Recurr. in months Bef./Aft.		Ratio	Duration in days Bef./Aft.		Symptoms A	B	C
19	5	2	F	21	Genital	1	--	--	14	3.5	+	?	+
7	60	28	M	45	Genital	1	13	13.0	18	7	+	+	+
18	2	12	F	29	Genital	1	12	12.0	14	3.5	+	+	?
8	7	22	M	45	Genital	0.5	4.5	9.0	35	9	+	+	+
17	8	18	F	28	Genital	0.5	4	8.0	8.5	3	+	+	+
4	36	15	M	34	Genital	1	7	7.0	9	5	+	+	+
10	10	5	M	29	Genital	0.5	3	6.0	14	7	+	+	0
16	24	12	F	21	Genital	1	5	5.0	10	2	+	+	+
21	18	27	F	32	Lowback	1	5	5.0	14	7	+	+	0
12	24	12	M	29	Genital	0.5	2	4.0	7	7	+	+	?
20	18	8	F	38	Genital	0.75	2.5	3.3	14	8	+	+	0
5	30	11	M	32	Genital	2.5	7	2.8	?	3	+	?	0
11	12	12	M	24	Genital	0.75	2	2.6	14	7	+	+	?
13	24	12	M	36	Genital	0.5	1	2.0	14	5	+	+	?
2	3	26	M	31	Genital	2.5	4.5	1.8	10	3	+	+	+
3	4	12	M	21	Genital	2.5	4	1.6	10	7	+	+	?
1	8	12	M	36	Genital	2	3	1.5	10	7	+	+	+
6	30	13	M	40	Genital	0.5	0.75	1.5	?	?	+	+	0
9	2	20	M	24	Genital	2	2	1.0	14	4.5	+	+	?
31	24	18	F	38	Labial	4	--	--	9	5	+	?	+
26	96	29	F	21	Lab+Face	1	12	12.0	18	10	+	+	0
25	120	11	F	20	Labial	0.5	5	10.0	18	8.5	+	0	0
14	156	12	M	30	Facial	3	27	9.0	?	7	?	?	?
24	240	30	F	25	Labial	0.5	4	8.0	14	3	+	+	+
28	60	16	F	30	Labial	0.5	4	8.0	16	6	+	+	+
15	60	5	M	24	Labial	1	6	6.0	21	7	+	+	?
23	216	11	F	31	Labial	1	6	6.0	10	10	+	+	+
29	120	16	F	32	Lab+Nose	1	6	6.0	14	5.5	+	+	+
22	60	11	F	25	Labial	2	5	2.5	8.5	?	0	0	0
27	84	8	F	21	Labial	0.75	0.75	1.0	14	7	+	+	?
30	120	18	F	43	Labial	0.5	0.5	1.0	14	7	+	+	0

Symptoms: A. Reduction of subjective symptoms. B. Reduction in intensity of subsequent attacks. C. Prevention of attacks by increased application at first symptoms. ? Indicates cases where information could not be reliably obtained.
*Patients listed according to the increase in time (months) between recurrences after treatment.

to treatment. Herpes simplex virus was isolated from patients vesicles and typed serologically. The sensitivity of the HSV isolates to Hu IFN-β was determined (10) in cultures of human fibroblasts FS11.

Frone-cream (produced by InterYeda Ltd, Israel, for Serono Inc.) is a preparation of human IFN-β from poly (rI):(rC)-induced foreskin diploid fibroblasts, purified to over 10^7 units per mg protein, and presented in a polyethyleneglycol base at 20,000 or 100,000 IU per gram of cream (11). This preparation is stable for over a year when stored at 4°C. After virus isolation, the patients were treated as follows: at the stage where papules, vesicules or crusts were present, Frone-cream was applied 4-6 times daily (about $2x10^4$ units) on the affected skin area. During remission periods, cream was applied twice daily. In a number of patients, application during remissions was limited to the time when some symptoms of itching, burning or numbness appeared, and was then done 6 times daily. Patients were evaluated for: a) improvement of symptoms as pain, itching, burning, fever, etc.; b) reduction of the duration of first treated episode or eventual recurrence; c) decrease in the dimension and number of lesions in eventual recurrence; d) decrease in the frequency of recurrences. These parameters were followed for up to two years (average 20 months), and compared to the history of each patient recorded in the same clinic for prolonged periods prior to treatment with IFN-β.

RESULTS

Genital Herpes

Thirteen males and 6 females, average age 31 years, were included in this study (Table 1). Except for one case with sacral lesions where HSV-1 was found, all patients had genital lesions with HSV-2 isolates. Alleviation of subjective symptoms was seen in 93% of the patients treated with Frone-cream (Table 1). The average interval between recurrent episodes was before treatment of 34.5 days (i.e. 10 episodes per year). During the treatment with Frone-cream (20,000 u per g), the average interval between recurrences increased to 149 days (2.4 episodes per year). In addition, the duration of eventual eruptive episodes was reduced from an average of 13.5 days before treatment to 5.7 days during Frone-cream treatment. Combining these values, the number of days with genital herpes eruptions was reduced from 103 days per year to 13.5 days per year. Furthermore, we noted that the severity of an eventual eruption (size and number of lesions) was reduced by Frone-cream in 95% of the cases. In 47% of the patients, a 1-2 days prophylactic treatment at the time when the first symptoms of an eventual eruption appeared, was sufficient to prevent the full-blow eruption (Table 1). When patients were classified according to the ratio of recurrence frequency before and after treatment (Table 2), the results were significantly better in women since 83% had an over 5-fold increase in disease-free intervals versus 30% of the men. Nevertheless, 73% of all patients had an over 2-fold increase in disease-free intervals (Table 2). The rate at which recurrence appeared was much reduced after the onset of treatment (Table 3). Three patients had no recurrence for 1 year or more (Table 1).

TABLE 2

RESPONSE TO FRONE CREAM MEASURED IN ELONGATION OF REMISSION BETWEEN HERPES ATTACKS

Remission Increase	All Cases of Herpes Total	Males	Females	Genital Herpes Total	Males	Females	Facial Herpes Total	Males	Females
5 fold and more	18 (58%)	6 (40%)	12 (75%)	9 (47%)	4 (30%)	5 (83%)	9 (75%)	2 (100%)	7 (70%)
2-4 fold	6 (19%)	4 (26%)	2 (12%)	5 (26%)	4 (30%)	1 (17%)	1 (8%)	0 (0%)	1 (10%)
less than 2 fold	7 (23%)	5 (33%)	2 (12%)	5 (26%)	5 (38%)	0 (0%)	2 (16%)	0 (0%)	2 (20%)
Total:	31	15	16	19	13	6	12	2	10

Facial Herpes.

Ten women and 2 men, suffering of recurrent labial herpes for many years were included in the study (Table 1). All patients had HSV-1 infections. Frone-cream treatment increased the disease-free intervals from 39 to 236 days, and reduced the duration of an eventual eruption from 14.8 to 6.9 days, on the average. Thus the total number of days with disease decreased from 100 to 10.3 per year during treatment. Three patients had no recurrence for 1 year or more. The subjective symptoms were strongly reduced in over 80% of cases. In 75% of the patients, the subsequent eruptions were reduced in size and severity. The prophylactic treatment at first signs of itching or numbness succeeded to block the eruption in 42% of the cases. A total of 75% of the patients showed a 5-fold or more increase in disease-free intervals (Table 2). No difference was seen between sexes, but there were only two men in this group.

In vitro sensitivity of HSV to IFN and clinical response.

The virus isolates were classified according to their sensitivity *in vitro* to IFN (Table 4). In general, HSV-2 isolates were more sensitive *in vitro* than HSV-1. There was no correlation between the *in vitro* sensitivity and the clinical results in terms of reduction of the frequency of recurrences. However, the number of failures in reducing the duration of an attack, and the absence of

TABLE 3

CUMULATIVE RATE OF RECURRENCE IN IFN-β TREATED AND UNTREATED HERPES

	Per Cent of Patients with Recurrence after (months)						
	1 mo.	2 mo.	3 mo.	4 mo.	5 mo.	6 mo.	1 year
1. All cases							
Untreated	74%	84%	97%	100%	100%	100%	100%
with IFN-β	13%	22%	32%	45%	64%	74%	80%
2. Genital herpes							
Untreated	74%	84%	100%	100%	100%	100%	100%
with IFN-β	10%	26%	42%	52%	74%	74%	84%
3. Female patients							
Untreated	87%	94%	94%	100%	100%	100%	100%
with IFN-β	12%	12%	19%	37%	62%	75%	75%

TABLE 4

In vitro SENSITIVITY OF HSV ISOLATE TO IFN AND CLINICAL RESPONSE

Case Nbr	Site	*In vitro* virus sensitivity to IFN	HSV type	Remission increase ratio	Eruption duration ratio	Prevention of eruption if IFN applied at first symptoms
1	Genit.	Sensitive	2	1.5	0.7	Yes
2	Genit.	" "	2	1.8	0.3	Yes
4	Genit.	" "	2	7	0.5	Yes
7	Genit.	" "	2	13	0.4	Yes
9	Genit.	" "	2	1	0.3	?
13	Genit.	" "	2	2	0.35	?
16	Genit.	" "	2	5	0.2	Yes
17	Genit.	" "	2	8	0.35	Yes
6	Genit.	Poorly sensitive	2	1.5	1	No
21	Sacral	" "	1	5	0.5	No
25	Facial	" "	1	10	0.5	No
26	Facial	" "	1	12	0.55	No
28	Facial	" "	1	8	0.4	Yes
14	Facial	Resistant	1	9	1	?
22	Facial	" "	1	2.5	1	No
24	Facial	" "	1	8	0.2	Yes

prophylactic effect, showed some correlation with the relative resistance of the virus to IFN in vitro (Table 4).

When Frone-cream or placebo-cream were applied during eruptions and the virus titers were measured in liquid harvested from individual vesicules, a clear antiviral effect of the IFN-β cream was observed in vivo. With placebo, titers of 10^3-10^4 virus were found for the first 3 days, which decreased to 10^1-10^2 at 6 days. With Frone-cream, titers decreased from 10^3 to 10^1 in 12 hours and were below detection at day 2. Thus, Frone-cream blocks efficiently virus replication in the lesions (in collaboration with Dr M. Isacsohn).

DISCUSSION

This preliminary study of the effect of IFN-β cream on recurrent herpes shows that a topical application of IFN is able to influence the rate of recurrence which on the average was reduced over 5-fold. Combined with a 2-fold reduction on the duration of eruptive episodes, an overall 10-fold decrease in the days of disease was achieved. This result should be very significant for the patient, in addition to the improvement in subjective symptoms which was observed in nearly all cases. The topical IFN-β treatment at the concentration used, was however not sufficient to cure the disease, and recurrences were not completely eliminated. Nevertheless, the fact that 25% of the patients had no recurrence for over 1 year is significant. It can be hoped that increasing the concentration of IFN-β in the cream, which can be achieved with the larger amounts of IFN-β available through genetic engineering of hamster CHO cells (12), could improve the results. Inhibition of HSV replication requires larger amounts of IFN than that of other viruses like EMC (13).

The increase in disease-free interval achieved in the majority of patients, suggests that topical application of IFN-β influences the reinfection of the ganglional nerve cells either by reducing the virus load in the skin, or by stimulating the immune system to destroy herpes virus infected cells (14). The preventive action of IFN-β cream applied at the first subjective symptoms, would indicate that IFN acts mainly by preventing virus multiplication in the skin. It is likely also that the penetration of IFN requires the skin abrasion which accompanies the herpes lesions, so that application during remissions may have little effect. A combination of IFN injections with topical treatment during eruptions could improve the results.

A double-blind placebo-controlled study is presently underway. Two other open studies with topical Frone treatment in Israel, support our present results: in labial herpes, application of a Frone solution (500,000 U/ml) on the buccal mucosa and of Frone-cream on the peribuccal area at the time when numbness was was felt, aborted the eruption in 5 out of 6 cases (15). In 15 female herpes genitalis patients, a one week intensive application of Frone-cream (10^5 units/day) eliminated recurrences for 8 months at least in 10 cases and increased the disease-free interval from 35 to 72 days in the other five cases. Duration of eruptive episodes was reduced from 7 to 3.5 days in this trial (Marcovici R., Peretz B.A. and Paldi E.). Treatment of labial and genital herpes by IFN-alpha ointment was also reported (16).

IFN-β (Frone)-cream seems to give better results on genital Herpes than topical acyclovir treatment (17), which had little effect on recurrences (18). IFN is also less likely to lead to drug-resistant viruses. In herpes keratitis, IFN does not seem to influence the recurrence rate (19) although IFN is effective in combination with an antiviral drug such as trifluorothymidine, iododeoxyuridine or acyclovir to prompt healing of keratitis lesions (19,20,15). Prevention by systemic administration of IFN-α, of herpes eruption in patients undergoing surgery for tic douloureux was demonstrated in a double blind trial (21), but without effect on recurrences (22). It would be interesting to test the IFN-β topical application in this situation as well, because of the simplicity of the treatment and the complete absence of side-effects. It will be also very interesting to try combinations of IFN-β with antiviral chemicals such as acyclovir or 2-deoxyglucose (23) for the topical treatment of recurrent herpes dermal infections.

REFERENCES

1. Baringer JR, Swoveland P (1983) Recovery of Herpes simplex virus from human trigeminal ganglions. N Eng J Med 288:648-650
2. Baringer JR (1973) Recovery of Herpes simplex virus from human sacral ganglions. N Eng J Med 291:828-830
3. Stevens J (1975) Latent Herpes simplex and the nervous system. Curr Topics Microbiol Immunol 70:31-50
4. DeThe G (1982) Epidemiologie des virus Herpes en Medecine humaine, In: Proceedings 17th Internl Cong on Herpes virus of Man and Animal, Develop biol Standard, Karger, S. Publisher, Basel, Vol 52, pp 13-27
5. Rapp F (1978) Herpes viruses, venereal disease and cancer. American Scientist 66:670-674
6. Glasgow LA (1970) Cellular immunity in host resistance to viral infections. Arch Intern Med 126:125-134
7. Revel M (1983) The Interferon system in man: Nature of the Interferon molecules and mode of action, In: Becker Y (ed.) Antiviral drugs and Interferons: The molecular basis of their activity, Martinus Nijhoff, Boston, pp 357-433
8. Levin S, Hahn T (1981) Evaluation of the human Interferon system in viral disease. Clin exp Immunol 46:475-483
9. Scott GM (1983) The toxic effects of Interferon in man: In: Gresser I (ed.) Interferon 5, Acad Press, New York, pp 84-114.
10. Lazar R, Breinig MK, Armstrong JA, Ho M (1980) Response of cloned progeny of clinical isolates of herpes simplex virus to human leucocyte interferon. Infect Immun 28:708-715

11. Schonfeld A, Nitke S, Schattner A, et al. (1984) Intramuscular interferon-beta injections in the treatment of condylomata acuminata. Lancet 1: 1038-1042

12. Chernajovsky Y, Mory Y, Chen L, Marks Z, Novick D, Rubinstein M, Revel, M (1984) Efficient constitutive production of human fibroblast interferon by Hamster cells transformed with the IFN-β_1 gene fused to an SV40 early promoter. DNA 3:297-308

13. Panet A, Falk H (1983) Inhibition by interferon of Herpes simplex virus thymidine kinase and DNA polymerase in infected and biochemically transformed cells. J Gen Virol 64:1999-2006

14. Munoz A, Carrasco L, Fresno M (1983) Enhancement of susceptibility of HSV-1 infected cells to natural killer lysis by interferon. J Immunol 131: 783-787

15. Isacsohn M, Berson B, Sternberg I, Morag A (1983) Human fibroblast interferon in treatment of viral diseases of the skin and mucous membranes. Isr J Med Sci 19:959-962

16. Ikic P, Smerdel S, Rajninger-Miholic M, Soos E, Jusic D (1975) Treatment of labial and genital Herpes with human leukocyte interferon. In: Proceed Symposium on clinical use of interferon. Yugoslav Acad Sci and Arts pp 195-202

17. Kinghorn GR, Turner EB, Barton IG, Potter CW, Burke C, Fiddian AP (1983) Effect of topical acyclovir cream in first and recurrent episodes of genital herpes. Antiviral Res 3:291-301

18. Barton IG, Kinghorn GR, Rowland M, Jeavons M, Al-Omer LS, Potter CW (1984) Recurrences after first episodes of genital Herpes in patients treated with topical acyclovir cream. Antiviral Res 4:293-300

19. Sundmacher R (1982) Interferon in ocular viral diseases. In: Gresser I (ed.) Interferon 4, Acad Press, New York, pp 177-200

20. Smetana O, Eylan E, Prialnick M, Savir M (1983) Effect of human fibroblast interferon on Herpetic keratitis. Isr J Med Sci 19:668

21. Pazin GJ, Armstrong JA, Lam MT, Tarr GC, Jannetta PJ, Ho M (1979) Prevention of reactivated Herpes simplex infection by human leukocyte interferon after operation on the trigeminal root. N Eng J Med 301:225-230

22. Haverkos HW, Pazin GJ, Armstrong JA, Ho M (1980) Follow-up of interferon treatment of herpes simplex. N Eng J Med 303:699-703

23. Blough HA, Giuntoli RL (1979) Successful treatment of Human Genital Herpes infections with 2-deoxy-D-Glucose. JAMA 241:2798-2801

APPLICATION OF HUMAN INTERFERON FOR THE TREATMENT OF ADENOVIRUS KERATOCONJUNCTIVITIS

MICHIKO KANEKO AND YUKIO UCHIDA

Department of Ophthalmology, Tokyo Women's Medical College, 10 Kawada-cho, Shinjuku-ku, Tokyo 162, Japan

INTRODUCTION

Evaluation of therapeutic effect of human interferon (IFN) on adenovirus keratoconjunctivitis still remains inconclusive[1)], though some investigators claimed favorable results[2,3,4,)]. In this report, we used human IFN-α and IFN-β in the form of eye drop for the treatment of adenovirus keratoconjunctivitis.

MATERIAL AND METHODS

Out of the patients with acute conjunctivitis which was diagnosed tentatively as adenoviral at Eye clinic of Tokyo Women's Medical College, for a period of 12 months in 1981, only those who were in the early stage of the disease (within 3 days after the onset) were selected and subjected to the trial. Conjunctival scrapings for virus isolation were taken from all patients, and their paired sera for antibody tests were obtained at the acute and convalescent stages. Three kinds of eye drops, IFN-α 1×10^5 IU/ml, IFN-β 1×10^5 IU/ml, and human albumin 1 mg/ml as a placebo were used. Both IFNs were natural types. The patients were divided into groups, each of which was composed of seven persons; three for IFN-α, three for IFN-β, and one for albumin. Selection of regimen was done randomly, and the patient received any one of these three drugs which was instilled four times a day for 2 weeks.

Symptoms such as discharge, tearing, pain, foreign body sensation, and photophobia, and signs such as lid-swelling, preauricular adenopathy, conjunctival hyperemia, follicles, and epithelial and subepithelial keratitis were recorded, and their severity was graded by scoring 0 to 3+. Judging from the total scores on day 3, day 7, and day 14, effects of application were evaluated in 3 categories as good, fair, and poor.

RESULTS

Out of 97 patients in this trial, 59 were confirmed virologically to have adenovirus infection, and were taken up for the assessment. Incidence of types of causative adenovirus was as follows, 39 type 8, 18 type 3, and 2 type 4.

In the group of cases with type 8 infection, the therapeutic efficacy of 3 drugs was compared in Table I. Significant differences were not seen among them. In cases with type 3 infection, there were also no differences among the 3 drugs.

The incidence and severity of subepithelial punctate corneal opacities observed in cases with type 8 and type 3 infection were shown in table II. Patients under 10 years old were excluded from the table, because subepithelial keratitis tends to be slight or absent in children. Differences in influence of drugs upon the condition were not seen.

COMMENT AND CONCLUSION

Contrary to our expectation, topical administration of IFN-α and -β was not superior to the inactive control, human albumin, in the treatment of adenovirus keratoconjunctivitis. The concentration of IFNs used here might not be high enough to suppress the disease, even in its early stages, although administration within 3 days after the onset has been reported to bring fevorable results by some investigators[2,4]. Experiments using IFNs of much higher concentrations are to be indicated.

TABLE I

EFFECT OF EYE DROPS ON KERATOCONJUNCTIVITIS CAUSED BY ADENOVIRUS TYPE 8

	Objective signs				Subjective symptoms			
Eye drops	good	fair	poor	total	good	fair	poor	total
Hu-IFN-α	9	4	3	16	3	8	5	16
Hu-IFN-β	9	5	3	17	4	7	6	17
Hu- Alb	3	2	1	6	1	3	2	6

TABLE II

DEVELOPMENT OF PUNCTATE SUBEPITHELIAL OPACITIES OF THE CORNEA
(children younger than 10y excluded)

	Cases of adenovirus type 8					Cases of adenovirus type 3				
Eye drops	no	slight	marked	total	%	no	slight	marked	total	%
Hu-IFN-α	2	8	6	16	87.5	2	3	0	5	60
Hu-IFN-β	0	11	3	14	100	3	2	1	6	50
Hu-Alb	0	4	1	5	100	1	0	2	3	67

REFERENCES

1. Sundmacher R et al (1982) Graefe's Arch Clin Exp Ophthalmol 218:139-140
2. Negoro Y et al (1980) Jpn J Ophthalmol 24:125-127
3. Romano Y et al (1980) J Interferon Res 1:95-100
4. Itoi M et al (1982) Folia Ophthal Jap 33:1668-1671

CLINICAL TRIAL OF RECOMBINANT LEUCOCYTE A INTERFERON FOR DENDRITIC KERATITIS

NAOHIKO TANAKA M.D., HIROSHI HATANO M.D.

Department of Ophthalmology, Yokohama City University School of Medicine. 3-46 Urafunecho Minamiku, Yokohama (Japan)

In recent years, the interferons can be produced by E-Coli and the highly purified these recombinant leucocyte A (rIFN-αA) containing high dose are available for clinical use.

A clinical trial was conducted to evaluate a therapeutic effect of rIFN-αA for the treatment of human herpes simplex keratitis. The interferon substance adopted for this study was jointly developed by Nippon Roche KK and Takeda Chemical Industries, Ltd., while its ophthalmic preparation was formulated by Senju Pharmaceutical Co.

Eighteen ophthalmic clinics* were participated to carry on present clinical study. The 36 eyes with typical dendritic keratitis were carefully selected by the clinical pictures of the cornea and were subjected to this study to evaluate the curative effect of high or low dose rIFN-αA. Two different concentrations of rIFN-αA were prepared for the sake of well-controlled study, that is, high dose (10^7/ml) and low dose (10^3/ml). Thus prepared ophthalmic solution was administered four times a day for two weeks period along with clinical observation of the size of dendritic ulcer by fluorescein staining. As a result of masked distribution of ophthalmic formula with high or low concentration of rIFN-αA, 20 eyes received high dose and 16 got low dose respectively.

No significant difference between two groupes of high and low dose were noted on the severity of the clinical sighns at the time of initial administration (Table 1). The clinical effect was determined based on how the dendritic ulcer was cured or the area of dendritic ulcer was decreased by rIFN-αA application. The residual rate of fluorescein staining of dendritic ulcer on each day of clinical observation was shown in figure (Figure 1). Each case was finally categorized in one of the five different judgements; remarkably effective, effective, slightly effective, Not effective and aggravated.

The rate of remarkably effective with high dose rIFN-αA was 90% compared to 37.5% with the low one (Table 2).

---

* Asahikawa Medical College (Prof. A. Hosaka), Hokkaido University (Prof. H. Matsuda), Tokyo Women's Medical College (Prof. Y. Uchida), Nihon University (Prof. S. Kitano), Tokyo Medical and Dental University (Prof. T. Tokoro), Kyorin University (Prof. H. Tokuda), Tokai University (Prof. D. Obazawa),

St. Mariannan University (Prof. S. Tane), Kitasato University (Prof. S. Ishikawa), Nagoya City University (Prof. A. Majima), Kyoto Prefectural University of Medicine (Prof. M. Itoi), Kansai Medical University (Prof. M. Uyama), Kinki Central Hospital (Dr. J. Hara), Niigata University (Prof. K. Iwata), Tokushima University (Dr. H. Shiota), Yamaguchi University (Prof. S. Kobayashi), Yokohama City University (Prof. N. Tanaka) and Shinkawabashi Hospital (Dr. E. Utsumi).

Table 1: Severity at the time of initial administration

Observation items		High Dose	Low Dose	Total	X^2 Test
Ulcer	-	1	0	1	N. S.
	+	3	3	6	
	2+	13	10	23	
	3+	3	3	6	
Multiple erosion	-	10	11	21	N. S.
	+	9	5	14	
	2+	1	0	1	
	3+	0	0	0	
Parenchymal edema	-	10	11	21	N. S.
	+	6	2	8	
	2+	4	2	6	
	3+	0	1	1	
Iritis	-	14	12	26	N. S.
	+	4	3	7	
	2+	2	0	2	
	3+	0	1	1	
Hyperemia	-	2	1	3	N. S.
	+	7	8	15	
	2+	7	6	13	
	3+	3	1	4	

Figure 1: Days before disappearance of gross fluorescein stains

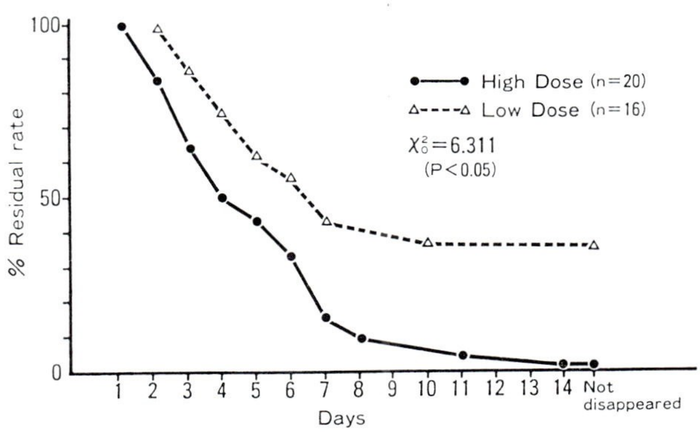

Table 2: Clinical efficacy

	Remarkably effective	Effective	Slightly effective	Not effective	Aggravated	Total
High Dose	18 (90.0 %)	2 (100 %)	0	0	0	20
Low Dose	6 (37.5 %)	4 (62.5 %)	2 (75.0 %)	0	4 (100 %)	16

$X_0^2=8.789$ (P<0.01) $X_0^2=6.502$ (P<0.05) $X_0^2=3.379$ (P<0.1)

Z=3.410 (P<0.01)

EFFECT OF HUMAN INTERFERON-β ON VIRAL PNEUMONITIS IN KIDNEY TRANSPLANT RECIPIENTS

KOTA TAKAHASHI, SATOSHI TERAOKA, TAKASHI YAGISAWA, KAZUO OTA AND SHIGEYASU KOBAYASHI*

Department of Urology, Kidney Center, Tokyo Women's Medical College, Shinjuku-ku, Tokyo, and *Basic Reseach Laboratories, Toray Industries Incorporation, Kamakura, Kanagawa, Japan

INTRODUCTION

Recently, a new immunosuppressive agent, cyclosporine has been administered to kidney transplant recipients leading to a marked improvement in graft survival. However, viral pneumonitis has proved to be one of the fatal complications of this treatment. Human fibroblast interferon-β (HuIFN-β) was therefore administered to kidney transplant recipients complicated with serious viral pneumonitis[1].

MATERIALS AND METHODS

Patients

Five patients received kidneys from 2 living-related and 3 cadaveric donors. The original disease was chronic glomerulonephritis in all cases. Viral infections including 1 case of herpes simplex virus (HSV) pneumonitis and 4 cases of cytomegalovirus (CMV) pneumonitis were observed in these patients (Table I).

Table I.
Kidney Transplant Recipients Complicated with Viral Pneumonitis Treated by HuIFN-β Therapy

Case	Age	Sex	Viral infection		Complication	HuIFN-β	Adverse Effect	Prognosis	Graft Function
1. CD53, T.E.	39	M	CMV	Pneumonitis	Diabetes Mellitus	29×10^6 IU	Fever	Cured	Good
2. CD58, N.S.	47	M	CMV	Pneumonitis	Acute Pancreatis	36×10^6 IU	Fever, Slight Hepatic Insufficiency	Cured	Good
3. LD136, M.H.	27	F	HSV	Pneumonitis Herpes Labialis	Wound Infection. Acute Renal Failure. Upper G-I Bleeding.	39×10^6 IU	Fever	Cured	Good
4. CD66, A.S.	52	F	CMV	Pneumonitis	Mitral Valve Insufficiency Atrial Fibrillation	34×10^6 IU	Fever	Cured	Good
5. LD157, S.S.	45	M	CMV	Pneumonitis	Non-A, non-B Hepatitis Duodenal Perforation	44×10^6 IU	Fever	Cured	Good

LD: Living Related Transplantation CD: Cadaveric Transplantation M: Male F: Female
CMV: Cytomegalovirus HSV: Herpes Simplex Virus

Methods of immunosuppressive and HuIFN-β therapy

The immunosuppressive regimen consisted of cyclosporine and a small dose of methylprednisolone after kidney transplantation. During the viral infection episode, a daily dosage of between 2×10^6 and 6×10^6 IU of HuIFN-β was administered by intravenous drip injection to each recipient for between 8 and 21 days with a mean of 13 days. Appropriate time for the first administration of HuIFN-β seemed to be when the value for the partial pressure of arterial oxygen (PO_2) fell below 60 mmHg. Therapeutic effects were followed by PO_2, chest x-ray examination and serum antiviral titer.

RESULTS

All 5 recipients were cured of viral pneumonitis and still now show good kidney function (Figure 1). These results were considered to indicate the usefulness of HuIFN-β in the treatment of opportunistic viral infections in kidney transplant recipients.

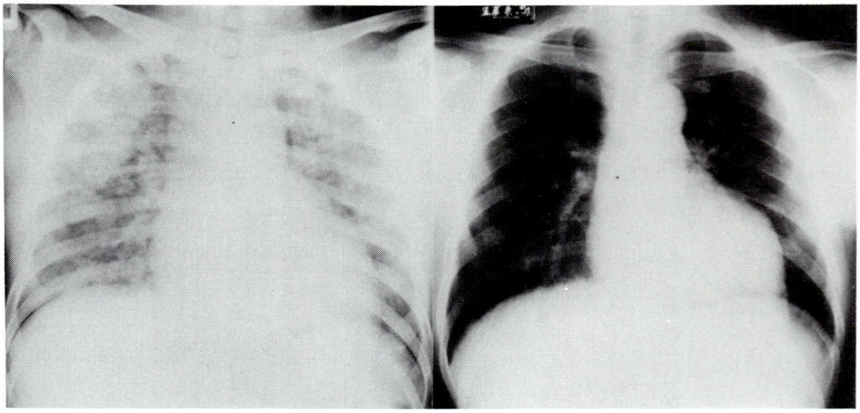

A B

Figure 1. Plain chest x-ray films in case 1 complicated with CMV pneumonitis. A: PO_2 42.4 mmHg. At beginning of HuIFN-β therapy on 100th day after kidney transplantation. B: Normal value after treatment.

REFERENCE

1. Kobayashi S, Iizuka M, Hara M (1982) In: Shioda H (ed) Preparation of human fibroblast interferon (HuIFN-β). Excerpta Medica, Amsterdam pp 286-294.

RECOMBINANT INTERFERONS FOR HERPES SIMPLEX KERATITIS

EMILY D. VARNELL, HERBERT E. KAUFMAN, JAMES J. SANITATO

Department of Ophthalmology, LSU Eye Center, Louisiana State University Medical Center School of Medicine, New Orleans, Louisiana 70112, USA

INTRODUCTION

Interferon has a slight but definite effect when used for the treatment of herpes simplex virus (HSV) keratitis.[1] This effect is not as great as that seen with the antimetabolite antivirals.[2] Naturally derived human leukocyte interferon is very difficult to obtain in large quantities with high titer and is quite expensive. Recent technology with genetic engineering has produced recombinant human leukocyte and fibroblast interferons that are available in large quantities and with very high titers.

The aims of our studies were: to compare recombinant human interferon alpha, subtype A and recombinant human interferon beta for efficacy against HSV keratitis in owl monkeys; to test the combination of recombinant human interferon beta and 1% trifluridine against HSV keratitis in owl monkeys; and to study the tolerance of recombinant human interferon alpha, subtype A eyedrops in human volunteers.

MATERIALS AND METHODS

Animal Trials

Animals. Adult owl monkeys (*Aotus trivirgatus*) were used.

Virus. McKrae herpesvirus type 1, 10^5 PFU/ml, was dropped onto anesthetized corneas after minimal scarification of the epithelium.

Treatments. Both types of interferon were prepared by Hoffmann-LaRoche, Inc., Nutley, New Jersey, U.S.A. Recombinant human interferon alpha subtype A was supplied as a lyophilized powder which was diluted with water and used at a concentration of 20 x 10^6 units/ml. Fresh interferon alpha was prepared daily. Recombinant human interferon beta was supplied frozen and was diluted for use to 20 x 10^6 units/ml. One percent trifluridine drops were prepared in normal saline. Two drops per eye were given at 8:00 and 12:00 a.m. and 3:00 p.m. until seven days after infection. Both eyes of each animal received the same treatment.

Evaluations. Slit lamp evaluations were made in masked fashion. Corneas were stained with fluorescein (Fluor-i-strips) and epithelial ulceration was graded as: 0 = clear cornea; 1 = ulceration of 1/4 of the epithelium; 2 = ulceration of 1/2 of the epithelium; 3 = ulceraton of 3/4 of the epithelium; 4 = complete epithelial ulceration.

Human Trial

Thirty one adult volunteers entered the double blind study after it was determined that they were free of eye disease. They were given two coded bottles, one for use in the morning and one for use in the evening.

The volunteers chose one eye to use for the study and always put the drops in that eye. Medicine was kept at refrigerator temperature. Each participant was examined daily Monday through Friday for the 21 days of the trial.

Recombinant human interferon alpha subtype A was supplied so that each drop contained 1.5 units. Three combinations of drops were studied: 1) interferon in the morning and evening; 2) interferon in the morning and placebo in the evening; and 3) placebo in the morning and evening.

RESULTS

Animal Trials

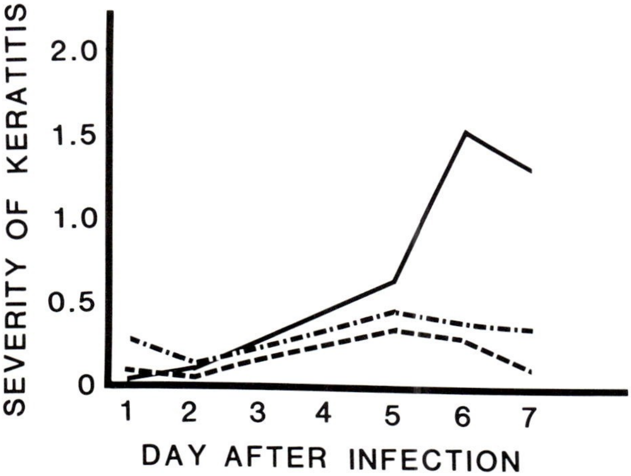

Figure 1. Owl monkeys treated from 1 day before infection with treatment continued three times a day. Solid line: control, 8 animals; dashed line: recombinant human interferon alpha subtype A, 7 animals; dot and dash line: recombinant human interferon beta, 8 animals.

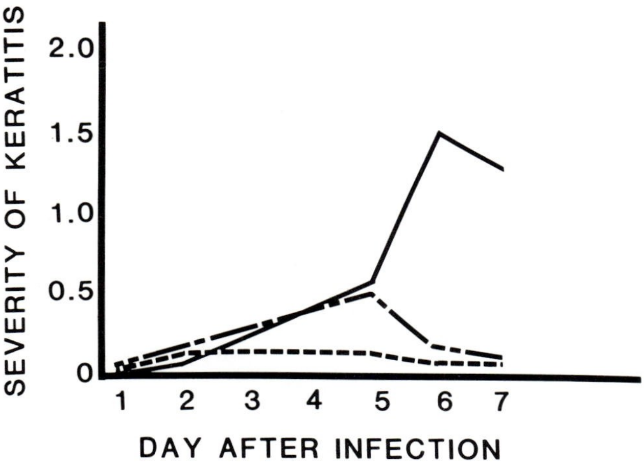

Figure 2. Owl monkeys treated from 1 day after infection with treatment continued three times a day. Solid line: control, 8 animals; dashed line: recombinant human interferon beta and trifluridine A, 6 animals; dot and dash line: trifluridine, 7 animals.

Human Trial

TABLE 1

INTERFERON TOLERANCE IN NORMAL HUMAN EYES

Treatment	No. eyes	Results
Interferon, AM and PM	10	Transient conjunctivitis in 2 eyes
		Transient conjunctivitis and punctate keratitis in 1 eye
Interferon, AM; placebo, PM	11	No changes
Placebo, AM and PM	10	Transient punctate keratitis in 1 eye

CONCLUSIONS

There are no significant differences between recombinant interferon alpha and beta on any day for treating herpetic keratitis in this owl monkey model, as determined by pairwise t-tests. The interferon-treated groups showed less severe disease than placebo-treated animals. The combination treatment (recombinant human interferon beta and trifluridine) produced a significantly better effect than trifluridine alone, similar to what has already been seen with human interferon produced from buffy coat[3] or recombinant human interferon alpha[4] combined with trifluridine. Recombinant human interferon beta is not as stable as recombinant interferon alpha and must be used immediately after preparation. Recombinant human interferon alpha subtype A is not toxic in the human eye at a total dose of 3.0 units per day, nor does it produce systemic side effects when used for 21 days.

REFERENCES

1. Sugar J, Kaufman, HE, Varnell ED (1973) Invest Ophthalmol 12(5):378-380.
2. Varnell ED, Kaufman HE, Sanitato JJ, Centifanto YM (1983) Invest Ophthalmol Vis Sci (Suppl) 24(3):215 (Abstract).
3. Sundmacher R, Cantell K, Neumann-Haefelin D (1978) Lancet 2:687.
4. Trousdale MD, Nesburn AB (1984) Invest Ophthalmol Vis Sci 25:480-483.

ACKNOWLEDGEMENTS

This work was supported in part by PHS grants EY02672, EY07073, and EY02377 from the National Eye Institute, National Institutes of Health, Bethesda, Maryland.

VII INTERFERON

Herpes Viruses and Virus Chemotherapy, R. Kono, editor

NOVEL INTERFERONS OBTAINED BY RECOMBINANT DNA TECHNIQUES: PROPERTIES AGAINST HERPES VIRUS INFECTIONS

NOWELL STEBBING, MELVIN D. TROUSDALE, ELEANOR N. FISH

Amgen, Thousand Oaks, CA (USA); Estelle Doheny Eye Foundation, Los Angeles, CA (USA); Hospital for Sick Children, Toronto (Canada)

INTRODUCTION

Although clinical efficacy of interferons (IFNs) against virus infections has been demonstrated the side effects are such that materials with better therapeutic index are needed. Molecular hybrids of IFN-αs have been constructed but none have been significantly more potent than natural subtypes (1). Complete gene synthesis methods have been used to construct novel analogs of human interferons and these also have been produced in E. coli (2). These analogs include a consensus of the known human IFN-α subtypes, designated IFN-αCon_1, and a variant of human IFN-γ, designated IFN-γ_{4A}. The IFN-α analog has a number of promising properties including very high specific activity (2) and pharmacological effects that should be clinically useful. Although conceived as an analog IFN-γ_{4A} now seems to correspond to the sequence of natural IFN-γ, which also lacks three residues from the N-terminus compared with the cDNA predicted sequence (3). These materials have been assessed for activity against herpes simplex virus (HSV) infections in cell cultures. Efficacy has been examined in HSV-1 infection of the rabbit eye. In addition, because IFN-αCon_1 proved to be effective in hamster cell cultures, efficacy was assessed against HSV-2 infections of hamsters. The results are compared to those of previous studies with other IFN preparations.

MATERIALS AND METHODS

Interferon Preparations

The structure of IFN-αCon_1 and IFN-γ_{4A} are indicated elsewhere (2); the materials were purified to homogeneity from E. coli harboring synthetic IFN genes. The specific activity of IFN-αCon_1 was 10^9 U/mg and that of IFN-γ_{4A} was $2x10^7$ U/mg. Natural IFN-α (Burroughs-Wellcome) and IFN-γ (Interferon Sciences) from peripheral blood leukocyte preparations were used as controls. All interferon titrations were assessed by cytopathic inhibition assays in HeLa cells infected with encephalomyocarditis virus (EMCV) calibrated against the NIH IFN standards (G023-901-527 and Gg23-903-530).

Cell Cultures

Activity of the interferons against HSV was assessed in the human T98G (neuroblastoma) cell line and hamster kidney cells (BHK). Cells were grown and antiviral effects determined as described elsewhere (4).

Ocular Infections and Treatments

New Zealand white rabbits were inoculated without scarification with 10^5 PFU/eye of McKrae strain HSV-1. Topical IFN doses were given for 7 or 14 consecutive days beginning 4 hours after inoculation. Each treatment group consisted of 6-9 rabbits.

Eyes were examined daily using a 0 (normal) to 4+ (most severe) grading system for corneal epithelial involvement and conjunctivitis. The average score for each group was calculated on each day and significance of differences between groups determined by the Newman-Keuls multiple comparison method.

Hamster studies

Six to 8 week old Syrian golden hamsters were infected i.p. with HSV-2 ($3x10^3$ $TCID_{50}$ = $100xLD_{50}$) or EMCV (10^3 PFU = $200xLD_{50}$) and treated with saline (controls) or IFN-αCon_1, 10^5 U or 10^6 U at 6 h prior to infection or 10 h after infection. At least 10 animals were included in each treatment group and survival was monitored.

RESULTS

Natural IFN-γ and IFN-γ_{4A} were equally effective against HSV-1 and -2 infection of T98G cells with 50% inhibition occurring at less than 100 U/ml. On a units basis IFN-αCon_1 was as effective as natural IFN-α against HSV-1 and -2 in T98G cells and this was comparable to effects against EMCV. IFN-αCon_1 was also effective against EMCV and HSV-2 in hamster cells infected with these viruses. Effects against HSV-2 in hamsters were therefore investigated.

Systemic HSV-2 infection of hamsters is rapidly lethal but a single treatement with IFN-αCon_1 (10^6 U) was highly effective and protected 90% of animals when given 6 h before infection and 45% of animals when given 10 h after infection. EMCV infection of hamsters was also responsive to IFN-αCon_1 but a 10-fold lower dose (10^5 U) produced the same degree of protection.

The activities of IFN-αCon_1 and IFN-γ_{4A} have not been assessed in rabbit cell cultures. However, previous studies have shown that efficacy against HSV-1 infection of the rabbit eye is unrelated to activity in cell cultures (5,6).

Rabbit eyes treated with IFN-αCon_1 for acute herpetic keratitis had less corneal epithelial involvement and conjunctivitis than did eyes treated with saline or IFN-γ_{4A} (Figure 1). Iritis and corneal stromal clouding were also decreased by IFN-αCon_1 treatment. In other studies, in which rabbits were treated in a similar manner, HSV was isolated from 3 of 10 trigeminal ganglia of IFN-αCon_1 treated rabbits, as compared to 10 of 12 trigeminal ganglia of placebo-treated rabbits. Efficacy of IFN-αCon_1, in terms of the symptoms investigated and virus isolates, was greater with 7 days of treatment than with 14 days of treatment. A dose-response study indicated that IFN-αCon$_1$ was as potent, on a units basis, as other human IFN-αs. No treatment schedule with IFN-γ_{4A} was found which had a demonstrable effect on HSV-1 ocular infections in rabbits.

DISCUSSION

Cell culture studies have generally shown that HSV-1 and -2 are less susceptible to human IFN-α treatment than are many other viruses (7). However, in some cell lines EMCV and HSV-2 show similar sensitivity (4). Although the same relative IFN sensitivity of different viruses occurs in different cell lines (7) there are instances of marked differences (8,9).

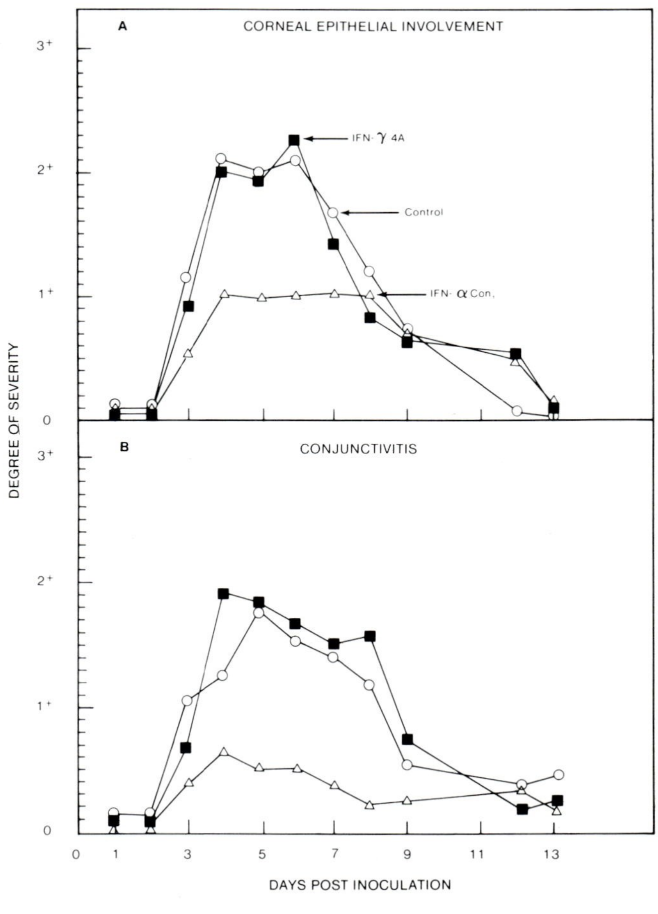

Fig. 1 Corneal epithelial involvement (A) and conjunctivitis (B) in rabbits following inoculation of HSV-1. Beginning 4 h after infection, eyes were treated topically 4 times a day for 14 consecutive days with either 10^6 U/eye/day IFN-αCon$_1$ (△), 10^6 U/eye/day IFN-γ_{4A} (■), or saline (0).

The activity of IFN-αCon_1 against HSV-1 infection of rabbit eyes indicates that potency is related to specific activity. Since IFN-αCon_1 is about 20 times more potent than other IFN-αs (2) this analog could have clinical advantages. The mechanisms of IFN action in the rabbit system are uncertain but appear to be indirect (5,6). The current studies indicate that a shorter treatment period (7 days) is better than 14 days. Thus extended or high dose treatments may reduce efficacy and this could explain why high doses ($15x10^6$ U/eye/day) have shown no effect with IFN-αA (10). The absence of an effect with IFN-γ_{4A} in rabbits is consistent with its greater species specificity.

Efficacy of IFNs is related to treatment regimens (11) but successful treatment of local, systemic and latent infections could require different treatment schedules. For IFNs, as for antimetabolites, the generation of resistant virus strains needs to be considered but may be less of a concern (12). The efficacy of IFN-αCon_1 in hamsters indicates a second animal model for further investigations of treatment regimens and mechanisms of action of human IFN-α against HSV.

REFERENCES

1. Stebbing, N (1983) Adv Exptl Med Biol 166:23-35

2. Alton K, Stabinsky Y, Richards R, Ferguson B, Goldstein L, Altrock B, Miller L, Stebbing N (1983) In: DeMaeyer E, Schellekens H (eds) The Biology of the Interferon System. Elsevier, Rotterdam, pp 119-127

3. Rinderknecht E, O'Connor BH, Rodriguez H (1984) J Biol Chem 259: 6790-6797

4. Fish EN, Banerjee K, Stebbing N (1983) Biochem Biophys Res Commun 112:537-546

5. Smolin G, Stebbing N, Friedlaender M, Friedlaender R, Okumoto M (1982) Arch Ophthalmol 100:481-483

6. Grabner G, Smolin G, Okumoto M, Stebbing N (1983) Curr Eye Res 2:785-790

7. Kramer MJ, Dennin R, Kramer G, Jones G, Connell E, Rolon N, Gruarin A, Kale R, Trown PW (1983) J Interferon Res 3:425-435

8. Stebbing N (1983) In: Smolin G (ed) Antimicrobial Agents in Ophthalmology. Masson Publishing, pp 151-161

9. Weck P, Apperson S, May L, Stebbing N (1981) J gen Virol 57:233-237

10. Sanitanto J, Varnell ED, Kaufman HE, Raju VK (1984) Invest Ophthalmol Vis Sci 25:874-876

11. Lee SE, Chiu H, Rinderknecht E, Sabo W, Stebbing N (1983) Cancer Res 43:4172-4175

12. Stebbing N (1979) J gen Virol 44:255-260

THERAPEUTIC ENDEAVOURS IN CHRONIC B+ve HEPATITIS

DAVID BRIGDEN

Clinical and Applied Research Division, Wellcome Research Laboratories, Langley Court, Beckenham, Kent (England)

INTRODUCTION

Chronic infection by the hepatitis B virus is a major afflication of mankind. The World Health Organisation estimate that there are between 170 and 200 million people infected in the world. The infection can and frequently does lead to premature death from cirrhosis or primary hepatocellular carcinoma[1]. Pioneering work into the possible use of antiviral therapy in chronic B+ve hepatitis by Merigan and his coworkers[2] concentrated on the use of Adenine arabinoside (Ara A) and Interferon. This work suggested that Interferon and Ara A were effective at permanently inhibiting viral replication in a proportion of patients and that combination therapy might offer an enhanced effect.

The objectives of antiviral therapy in chronic B positive hepatitis can be defined as follows:-

1. the suppression of virus replication during treatment.
2. The permanent suppression of virus replication and thus the production of the non infective state.
3. An improvement in the liver pathology.
4. The reduction in mortality from cirrhosis and primary hepatocellular carcinoma.

The suppression of virus replication is demonstrated by a reduction in the level of viral DNA polymerase and viral DNA in the circulating blood. These measures of virus replication can return after the end of therapy or remain permanently suppressed. Permanent suppression is confirmed if 'e' antigen is lost and is further reinforced if surface (s) antigen also disappears. The loss of these antigens may or may not be accompanied by the development of the corresponding antibodies. Ultimately confirmation of the success of treatment must be demonstrated by the loss of core (c) antigen and the improvement in the inflamatory liver disease.

This paper describes the approach that we have taken at the Wellcome Research Laboratories in collaboration with investigators in London University (quoted in the text) to explore the use of Wellferon (lymphoblastoid interferon) and acyclovir (Zovirax).

METHODS

Wellferon is produced from lymphoblastoid cells (Namalwa cells) in deep cell culture and purified by affinity chromatography and trichloroacetic acid precipitation producing highly purified mixture of at least 8 different alpha interferons[3]. Acyclovir was used as the sodium salt (Zovirax i.v.) and was infused intravenously at the doses quoted.

Wellferon (Lymphoblastoid Interferon)

Initial pilot studies were conducted in patients who had evidence of chronic B positive hepatitis for six months or more and who had raised DNA polymerase. Clear evidence of prompt depression of DNA polymerase was seen[4]. A controlled trial was then established to compare the results in patients on Adenine arabinoside monophosphate (Ara-AMP) and Wellferon. The protocol called for three arms to the study, the first consisting of patients treated with Ara-AMP at a dose of 10 mg/kg/day by IM injection for four weeks the second arm consisted of patients treated with the same dose of Ara-AMP but for 8 weeks and the third arm consisted of patients treated with Wellferon by IM injection at a dose of 10 mega units/square meter daily for 5 days followed by the same dose three times/week for 12 weeks. Forty-five patients were to be randomised between the three arms and follow up would proceed for at least one year. Early results were published by Lok et al.[5] All patients showed significant depression of their DNA polymerase. Between 20 and 25% of the Ara-AMP patients showed permanent suppression of their markers of virus replication at 6 months whereas 45% of the Interferon patients did. Furthermore 36% of the interferon patients had also lost 'e' ag by this time whereas no such findings were seen in the Ara-AMP patients. Further information is now available on all the patients entered into the trial although follow-up is not yet complete. Fifteen % of the Ara-AMP patients can be considered responders as measured by loss of 'e' ag whereas 31% of the interferon treated patients responded by the same criterion. (Details of the responders in each group can be seen in Fig. 1). All the Ara AMP patients were in the short treatment group. It is also noteworthy that in the interferon group the responses were much closer in time to the treatment period.

Several larger controlled clinical trials mainly in comparison with no treatment are now in hand though because of the long period of follow up required in these studies it will still be some considerable time before a full evaluation of the role of Wellferon in this disease can be made.

ACYCLOVIR (ZOVIRAX)

Although acyclovir is a specific antiherpes drug it seemed sensible to test a seemingly safe antiviral drug in the treatment of chronic B+ve hepatitis. Consequently pilot studies were set up at the Royal Free Hospital in London by Dr. Howard Thomas. The results[6] showed that at high intravenous doses (15 mg/kg every 8 hours) reductions in the DNA polymerase and viral DNA in the plasma were seen. In a study at King's College Hospital in which 14 patients were treated by continuous infusion of 45 mg/kg every 24 hours for 21 days Prof. A. Edelston (Personal communication) showed that 9/14 patients had a significant reduction in DNA polymerase and 5 of these (36%) lost 'e' ag. These results suggest that acyclovir is less effective than interferon at promptly switching off viral replication but the ability to induce the loss of 'e' ag seems to be not very dissimilar from the results produced by interferon. Unfortunately to give intravenous acyclovir requires in-patient treatment so it would seem desirable to develop a form of therapy that could safely

Fig. 1.

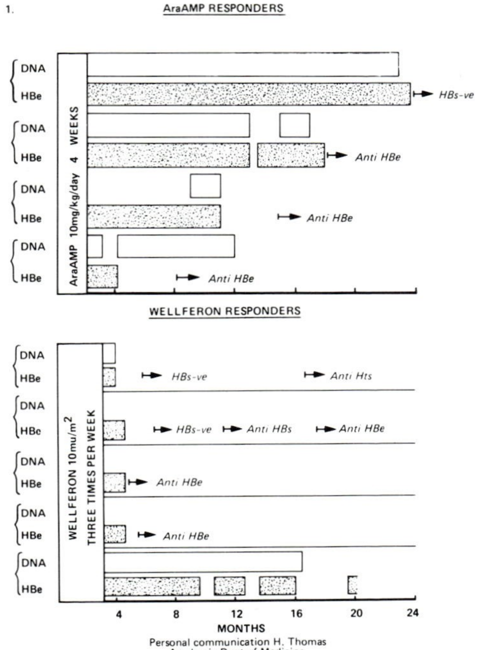

Personal communication H. Thomas
Academic Dept of Medicine,
Royal Free Hospital, London.

Fig. 2.

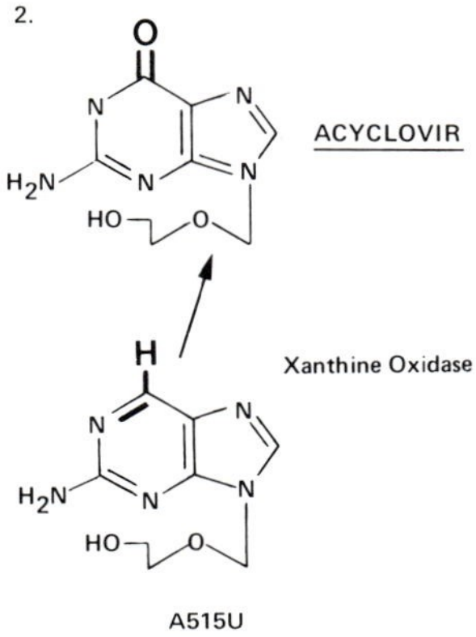

Fig. 3.

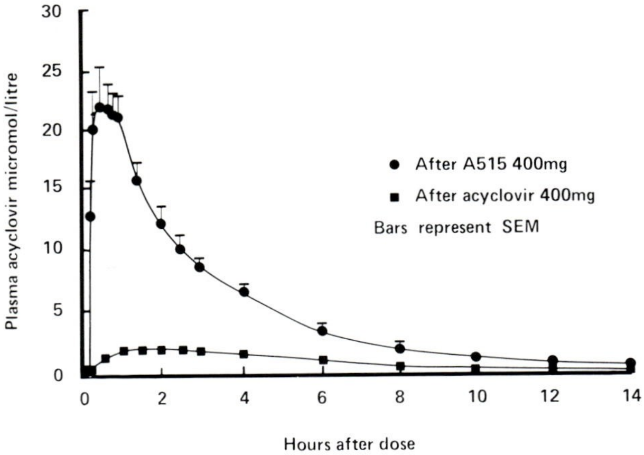

After Whiteman et. al. (in Press)

and conveniently be used in the out-patient clinic. Unfortunately oral acyclovir is only partially absorbed from the GI tract. Whilst plasma levels adequate for the treatment of Herpes simplex infections are achieved by oral dosing the levels are not high enough for the potential treatment of less sensitive viruses. Recently, however a prodrug of acyclovir has been developed that relies on xanthine oxidase to convert it to acyclovir[7] (fig. 2). Studies in normal human volunteers have shown that it is efficiently absorbed and converted to acyclovir[8] (fig. 3). Initial studies of this prodrug are now underway in patients with chronic B+ve hepatitis.

DISCUSSION

What progress towards the objectives has been achieved? Suppression of virus replication has clearly been demonstrated with a number of drugs. That this results in a permanent suppression combined with seroconversion in a proportion of patients is also clear. However, drug regimes need to be optimised and new drugs need to be developed. Whether the production of the non-replicative state confirs on the subject not only a reduction in their infectivity but also an improvement in their liver pathology will only be known when the long term follow-up of the patients currently in the clinical trials is complete. Success so far is only limited but it must give us hope that effective therapeutic regimes can be developed for the future.

REFERENCES

1. Beasley RP, Hwang L-Y, Lin C-C, Chien C-S, (1981) Hepatocellular carcinoma and hepatitis B virus. A prospective study of 22,707 men in Taiwain. Lancet ii: 1129-1133

2. Scullard GH, Pollard BB, Smith JL, et al (1981) Antiviral treatment of chronic Hepatitis B virus infection 1. Changes in viral markers with Interferon combined with Adenine Arabinoside J Infect Dis 143: 772-783

3. Finter NB, Fantes KH (1980) The purity and safety of Interferons prepared for clinical use: The case for lymphoblastoid Interferon. In I Gresser (Ed) Interferon 2, Academic Press, Oxford, pp 65-80

4. Weller IVD, Fowler MJF, Monjardino J, et al. (1982) Inhibition of Hepatitis B viral replication by lymphoblastoid interferon. Phil Trans Roy Soc, London Series B 299: 128-130

5. Lok ASF, Karayiannis P, Brown D, et al (1983) A randomised study of the effect of adenine arabinoside monophosphate (4 or 8 week course) versus lymphoblastoid Interferon on Hepatitis B virus replication. Hepatology 3: 865

6. Weller IVD, Carreno V, Fowler MJF et al. (1983) Acyclovir in hepatitis B antigen-positive chronc liver disease: inhibition of viral replication and transient renal impairment with i.v. bolus administration J Antimicrob Chemother 11: 223-231

7. Krenitsky TA, Hall WW, de Miranda P. et al. (1984) 6-Deoxyacyclovir: A xanthine oxidase-activated prodrug of acyclovir Proc Natl Acad Sci USA 81: 3209-3213

8. Whiteman PD, Bye A, Fowle ASE et al. Tolerance and pharmacokinetics of A515U an acyclovir analogue, in healthy volunteers (In press)

INTRALESIONAL HUMAN FIBROBLAST INTERFERON IN PATIENTS WITH EPIDERMODYSPLASIA VERRUCIFORMIS

MICHIHITO NIIMURA
Department of Dermatology, Jikei University School of Medicine,
19-18 Nishishimbashi 3-Chome, Minato-ku, Tokyo 105 (Japan)

INTRODUCTION

Epidermodysplasia verruciformis is a rare disease, and its warty lesions are caused by the human papilloma viruses. The wide spread warts begin at childhood and persist throughout life, and often associated with cutaneous malignancies. Up until now, there has been no effective treatment for these warty lesions. While the warts are benign, there is clear cut evidence that the malignancies begin in virally infected areas. Interferon has been reported to have therapeutic efficacy against viral diseases, and we decided to examine the effects of systemic and intralesional interferon in five patients with epidermodysplasia verruciformis.

MATERIAL AND METHODS

We tried two kinds of interferons. One is human fibroblast β interferon provided by Toray Industries Inc. Patients received 3 milion units of β interferon once daily or once every two days, intravenously for ten injections totalling 30 milion units for each course. Some patients also received intralesional β interferon. Intralesional injections contained one milion units per ml and were injected into each warts in volumes of 0.05 to 0.1 ml daily or every other day. The other interferon used was recombinant αA interferon kindly provided by Takeda Roshe company. Patients received 9 milion units a day intramuscullary, for eleven days totalling 99 milion units.

There were five patients with epidermodysplasia verruciformis, two females and three males (Table 1.). Patient No.3 has multiple skin cancers and intraperitoneal metastases (Fig.1.), and patient No.5 shows the typical reddish scaling macules of epidermodysplasia verruciformis, as well as the presence of common warts on the extremities (Fig. 2.) Patients first received courses of systemic interferon beta, then received intramuscular interferon β, after that, two patients received intralesional interferon β. With a 3ml dose limitation, we injected each and every lesion within a

Table 1. INTERFERON IN PATIENTS WITH EPIDERMODYSPLASIA VERRUCIFORMIS

case	age, sex		IFN-β (i.v)	IFN-α (i.m)	IFN-β (i.l)
1. Y.S.	22	f	60m.u.	297m.u.	582m.u.
2. Y.T.	38	f	60m.u.	403.2m.u.	510m.u.
3. Y.O.	38	m		99m.u.	
4. K.Y.	43	m		75.6m.u.	
5. H.Y.	41	m	30m.u.	106.2m.u.	

m.u.: milion units

selected area. This was repeated once every other day for six treatments. As most patients had thousands of lesions, total intralesional thrapy was painful and prolonged, requireing hospitalizations of up to two years.

RESULTS AND DISCUSSION

Patients received what we feel are high doses of both α and β interferons systemically (Table 1.), but unfortunately, no visible beneficial results were noted.

We previously reported a double blind study of intralesional interferon in common warts. More than 81% of the interferon treated warts were either cured or responded effectively to therapy. Only 17% of the placebo-treated lesions responded in this fashion. A statistical analysis of these data confirmed the effectiveness of intralesional interferon therapy in common warts (Table 2.)[1]. The average number of interferon injection until cure was 5.9. After our success with intralesional interferon in common warts, we decided to try it in the warty lesions of epidermodysplasia verruciformis.

This hardship has been rewarded with visible clearing, if not total cure (Fig. 3.). Although systemic interferon was offen associated with many side effects, intralesional interferon's side effects were minimal. Some patients developed low grade fever but no patient showed any bone marrow suppresion.

The histologic findings of the warty lesion of epidermodysplasia verruciformis show numerous vacuolated cells in the upper stratum Malpigii and granular layer, and many viral particles are found in the nuclei of the cells of granular layer by electron microscopic examination. These particles were further identified as human papilloma virus type 5.

The histological findings after the intralesional injection revealed disappearance of cellular clear degenaration, and no virus was seen by the electron microscope. Using the monoclonal antibodies, OKT-4 and OKT-8, most of the infiltrating lymphocytes reacted with OKT-4, which is a herper/inducer group. Paraffin-embedded biopsy specimens were stained by the peroxidase and anti-peroxidase technique with anti-papilloma virus immune serum. This serum stains tissue infected with papilloma viruses of any type. After the first injection the area was rebiopsied and we were surprised to see the total disappearance of viral antigens.

CONCLUSION

We treated five patients with epidermodysplasia verruciformis with interferon and concluded that although systemic interferon is not effective against warty lesions of epidermodysplasia vrruciformis, intralesional beta interferon was quite effective, although its administration was plrolonged and painful. We do not know how interferon acts on warts, or why the virus particles disappear so quickly. It has been generally accepted that in cells

Table 2. INTRALESIONAL HUMAN FIBROBLAST INTERFERON IN COMMON WARTS

		Placebo					
	Final score	+++	++	+	±	-	Total
Interferon	+++	3	2	1	25	3	42
	++	0	1	3	6	0	10
	+	3	0	0	0	0	3
	±	1	1	2	4	1	9
	-	0	0	0	0	0	0
	Total	7	4	14	35	4	64

+++: cured ±: unchanged Z =5.6120
++: markedly improved -: worsened (P 0.001)
+: improved

pretreated with interferon, viral growth is blocked at the level of gene expression. There is also evidence that interferon may block the maturation and release of certain viruses. In addition, local inhibition of cell growth and local immunododulation may be among the mechanism involved.

REFERRENCE

1. Niimura M (1983) J Dermatol 10:217-220

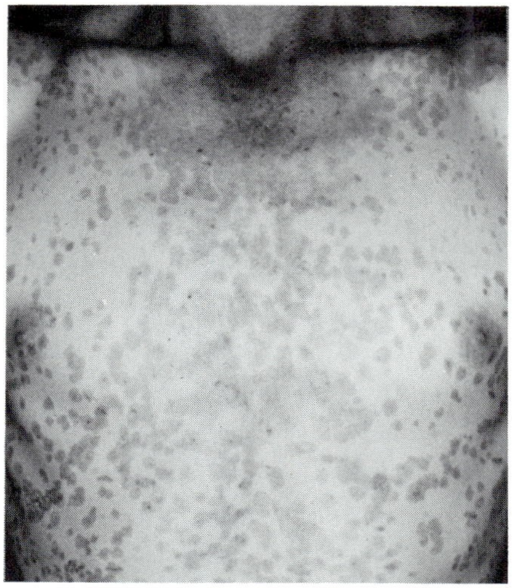

Fig. 1. Case No.3

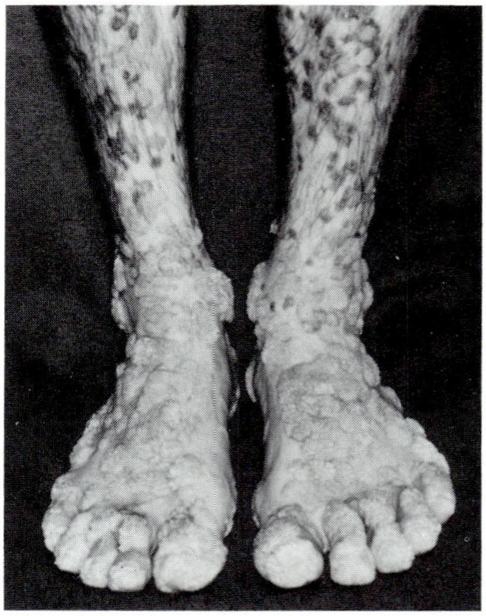

Fig. 2. Case No.5

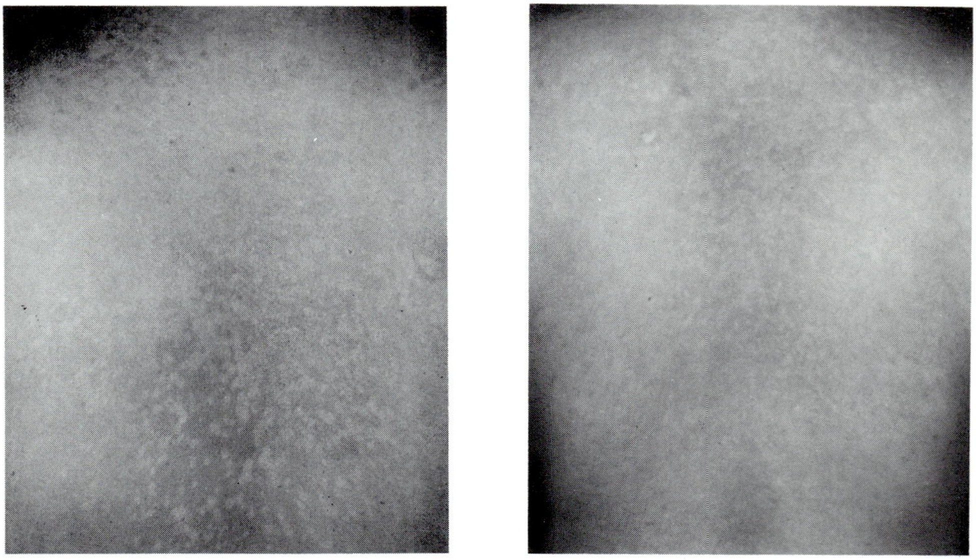

Fig. 3. Case No.1, before after intralesional interferon

Herpes Viruses and Virus Chemotherapy, R. Kono, editor

INTERFERON TREATMENT OF HERPES SIMPLEX VIRUS INFECTION AND PAPILLOMAS.

GEORGE J. PAZIN, M.D.

Department of Medicine, University of Pittsburgh School of Medicine, 969A Scaife Hall, Pittsburgh, Pa. 15261, U.S.A.

Our investigations of interferon treatment of oral and genital herpes and warts have involved close collaboration between infectious disease specialists (Drs. M. Ho, G.J. Pazin and I.D. fellows) and virologists (Drs. J.A. Armstrong and M.C. Breing), who share interests in herpes simplex virus (HSV) infections, interferon (IFN) and sexually transmitted disease research, and neurosurgeons (Dr. P. Jannetta and associates), who perform an operation that reactivates HSV in trigeminal ganglia of human beings.

INTRODUCTION

In 1978, we reported that microvascular decompression of the trigeminal root (MVDC-V), an operation for relief of trigeminal neuralgia, reactivated latent HSV in a highly predictable manner (1). In essence, we had an experimental model of herpesvirus reactivation in generally healthy humans.

In this presentation, I will review our published study of human interferon in prevention of HSV reactivations in this clinical - "experimental" setting (2) and will also present our recently completed sequel. In addition, our ongoing study of interferon treatment of initial genital herpes in non-pregnant women will be described and I will briefly summarize our experience treating papillomas.

INTERFERON-POST NEUROSURGICAL HSV REACTIVATION STUDIES.

MATERIALS AND METHODS

Subjects Patients with a history of herpes labialis who were scheduled for MVDC-V and had no significant underlying diseases were invited to participate. If informed consent was obtained, they were randomly assigned to interferon or placebo treatment. In study #1, patients received placebo or 70,000 units/kg, approximately 5.0 million units, human leukocyte interferon (Cantell variety) divided in two intramuscular injections daily for 5 days, beginning the day before surgery. In study #2, patients received the same dosages of interferon, but they were randomly assigned to receive 3 injections of interferon only before surgery (group 1), 7 injections of interferon only after surgery (group 2) or 10 injections of placebo before and after surgery (group 3). Placebo injections were added as necessary to maintain the double blind study design.

Stimulus to reactivation. The operation has been described in detail (1). Briefly, a blood vessel compressing the trigeminal nerve root was microneurosurgically displaced from the root and teflon or muscle was positioned between the blood vessel and nerve root. All patients received high dosage corticosteroids perioperatively to reduce edema.

Surveillance for reactivation. Daily, before and after surgery the patients were examined for herpes labialis. All typical and suspect lesions were cultured. Throat wash specimens were also cultured for HSV daily.

RESULTS

Study #1. Tables 1 and 2 present the effect of interferon before and after surgery on post-operative reactivation of endogenous HSV.

TABLE 1. HERPES REACTIVATION AFTER OPERATION

Group	No. Pts.	Lesions	+ Throat Wash	Total
Interferon	19	5 (26%)	8 (42%)	9 (47%)
Placebo	18	10 (56%)	15 (83%)	15 (83%)
Totals	37	15 (41%)	23 (62%)	24 (65%)
p value		>0.05	<0.05	<0.049

TABLE 2. CUMULATIVE TW CULTURE RESULTS

Group	Patient-culture days	Positive cultures	
Interferon	134	12 (9%)	P<0.001
Placebo	127	53 (42%)	
Totals	261	65	

Study #2. Results of interferon treatment only before <u>or</u> only after surgery are presented on Table 3.

TABLE 3

Group	No. Patients	Overall Reactivation Rate	
IFN "before"[a]	11	10/11 (91%)	
IFN "after"	23	13/23 (57%)	NS
Placebo	21	12/21 (57%)	
	55	35/55 (64%)	

[a]The "before surgery" group was discontinued when initial analysis after 30 patients indicated reactivation in that group was statistically significantly increased compared to concomitant controls.

CONCLUSIONS

Although transient fever, changes in neutrophil and lymphocyte counts and modest elevations of liver function tests were documented (see reference 2), natural Cantell human leukocyte interferon was well tolerated.

Three injections of interferon (∿7.5 million units - average total dosage) administered before surgery not only did not reduce reactivations, it appeared to enhance reactivation. Increased fever in patients receiving IFN before surgery may contribute to increased reactivation.

Seven injections of interferon ($\sim$17.5 million units) administered only after surgery did not reduce post-operative reactivation rate.

However, $\sim$25 million units of interferon administered in 10 doses over 5 days, beginning the day before surgery and continuing on the day of surgery and for 3 days thereafter, significantly and dramatically decreased the frequency and duration of post-operative reactivation.

INTERFERON-INITIAL GENITAL HERPES IN NON-PREGNANT WOMEN STUDY.

Encouraged by results of IFN in post-operative reactivation of oral herpes, we began a study of initial genital herpes in women in November 1980. Goals are to determine whether IFN can ameliorate initial genital herpes in women, to determine whether IFN can prevent establishment of ganglionic latency and to learn about genital herpes in patients of our region. Patients receive $\sim$36 million units Cantell IFN or placebo in 12 injections over 14 days. The first episode is carefully documented and patients are followed twice monthly for one year for recurrences or asymptomatic reactivations.

The code of this double blind study has not been broken so no data are available regarding efficacy. However, we have observed that initial genital herpes in women of our region is often ($\sim$35-40%) caused by type 1 HSV, and like others, we are observing fewer recurrences in these patients. Also approximately one-third of our patients have neutralizing antibodies upon enrollment and thus have initial "non-primary" genital herpes which is milder and shorter in duration. These factors will complicate data analysis and may require enrollment of more patients. We have also noted that source contacts of genital herpes are frequently asymptomatic and genital herpes, in contrast to other sexually transmitted diseases, is often acquired in "closed" relationships confined to 2 persons for 6 months or more.

INTERFERON-PAPILLOMA STUDY

Our investigations in this area have been confined to intensive studies in a single patient who is noteworthy because he has extensive chronic warts refractory to standard treatments. He also has atopic eczema with hyperimmunoglobulin E associated with decreased natural killer (NK) cell activity and decreased in vitro NK cell responsiveness to interferon and has idiopathic thrombocytopenia.

Studies of our patient's NK cell responses to parenteral interferon treatment have been reported (3). We have also reported (4) that no significant clinical responses of his warts were observed with systemic interferon, but intralesional injections to interferon (1.2 million units per injections time 8-32 injections) resulted in complete and persistent resolution of 5 separate warts. More noteworthy, we performed a double blind, dose-response study. The results presented on Figure 1 demonstrated that 1.9 x 10^3 units per injection was indistinguishable from placebo, injections of 3.8 x 10^4 units were the threshhold level for response and after 10-20 injections, $\geq$7.6 x 10^4 units per injection produced readily apparent responses. The dosages necessary to produce demonstrable clinical responses in our patient suggest that responses to systemic therapy are not likely unless other hosts respond in a more dramatic fashion.

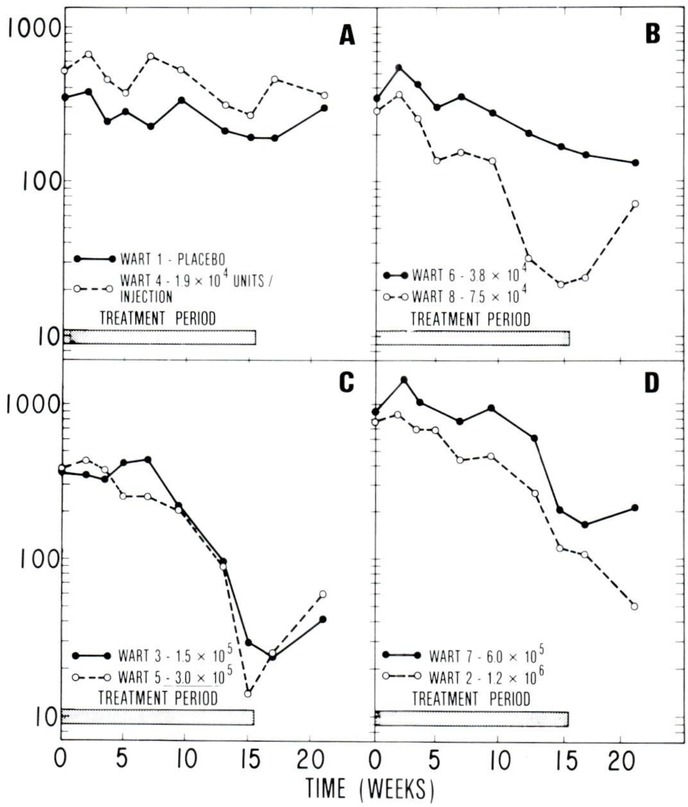

Figure 1. Effect of varying dosages of interferon administered intraletionally on on volume of warts (mm^3)

REFERENCES

1. Pazin GJ, Ho M, Jannetta PJ (1978) J Infect Dis 138:405
2. Pazin GJ, Armstrong JA, Lam MT, et al (1979) N Engl J Med 301:225
3. Ho M, White LT, Haverkos HW, et al (1981) J Infect Dis 144:605
4. Pazin GJ, Ho M, Haverkos HW, et al (1982) J Interferon Res 2:235

TREATMENT OF COMMON WARTS WITH INTRALESIONAL INJECTION OF HUMAN FIBROBLAST INTERFERON

SANAE HORIUCHI, SHUICHI NAITO, TORU BABA AND KENICHI UYENO
Department of Dermatology, Institute of Clinical Medicine, the University of Tsukuba, Sakuramura, Niiharigun, Ibarakiken 305 Japan

INTRODUCTION

While we have applied interferon (IFN) to a treatment of malignant skin tumors,[1] we also clearly demonstrated effectiveness of human fibroblast interferon (Hu IFN-β) against common warts in 1981.[2] Since then, we have used IFN-β for the treatment of common warts. In this paper, we will describe the mechanisms of its effectiveness from clinical point of view as well as summarize its therapeutical effect on common warts.

MATERIALS AND METHODS

Interferon. Hu IFN-β used in the treatment was a product of Toray Industries Inc..

Injection. Intralesional injection was performed.

RESULTS AND DISCUSSION

Interval of injection. The following experiments revealed that once a week injection might provide a sufficient clinical result. We prepared two groups of common warts. Lyophilized IFN 3×10^6IU was resolved into 3 ml of 1% procaine hydrochloride to be 1×10^6 /ml. Every wart received 1×10^5IU of IFN-β . One group was given once a week injection. The other group received twice a week injection. Clinical improvemnet was sufficiently obtained in both groups. In addition, total doses of the IFN required were almost the same.

The relation of dose of IFN-β required to the size of the wart. In order to study the relation between dose of IFN-β required for the treatment and the size of the wart, intralesional injection of IFN-β was performed into various sizes of the warts on 5 patients with many warts. The bigger wart required the more amount of the IFN. Similar analysis on 166 warts which had been randomly treated by the IFN exhibitted an identical result. These results might suggest that IFN-β acts locally against the warts.

Induction of erythema by the IFN injection. Intralesional

injection of IFN-β led to appearance of erythema around the warts in some cases. However, as shown in Table 1, its percent was smaller and the warts which produced erythema did not show significant difference in cure rate and in total doses of the IFN required for the treatment in comparison with those which did not produce erythema. This result seem to indicate that appearance of erythema may not be an essential phenomenon for treatment of common warts by IFN-β.

TABLE 1
Appearance of erythema around the warts.

	Erythema	No Erythema
No. of lesions	31 (38 %)	48 (62%)
cure rate	98.2 %	92.3 %
Total dose of IFN - β (IU)	$79.3 \times 10^4 \pm 29.3 \times 10^4$	$84.4 \times 10^4 \pm 23.3 \times 10^4$

Histological study on the warts with erythema revealed that neither invasion of lymphocytes nor necrosis of keratinocytes was found in the epidermis. The dermis showed slight mononuclear cell infiltration and delatation of blood vessels. Accordingly, the erythema may not be produced in association with the epidermal changes. Furthermore, a few times of the injection was required before we noticed decreasing a size of the wart. Thus, IFN-β may not provide acute changes to keratinocytes.

Therapeutical effect of IFN-β on common warts. We have treated 206 common warts on 52 cases. As shown in Fig. 1, common warts completely disappeared by intralesional injection of IFN-β. As can be noted from the data summarized in Table 2, the clinical response of common warts to the IFN therapy were remarkably encouraging. The treatment produced a significant clinical improvement in 98% of the warts.

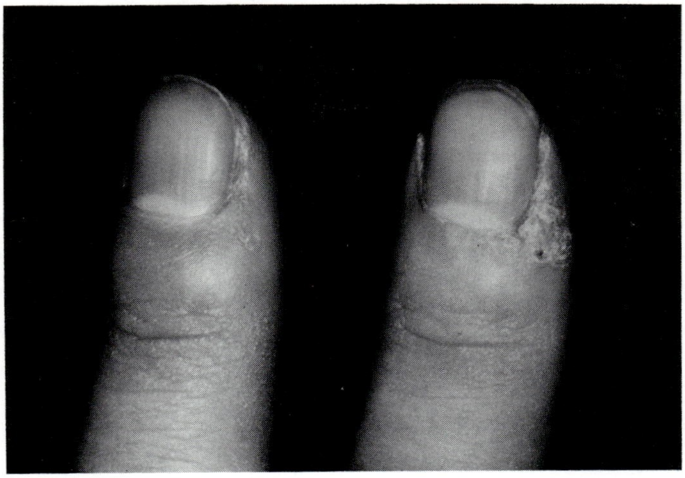

Fig. 1. Treatment of common wart by intralesional injection of IFN-β. left : after treatment, right : before treatment

TABLE 2
THERAPEUTICAL EFFECT OF IFN-β ON COMMON WARTS

Clinical response to treatment	No. of lesions	Cure rate %
Excellent	189	92
good	12	6
Fair	5	2
Poor	0	0
Total	206	

Local concentration of IFN-β. At this experiment, 1.5 x 10^6IU of IFN-β was injected into normal skin of healthy volunteers. Then, we kinetically collected skin specimen from the injection sites and prepared tissue extracts. IFN activity in the tissue extracts were measured by the method of CPE 50. The IFN activity in the tissue extracts decreased with time, but was clearly detected even at 72 hr after the injection. IFN activity could not be detected in the blood (below 6 IU) at this time. Therefore, IFN-β may stay in skin tissue relatively for a long time. Intralesional injection of IFN-β did not show any marked side effects. We also tried to use IFN-α against small number of common warts. However, even by local injection, the patients complained of fever, headache and discomfort. In addition, leukopenia was found. This difference may be partly due to the above character of IFN-β. In the present study, we demonstrated effectiveness of local use of IFN-β against common warts. One of the clinical benefit of this treatment, which we should pay attention, is that the warts can be cured without intense inflammation. Thus, this treatment would be useful especially against warts on the face, on the finger tip, or on the nail bed. The mechanisms of suppression of a common wart by IFN-β still remains unknown. However, the present study revealed that the amount of IFN-β required for the treatment depended on the size of the warts. And erythema induced by the IFN injection was not directly related to effect of the treatment. Consequently, we presume that direct effect of IFN-β on keratinocytes, especially on those affected by the virus, might play a main role in suppression of the warts by the IFN. On the other hand, we also found elevation of cutaneous delayed type hypersensitivity, when large dose of IFN-β was intramuscularly injected. Thus, further study would be necessary to know whether some immunological mechanisms might participate in suppression of the wart by IFN-β.

REFERENCES

1. Uyeno, K., Ohtsu, A.: Interferon treatment of viral warts and some skin diseases. Proceedings of the International Conference on Clinical Potentials of Interferons in Viral Diseases and Malignant Tumors. University of Tokyo Press, pp. 149-165, 1982

2. Niimura, M., Uyeno, K.: Clinical application of human β-IFN for viral wart treatment. Proceedings of Symposium on Immunobiology and Treatment for Cancer. Kyung Hee University Press. pp. 31-36, 1981

RECOMBINANT INTERFERON-ALPHA 2 FOR PREVENTION AND TREATMENT OF RESPIRATORY VIRAL INFECTIONS

FREDERICK G. HAYDEN
Departments of Internal Medicine and Pathology, University of Virginia Medical Center, Box 473, Charlottesville, Virginia 22908 (U.S.A.)

INTRODUCTION

Experimentally induced rhinovirus infections have been prevented by intranasal administration of either leukocyte-derived human interferon (HuIFN-α) (1) or recombinant DNA produced interferon-alpha2 (IFN-α2) (2-4). Protection appears to occur in a dose-dependent fashion, such that high dosages (22-46x10^6 IU/day) protect against both laboratory documented infection and colds (2,3); lower dosages (2-10x10^6 IU/day) generally modify the frequency and/or severity of illness (4). Protection has also been associated with once daily administration (3). Because of these encouraging results, several groups have conducted tolerance and efficacy studies of intranasal IFN-α2 in naturally occurring respiratory viral infections. This paper summarizes the results of clinical studies conducted at the University of Virginia and focuses particularly on the toxicity of intranasal IFN-α2 and its potential practical applications involving shortterm, episodic use. All the studies which will be discussed were randomized, double blind, and placebo controlled in design.

FIELD PROPHYLAXIS STUDIES

In the first field study, conducted in September, 1982, volunteers were given IFN-α2 10x10^6 IU (specific activity $10^{8.0}$ IU/mg protein) or placebo (vehicle containing human serum albumin, phosphate buffers, and 0.002% thimerosal preservative) once daily by intranasal spray (5). The population consisted of 304 working adults who self-administered the drug at work under the observation of a study nurse during the week and at home on weekends. The volunteers recorded the presence or absence of respiratory and constitutional symptoms, and if respiratory symptoms occurred, nose and throat swabs were collected for virus isolation. During the three week treatment period, 13 (8.5%) placebo treated volunteers compared to none of the IFN-α2 treated had laboratory documented rhinovirus colds ($p<0.001$). During the four week period after termination of IFN-α2 exposure, rhinoviruses were isolated from five placebo and three IFN-α2 recipients, and the first posttreatment isolate from an IFN-α2 subject occurred 11 days after cessation of treatment. These results indicated no rebound in infections after administration was stopped.

This study and one conducted at the University of Rochester, which used the same total dosage in two divided doses (6), documented for the first time that intranasal IFN-α2 was effective in preventing naturally occurring rhinovirus infections. However, both of these studies were terminated one week earlier than planned because of the unexpected occurrance of nasal irritation in IFN-α2 recipients. Nasal intolerance confounded symptom analysis, such that the number of illness episodes during the three week treatment period was actually higher in the IFN-α2 group (64 placebo vs 94 IFN-α2, $p<0.001$). These episodes occurred principally in the second and third weeks of IFN- 2 administration and were largely due to complaints of nasal obstruction. Episodes more typical of colds, with three or more days of rhinorrhea, tended to occur less frequently in the IFN-α2 group (20 versus 15) and episodes with three or more days of cough occurred significantly less often (8 versus 1, $p<0.05$), which indicated a real clinical benefit.

TABLE I

TOXICITY ASSOCIATED WITH INTRANASAL IFN-α2 $10X10^6$ IU/DAY.

	IFN-α2 (n=151)	Placebo (n=153)
No. (%) subjects with irritative symptoms	40 (27)*	8 (5)
No. (%) symptomatic subjects with abnormal exam	39 (98)*	4 (50)
Erythema	25	1
Erosions/ulcerations	28	1
Bleeding sites	24	2
No. (%) subjects with WBC <4,000/mm^3	16 (11)*	2 (1)

*$p<0.01$, placebo vs IFN-α2.

As shown in table 1, 27% of IFN-α2 recipients compared to only 5% of placebo complained of nasal irritative symptoms, including nasal obstruction, dryness, and blood tinged nasal mucus ($p<0.01$). Nearly all symptomatic IFN-α2 recipients had abnormal examinations. Most of these abnomalties resolved within two weeks of stopping intranasal adminstration, but one-third of those with ulcerations required more than 2 weeks for complete healing. Eleven percent of IFN-α2 recpients developed transient leukopenia (WBC 3-4,000 cells/mm^3), which indicated that high dosages of intranasal IFN-α2 may be associated with systemic side effects.

In an effort to identify a dosage regimen which would be acceptable for longterm administration to healthy adults, a second study was conducted in this population in April, 1983, at a dosage of $2x10^6$ IU/day in divided dosages (7). Although planned for four weeks, drug administration was stopped early because of the frequent occurrance of nasal irritation and the consequent concern of sensitization to either IFN-α2 or the thimerosal preservative. Over 80% of the volunteers in the second study had participated in the first field trial, so that the effects of a second IFN-α2 exposure could be assessed. As shown in table 2, no differences were observed in the proportions of IFN-α2 recipients in the second study who reported blood tinged nasal mucus or nasal dryness based on their prior exposure histories. The results indicated no evidence of cummulative toxicity to a second IFN-α2 exposure.

TABLE II

ADVERSE SYMPTOMS DURING INTRANASAL IFN-α2 ($2X10^6$ IU/DAY).

Symptom	Treatment	% with symptom	% symptomatic with prior exposure to		
			IFN-α2	Placebo	Neither
Blood tinged mucus	HuIFN-α2	44	48	38	43
	Placebo	15	17	13	15
		($p<0.001$)			
Nasal dryness	HuIFN-α2	34	37	29	36
	Placebo	11	17	7	10
		($p<0.001$)			

The low prevalence of viral infections during this abbreviated study did not allow an adequate assessment of efficacy. Laboratory documented viral infections occurred in 6 IFN-α2 (3 parainfluenza, 1 influenza B, 1 adeno, 1 rhino) and 3 placebo (1 parainfluenza, 1 influenza B, 1 adeno) recipients. No beneficial effects on illness episodes associated with rhinorrhea, cough, or feverishness were detected, and IFN-α2 recipients had significantly more episodes in which nasal stuffiness was the principal respiratory complaint (3 versus 14, $p<0.01$).

Some information on the antiviral activity of this dosage is available from studies conducted at the University of Adelaide (RM Douglas, personal communication) and the University of Michigan (8), which have found that IFN-α2 $2x10^6$ IU/day in divided dosages is protective against naturally occurring rhinovirus infections with an approximate 75% efficacy. However, studies at this dosage have not found protection against parainfluenza, corona, or other respiratory viral infections. These studies have also found significantly higher rates of nasal irritation in IFN-α2 than placebo recipients during 4 week periods of administration. In the University of Michigan, study the cummulative incidence of blood-tinged nasal mucus was 50% in IFN-α2 recipients, and mucosal erosions or ulcerations were detected in approximately 20% (8).

In summary, the occurrance of local intolerance indicates that IFN-α2 in this dosage and formulation is not feasible for longterm prophylaxis of respiratory infections in healthy adults. Tolerance and efficacy studies are needed in high risk populations, such as those with asthma, chronic obstructive, pulmonary disease, or serious cardiac disease, in whom the clinical consequences of respiratory viral infections are greater than in healthy adults.

SHORTTERM APPLICATIONS

One strategy for preventing respiratory viral infections with IFN-α2 is shortterm use after exposure to respiratory illness. Because of the relatively high transmission rate of colds in families, postexposure prophylaxis of family contacts is a logical approach for prevention. A preliminary report from a group of Swiss workers has indicated that recombinant leukocyte A interferon given at a dosage of $1.5x10^6$ IU/day for 5 days after exposure was not effective in reducing illness episodes but tended to reduce the burden of illness in family contacts (9). In addition, field studies have been recently conducted at the University of Virginia and the University of Washington to determine the efficacy and tolerance of intranasal IFN-α2, when used by adult and teenaged contacts of ill family members in a dosage of $5x10^6$ IU/day for 7 day periods. Preliminary analysis has found that repetitive, shortterm use of intranasal IFN-α2 is not associated with clinically important intolerance.

Another alternative to longterm or seasonal prophylaxis is treatment of established infection. Studies of the therapeutic activity of intranasal IFN-α2 have been conducted in volunteers with experimental rhinovirus infections at the University of Virginia (10). Seronegative adult volunteers were inoculated with rhinovirus type 39 on the first day of the study and treatments were begun with intranasal IFN-α2 ($9x10^6$ IU 3 times/day for 5 days) at 28 hours after virus challenge. The results of these studies are summarized in table 3. IFN-α2 administration was associated with a greater than 50% reduction in the proportion of virus positive days, and similarly, the median duration of virus shedding was significantly reduced compared to placebo. Studies of quantitative virus shedding found that IFN-α2 administration was assoicated with marked reductions of titers in nasal secretions by the third day of administration. These results suggest that therapeutic use might reduce transmissibility of rhinovirus infections.

However, approximately three-quarters of the volunteers in each of the treatment groups developed clinical colds, which indicated that a relatively high dosage of IFN-α2 given late in the incubation period did not prevent rhinovirus colds. Peak nasal symptom scores (days 2 and 3 postchallenge) were significantly reduced in IFN-α2 recipients (10), and trends toward reduced quantities of nasal mucus and associated use of nasal tissues were present in the IFN-α2 group (table 4). Further studies in natural colds are needed to determine the therapeutic effects of IFN-α2 in reducing the morbidity associated with common colds, both the respiratory symptoms and complications such as tracheobronchitis, sinusitis, otitis media, and exaccerbations of underlying airways disease.

TABLE III

INFECTION AND ILLNESS IN EXPERIMENTAL RV39 INFECTION.

	IFN-α2 (n=15)	Placebo (n=14)	
Laboratory documented infection (%)	80	93	
Virus positive days (% of total)	31	68	($p<0.01$)
Duration of shedding (median no. days)	3.8	8.2	($p<0.03$)
Colds (%)	73	79	
Nasal symptoms (score/9 days)*	16±11	20±9	
Nasal mucus weights (grams/4.5 days)*	8±8	17±16	($p<0.1$)
Nasal tissue counts (no./4.5 days)*	19+13	40+44	($p<0.1$)

*Values listed as mean ±S.D.

MECHANISMS OF INTOLERANCE

Studies by various groups have provided consistent evidence that topical IFN-α2 is associated with nasal mucosal irritation, although the causes of this local intolerance have not been resolved. Nasal tolerance studies incorporating detailed histologic analysis of punch nasal biopsies have determined that IFN-α2 exposure is associated with alterations in the histology of the nasal mucosa (table 4) (11). In this study the most common histopathologic alteration was an increase in the number of mononuclear cells in the submucosa 58% of IFN-α2 treated volunteers developed moderate or marked submucosal chronic inflammation after 28 days of exposure.

TABLE IV.

Histology of nasal biopsies after 28 days of intranasal IFN-α2 (8.5×10^6 IU/day).

	Pretreatment		Posttreatment	
	IFN-α2 (n=26)	Placebo (n=26)	IFN-α2 (n=26)	Placebo (n=26)
Epithelial inflammation (moderate or severe)	0	0	5(19%)*	0
Epithelial ulceration	0	0	4(15%)	0
Submucosal inflammation (moderate or severe)	0	0	15(58%)†	0

*$p=0.05$, posttreatment HuIFN-α2 vs pretreatment or vs placebo.

†$p<0.0001$.

A second study, which utilized recombinant leukocyte A interferon at a dosage of 9×10^6 units/day, was conducted to determine the nature of the inflammatory cells involved in this histologic response and the kinetics of their appearance (12). Preliminary analysis has found that approximately one-half of the IFN-α2 recipients developed increases in lymphocytic infiltration in postexposure biopsies, compared to preexposure, after 4 or 10 days of treatment. The clinical significance of these observations remains to be determined, but the results suggest that the histologic changes are secondary to the immunologic activity of IFN-α2 and are linked to the clinical intolerance observed. Comparable studies using other interferons including HuIFN-α (leukocyte) and also histologic studies during the course of naturally occurring respiratory viral infection, particularly those marked by brisk interferon responses such as influenza A virus infection, would provide some perspective on these findings.

REFERENCES

1. Scott GM, Phillpotts RJ, Wallace J, Secher DS, Cantell K, and Tyrell DAJ (1982) Br Med J 284:1822-1825

2. Scott GM, Wallace J, Greiner J, Phillpotts RJ, Gauci CL, and Tyrell DAJ (1982) Lancet 2:186-188

3. Hayden FG and Gwaltney JM Jr (1983) J Infect Dis 148:543-550

4. Samo TC, Greenberg SB, Palmer JM, Couch RB, Harmon MW, and Johnson PE (1984) J Infect Dis 150:181-188

5. Farr BM, Gwaltney JM Jr, Adams KF, and Hayden FG (1984) Antimicrob Agents Chemother 26:31-34

6. Betts RF, Erb S, Roth F, Reichmen RC, Treanor J, Beutner K, and Dolin R (1983) 13th Internat Cong Chemother, no. SE4.7/1-5

7. Hayden FG, Gwaltney JM Jr, and Johns ME (1984) Antiviral Res [in press]

8. Shope TC, Schwartz SA, Monto AS, and Albrecht JK (1984) Abstr 24th Interscience Conf Antimicrob Agents Chemother, Amer Soc Microbiol, no. 1022

9. Herzog C, Just M, Berger R, Havas L, and Fernex M (1983) Lancet 2:962

10. Hayden FG and Gwaltney JM Jr (1984) J Infect Dis 150:174-180

11. Hayden FG, Mills SE, and Johns ME (1983) J Infect Dis 148:914-921

12. Winther B, Innes DJ, Mills SE, and Hayden FG (1984) Abstr 24th Interscience Conf Antimicrob Agents and Chemother, Amer Soc Microbiol, no. 919

VIII ANTIVIRAL AGENTS AGAINST OTHER VIRUS INFECTIONS

Herpes Viruses and Virus Chemotherapy, R. Kono, editor

ANALYSIS OF CIRCUMSCRIBED INFLUENZA VIRUS EPIDEMICS USING MONOCLONAL ANTIBODIES

J S OXFORD

National Institute for Biological Standards and Control, Holly Hill, Hampstead, London NW3 6RB, UK.

INTRODUCTION

This paper reviews our studies on the genetic and antigenic characteristics of influenza B viruses isolated during single outbreaks in three boarding schools. Such school communities represent a relatively homogeneous collection of susceptible persons with experimentally established levels of anti-influenza antibody and with reduced opportunities for the introduction of new viruses once an outbreak has commenced and are thus suitable for detailed investigations of the evolution of single epidemics. A particular reason for our interest in influenza outbreaks in these boarding schools has been the lack of efficacy of inactivated influenza vaccine in preventing epidemics(1). The use of the antiviral compound amantadine has also been investigated in these school populations(2). We considered that any biochemical and antigenic heterogeneity detected among viruses during an outbreak could ameliorate the protective effects of either antiviral drugs or influenza vaccine.

MATERIALS AND METHODS

Virus isolation procedures.

In order to avoid arbitrary selection of a single plaque as representative of a possibly heterogeneous virus population, clinical specimens were not plaque-purified. Only infected egg allantoic fluids were used for serological investigations unless otherwise stated since we have recently described antigenic differences between influenza B viruses cultivated in MDCK cells or in eggs(3).

Christ's Hospital, Horsham, UK, from which the majority of viruses were isolated, is a boarding school for some 800 boys aged between 11 and 18 years(1). The school is entirely contained within its own grounds on a site approximately 2 miles from the nearest town. An outbreak of influenza caused by influenza B virus occurred at the school in 1982. There were 182 cases of

TABLE 1. Epidemiological and virological characteristics of influenza A and B virus epidemics in semi-closed communities

	Location and date of epidemic	Causative virus	No. of persons in the school	No. of viruses examined	Approximate no. of clinical cases	Antigenic and biochemical analysis of viruses
1.	Christ's Hospital School, Horsham, (1980)	Influenza A (H3N2)	800	110	200	30 antigenic groups. Most viruses in two antigenic groups. Viruses biochemically related.
2.	Christ's Hospital School, Horsham, (1982)	Influenza B	800	53	182	13 antigenic groups. Most viruses in two antigenic groups. Viruses biochemically related.
3.	St Edmunds School, Guildford, (1982)	Influenza B	190	6	?	4 antigenic groups. Viruses biochemically related.
4.	Christ's Hospital School, Horsham, (1984)	Influenza A (H1N1) (H3N2) (H3N2 + H1N1)	800	47	260 246 10 16	H1N1 and H3N2 viruses antigenically heterogeneous. Some persons were infected with both viruses.

The above studies have been carried out in collaboration with Drs J Smith and E Grilli, PHLS Laboratories, Guildford.

clinical influenza, including 21 for which there was no laboratory evidence of infection with influenza viruses. A total of 53 viruses were studied in detail, 51 from clinical cases and two from boys without symptoms (Table 1).

RESULTS

Antigenic analysis of influenza B viruses from Christ's Hospital School

Twelve monoclonal antibodies prepared against the HA of influenza B/Oregon/5/80[4] were used to analyse in detail the antigenic composition of 53 viruses isolated during the epidemic. Surprisingly, the viruses could be divided into 13 unique antigenic groupings. The number of virus isolates in each antigenic group varied from 1 to 16 but over half the isolates fell into two of the groups (III and IV). Most antigenic groups were detected sporadically during the course of the epidemic but viruses of two groups, namely III and IV were isolated throughout the outbreak and constituted approximately half of the isolates.

A group of six influenza viruses from a similar epidemic at another school, St Edmund's, was analysed using the same panel of monoclonal antibodies. These viruses were also antigenically heterogeneous and, moreover, formed four different serological groupings which were distinguishable from the viruses isolated at Christ's Hospital school.

Biochemical analysis of school viruses

The RNAs of representative viruses from the different schools were compared. Markedly different electrophoretic migration characteristics were noted for the majority of genes for viruses isolated in the different schools, but viruses from the same school were related and showed few differences. Thus, RNAs 1, 2, 3 and 6 migrated differently for a representative virus isolated at Rugby School, compared to three viruses from Christ's Hospital School and three viruses of St. Edmund's School. Oligonucleotide maps of RNA and RNA:RNA hybridisation (S.Klimov, unpublished data) of representative viruses from Christ's Hospital also confirmed the genetic relatedness of viruses from a single school.

DISCUSSION

Several explanations for the marked antigenic heterogeneity in the HA of these influenza B viruses from Christ's Hospital School are possible and include the artefactual induction or selection of antigenic mutants during laboratory manipulation of the viruses which would therefore have no relevance to the natural epidemiology of the virus, or the introduction into the school of several antigenically different virus isolates from some outside source during the outbreak. Genetic variation may occur during laboratory passage of influenza virus, as for example, demonstrated by Brand & Palese[(5)] and tissue cultures or eggs exert strong selective pressures[(3)]. However, biochemical analysis of polypeptides of 53 influenza B viruses from Christ's Hospital School only detected three viruses with changes in electrophoretic properties of NP or NS1 polypeptides which could be attributed to the results of random mutation. Also antigenically and biochemically quite distinct influenza B viruses were isolated in the three different schools and this would not be anticipated if random laboratory-induced mutations reached a significant level. Certain viruses were reisolated from throat swab material and were antigenically identical on each isolation. As regards the second hypothesis, if new viruses were introduced into the school during the outbreak from outside then a distinct change in prevalence of antigenic varieties of virus might be detected during the evolution of the epidemic. In fact a more or less random distribution of antigenic variants with time was noted and most viruses (such as those in groups III and IV) were present throughout the outbreak. Furthermore, no evidence of introduction of new viruses was detected when viruses of Christ's Hospital School were examined biochemically by analysis of polypeptides and virion RNAs. Rather, the viruses of an individual school formed a biochemically closely related group, distinguishable from viruses in the community or viruses from the other two schools.

We suggest, therefore, the working hypothesis that a variety of antigenic mutants in a dynamic equilibrium could be shed by a single person (including the person who initiated the epidemic) and these mutants would be selected according to the varying immune status of persons in the school ('clonal expansion') as they progressively become infected. This explanation would simultaneously concur with current concepts of genetic heterogeneity even in cloned RNA virus populations[6] and the limited antibody repertoire to influenza HA in children and young adults[7,8] thus potentially allowing new antigenic variants, even with a mutation change in a single epitope of HA, to escape neutralization and to spread. The data is not restricted to influenza B virus, since we have investigated outbreaks of influenza A (H1N1) and (H3N2) viruses in the same school with essentially similar results.

There has been an assumption in the past that limited outbreaks of influenza would be associated with a single influenza antigenic variant. Our present studies indicate that this assumption is an over simplification, and that the evolution of even small and confined epidemics of influenza is more complex than previously considered. It will be of particular interest now to correlate particular antigenic groupings with other phenotypic and genetic properties of the viruses including resistance or sensitivity to amantadine, and virulence, which could effect both antiviral or vaccine induced 'immunity' to influenza virus infection.

REFERENCES

1. Hoskins TW, Davies JR, Smith AJ, Miller CL, Allchin A (1979) Assessment of inactivated influenza A vaccine after three outbreaks of influenza A at Christ's Hospital. Lancet i:33-35

2. Payler DK, Purdham PA (1984) Influenza A prophylaxis with amantadine in a boarding school. Lancet i:502-504

3. Schild GC, Oxford JS, De Jong JC, Webster RG (1983) Evidence for host cell selection of influenza virus antigenic variants. Nature, London 303:706-709

4. Oxford JS, Hiyam Abbo, Corcoran T, Webster RG, Smith AJ, Grilli EA, Schild GC (1983) Antigenic and biochemical analysis of field isolates of influenza B virus: evidence for intra- and inter-epidemic variation. Journal of General Virology 64:2367-2377

5. Brand CM, Palese P (1980) Sequential passage of influenza virus in embryonated eggs or tissue culture: emergence of mutants. Virology 107:424-433

6. Holland J, Spindler K, Hordyski F, Grabau E, Nichol S, Van de Pol S (1982) Rapid evolution of RNA genomes. Science 215:1577-1585

7. Yewdell JW, Webster RG, Gerhard WH (1979) Antigenic variation in three distinct determinants of an influenza A haemagglutinin molecule. Nature, London 279:246-248

8. Natali A, Oxford JS, Schild GC (1981) Frequency of naturally occurring antibody to influenza virus antigenic variants selected in vitro with monoclonal antibody. Journal of Hygiene 87:185-190

ANTIRHINOVIRUS CHALCONES

HIDEO ISHITSUKA, YASUYUKI NINOMIYA AND YASUJI SUHARA
Nippon Roche Research Center, Kajiwara 200, Kamakura City, Kanagawa, Japan

INTRODUCTION

Human rhinovirus (HRV) is the major causative agent of the common cold. HRV can be divided into over 115 serotypes. This serorogical diversity makes the control of the infection by vaccine seem unlikely. Therefore, chemotherapy and chemoprophylaxis against HRV infection have deserved serious considerations. For several years we have screened microbial and natural products for antirhinovirus activity. Ro 09-0179 (4',5-dihydroxy-3,3',7-trimethoxyflavone), a potent anti-picornavirus agent, was isolated from, *Agastache rugosa* Kuntze (1). The discovery of this agent led to the synthesis of a series of analogs. Among hundreds of compounds prepared and evaluated, Ro 09-0410 (4'-ethoxy-2'-hydroxy-4,6'-dimethoxychalcone) (2) (Fig. 1) emerged as an agent exclusively active against HRV. Ro 09-0410 inactivated HRV with a unique mode of action, stabilization of HRV virion (2,3). In this report we describe some characteristic properties of Ro 09-0410 in detail.

MATERIAL AND METHODS

Cells

HeLa cells (Bristol strain) were grown in Eagle's minimum essential medium (MEM) containing 10% calf serum, 1% tryptose phosphate broth, 100 μg of streptomycin sulfate and 50 units of penicillin G/ml.

Viruses

HRV type 2 (HGP) and its subline resistant to Ro 09-0410 (2) were used. For preparation of [^{3}H] and [^{14}C]HRV type 2, the virus was gorwn with an ^{3}H-labeled amino acid mixture and a ^{14}C-labeled amino acid mixture, respectively, and were purified (3). The virus titer was assayed by a plaque assay method described elsewhere (2).

Fig.1

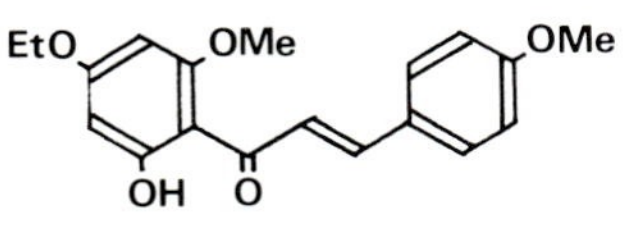

Ro 09-0410

4'-ethoxy-2'-hydroxy-4,6'-dimethoxychalcone

Virus inactivation

HRV type 2 (10^6-10^7 PFU/ml) was incubated with or without Ro 09-0410 in MEM containing 2% fetal calf serum and 20 mM HEPES buffer (pH 7.2) at 33°C. Thereafter, the virus suspensions were diluted and assayed for their residual virus titer. For the acidification, the pH of the virus solution was adjusted to pH 5 by addition of 0.3 vol of 0.2 M acetate buffer (pH 5), and then the mixture was incubated at 33°C for desired periods. The incubation was terminated by adding 0.3 vol of 1 M HEPES buffer (pH 7.2). The heat treatment of the virus solution was carried out at 56°C.

Compounds

Ro 09-0410 and [4'-ethoxy^{3}H]Ro 09-0410 (20 Ci/mmol) used in this report were synthesized by the method descirbed elsewhere (7).

RESULTS AND DISCUSSION

Specific activity to rhinovirus infection

Ro 09-0410 was active exclusively against HRV, but not against other viruses. Among 53 serotypes of HRV so far tested, 46 types were susceptible to this compound. The mean MIC was about 0.03 μg/ml, while the cytotoxic dose 50%, at which growth of HeLa cells was inhibited by 50%, was about 30 μg/ml.

Virus inactivation

The most interesting feature of Ro 09-0410 was that this compound inactivated HRV directly. As shown in Fig. 2, when incubated with the compound, HRV type 2 was inactivated by 99.8% at a dose of 50 ng/ml, while a subline of the virus resistant to Ro 09-0410 was inactivated only slightly. Virus inactivation was time and temperature dependent (2). Interestingly, infectivity, reduced by exposure to the agent, completely regained the original level by extraction of the agent with chloroform (Fig. 2). These results suggested that the virus inactivation was associated with interaction of the agent with the virus particles.

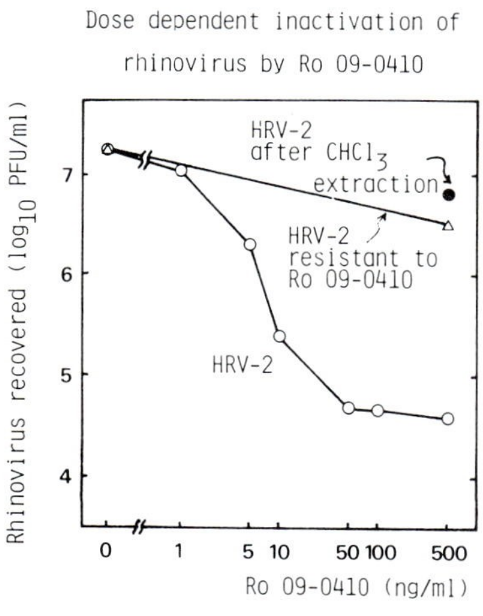

Fig. 2. HRV was incubated with Ro 09-0410 at 33°C for 2 hr. Point (●) shows remaining virus titer of HRV-type 2 after chloroform extraction.

Binding of Ro 09-0410 to a specific site of rhinovirus

The specific interaction of Ro 09-0410 with HRV was confirmed using radiolabeled Ro 09-0410 and HRV. After exposure of ^{14}C-HRV type 2 to ^{3}H-Ro 09-0410 at a dose of 0.042 μg/ml, the amount of the agentbound to the virus was assayed by a sucrose gradient centrifugation. As Fig. 3 shows, a distinct peak of ^{3}H-Ro 09-0410 was observed at the position of ^{14}C-HRV particles. Extraction of ^{3}H-Ro 09-0410 by chloroform from the peak fraction of ^{14}C-HRV, which was inactive, restored the infectivity to the original level (data not shown). These suggest that HRV was inactive while bound to the agent.

Fig.3 Specific binding of ^{3}H-Ro 09-0410 to ^{14}C-HRV-2

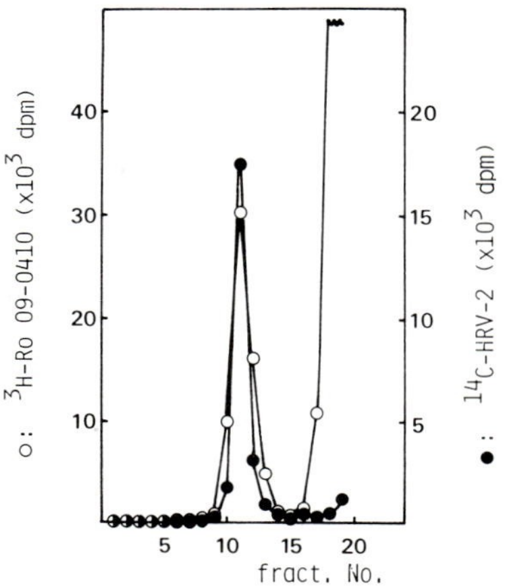

Further studies on the binding revealed that 1) Ro 09-0410 bound to the virion of susceptible HRV strains but not to that of resistant strains or other picornaviruses, 2) the binding occurred with intact HRV particles but not degraded HRV particles caused by pH 5 or 56°C treatment, and 3) Ro 09-0410 once bound to the intact virions remained bound even after treatment of the complex at pH 5 or 56°C. Ro 09-0410 was suggested to bind tightly to some specific site on the capsid of the intact HRV.

The mode of action of Ro 09-0410 have been compared with that of other agents such as 4',6-dichloroflavan (5) and RMI-15,731 (6), which are also active exclusively against HRV. These two agents were found to inactivate HRV directly through the same mode of action as that of Ro 09-0410, although their inactivation activity was lower than that of Ro 09-0410. All these agents bound to or interacted with the same site on the viral capsid of HRV type 2, though their chemical structures are quite different. These results suggest that the binding site is one of targets for design of new antirhinovirus agents.

Stabilization of HRV type 2 by Ro 09-0410

It is of interest to investigate how Ro 09-0410 bound to HRV makes the virus inactive. One explanation is that Ro 09-0410 stabilizes the virus particles in such a way that the virus resists uncoating process. In order to ascertain this possibility we made the following experiment. ^{3}H-HRV type 2 pretreated with Ro 09-0410 at 0.5 µg/ml for 60 min was incubated at pH 7 and 33°C, at pH 5 and 33°C, or at pH 7 and 56°C for 15 min. Thereafter, the size of the virus particles was examined by a sucrose gradient centrifuation. Upon incubation at pH 7 no difference was observed between the patterns of the radioactivity for the virus pretreated with or without Ro 09-0410. On the other hand, when the virus was treated at pH 5 or 56°C, the intact particle was completely lost, concomitant with the appearance of smaller particles. In contrast, the virus pretreated with Ro 09-0410 remained apparently intact upon incubation at pH 5 or 56°C, and the patterns of the radioactivity were the same as that of the virus kept at pH 7 and 33°C. These results clearly indicate that HRV was apparently stabilized by Ro 09-0410 to such an extent that Ro 09-0410 arrested the conformational change caused by the treatment at pH 5 or 56°C.

Fig. 4.

Antiviral mechanism of Ro09-0410

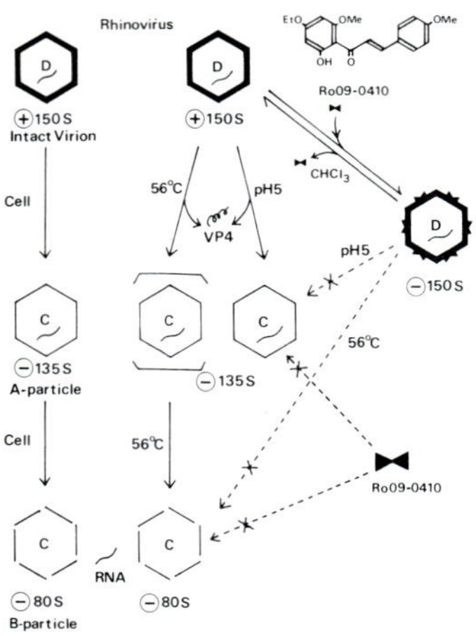

The mechanism of the inactivation of HRV by Ro 09-0410 is illustrated in Fig. 4. Instability of HRV at acidic pH is the most common characteristic property that distinguishes HRV from other human picornaviruses. Acid causes changes in the virion size from 150S to 135S and antigenicity from "D" to "C." Ro 09-0410 arrested these alterations through apparent stabilization of the virus conformation. Infection with HRV accompanies the same type of alteration in the infected cells as that observed by treatment at pH 5. Therefore, HRV, when bound to Ro 09-0410, may not be able to undergo such process in the infected cells.

In toxicological studies, Ro 09-0410 produced no adverse effects when administered to rodents by either the i.p. or p.o. route at a dose of 1 g/kg daily for 2 weeks. We have synthesized several analogs of Ro 09-0410, which are more active against HRV and more bioavailable than Ro 09-0410 (7). Ro 09-0410 and its analogs may have therapeutic value for the treatment of the common cold.

REFERENCES

1. Ishitsuka H, Ohsawa C, Ohiwa T, Umeda I, Suhara Y (1982) Antimicrob Agents Chemother 22:611-616

2. Ishitsuka H, Ninomiya Y, Ohsawa C, Fujiu M, Suhara Y (1982) Antimicrob Agents Chemother 22:617-621

3. Ninomiya Y, Ohsawa C, Aoyama M, Umeda I, Suhara Y, Ishitsuka H (1984) Virology 134:269-276

4. Suhara Y, Fujiu M, Umeda I, Suzuki Y, Ohtsuka T, Shirai H, Ninomiya Y, Ishitsuka H (1982) Proc 103th Annu Meet Japn Pharm Assoc page 388

5. Bauer DJ, Selway JWT, Batchelow JF, Tisdale M, Caldwell IC, Young DAB (1981) Nature (London) 292:369-370

6. Ash RJ, Parker RA, Hagan AC, Mayer GD (1979) Antimicrob Agents Chemother 16: 301-305

7. Ishitsuka H, Ninomiya Y, Aoyama M, Shimma N, Ohtsuka T, Kamata M, Fujiu M, Suhara Y (1984) Proc 6th Internat'l Congr of Virology page 245

RIBAVIRIN AEROSOL TREATMENT OF INFLUENZA AND RESPIRATORY SYNCYTIAL VIRUS INFECTIONS

VERNON KNIGHT and BRIAN E. GILBERT, Baylor College of Medicine, Houston, Texas.

Recently in clinical trials by ourselves and others ribavirin administered in small-particle aerosol was shown to be efficacious in the treatment of infections caused by respiratory syncytial virus, influenza virus A(H1N1), A(H3N2) and B. The purpose of this report is to summarize the evidence for those beneficial effects.

Production and administration of ribavirin aerosol. Aerosol was continuously produced from a Collison generator at a rate of 12.5 lpm with a mean particle size of 1.6 μm diameter. Respiratory tract scans with ^{99}technetium pyrophosphate aerosol revealed uniform deposition of particles throughout the respiratory tract in accord with predicted patterns of deposition (1). About 70 percent of inhaled aerosol was estimated to deposit within the respiratory tract. The aerosol concentration of ribavirin was about 190 μg per liter which led to an estimated deposited dose of 50 mg of ribavirin per hour in adults. Infants and children exchange smaller volumes of air and this difference is roughly proportional to weight. Thus hourly doses in adults, infants and children were about 0.82 mg/kg/hr.

Respiratory syncytial virus infection. This virus causes regular fall and winter outbreaks of respiratory illness, the most severe of which are lower respiratory tract disease with bronchiolitis or pneumonia or both. The disease may occur in very young infants and is the most important viral respiratory disease in the first six months of life. Bronchiolitis, inflammation of small airways, is associated with interference with expiration so that hyperinflation of lungs may occur. Respiration is difficult and inefficient which interferes with sucking, breathing, sleeping and general well-being. Severely ill infants develop major reductions in arterial oxygen tension which may persist weeks or months after recovery from the acute process.

We made a controlled study of the effect of treatment with ribavirin aerosol administered by oxy-hood in the treatment of bronchiolitis in infants (12 treated, 14 control) (2). In severely ill patients the aerosol generator was connected to a respirator. Detailed clinical, hematologic, biochemical and virologic studies were made. There was a clear trend of more rapid recovery in patients treated for five days, 12 hours per day, which reached significance on the third day of double-blinded observations ($P = 0.04$). There was no laboratory or clinical evidence of toxicity in any of the patients. Hall and her associates also made a study of ribavirin aersol treatment of respiratory syncytial virus infection in infants (16 treated, 17 placebo) (3). However, in her study, all of the patients had pneumonia associated with RSV infection, with or without bronchiolitis, and were treated for 20 hours daily, for up to six days, with a mean treatment period of 4.9 days. The rate of recovery from illness of treated patients in Hall's study was similar to that in the previous study. In addition, Hall found a significant reduction in the titer of RSV in secretions at the end of treatment in treated patients compared to controls. Moreover, it was found that arterial oxygen tension returned more toward normal in treated than in control patients. Thus, a physiologic abnormality of major significance exhibited drug-induced improvement. There was no intolerance or toxicity observed in this study.

Gelfand treated two patients with viral pneumonia complicating severe combined immune deficiency disease (4). In one case, a 5 1/2 month old boy, the etiology was RSV and in the other, an 8 month old boy, parainfluenza type 3. In both cases virions disappeared from respiratory secretions within a few hours of start of treatment and dramatic recovery occurred. Following five days of treatment of the patient with parainfluenza type 3 infection relapse occurred with reappearance of virus in secretions. Retreatment was again successful and a total of six treatments were administered before a successful bone marrow transplant resulted in recovery. The second patient with RSV infection had a successful marrow transplant after the first course of treatment.

Treatment of influenza A with ribavirin aersol. The first studies with ribavirin aerosol administered by face mask were in the treatment of influenza in college students (5). In that study 14 randomly selected students acutely ill with influenza were treated and 17 others served as controls. The infection was caused by influenza A/England/333/80(H1N1). The treatment was shown to be effective by shortening of the period of sustained fever (37.4°C or higher) (22.8 hours, treated patients; 38.1 hours, control patients; P = 0.008), more rapid reduction in height of fever in treated patients (36.9°C treated, 37.4 control on day 2; P =0 .003), more rapid clearance of virus from secretions which after 17-18 hours of treatment and later was significantly less in treated patients (P = 0.008) and more rapid disappearance of systemic illness (P = 0.004, day 1). In addition, a critically ill, 61 year old man with severe pneumonia and a high titer of influenza virus A/Bangkok/79(H3N2) in his tracheal exudate was treated with ribavirin aerosol and recovered within a five day period. In the following year a study of the effect of ribavirin aerosol in the treatment of influenza B virus infection was made (6). The results were very similar to those described above resulting from influenza A(H1N1) virus infection, namely, more rapid disappearance of fever and symptoms and more rapid reduction of virus shedding from treated patients as compared to controls.

These studies reveal a major therapeutic effect of ribavirin aerosol against respiratory syncytial and influenza virus infections. In addition, small-particle aerosol treatment may be effective in treatment of influenzal pneumonia.

REFERENCES

1. Knight V (1973), Lea and Febiger, Philadelphia, Chapter 1 p. 1-9.

2. Taber LH, Knight V, Gilbert BE, McClung HW, Wilson SZ, Norton HJ, Thurston JM, Gordon WH, Atmar RL and Schlaudt WR. (1983) Pediatrics 72:613-618.

3. Hall CB, McBride JT, Walsh EE, Bell DM, Gala C, Hildreth S, Ten Eyck LE and Hall WJ. (1983) N. Eng. J. Med. 308:1443-1447.

4. Gelfand EW, McCurdy D, Rao CP and Middleton P. (1983) Lancet 732-733.

5. Knight V, McClung HW, Wilson SZ, Waters BK, Quarles JM, Camerson RW, Greggs SE, Zerwas JM, and Couch RB. (1983) 249:2671-2674.

6. McClung HW, Knight V, Gilbert BE, Wilson SZ, Quarles JM, Divine GW. (1983) JAMA 249:2671-2674.

IX CURRENT STATUS AND FUTURE PROSPECTS

CURRENT STATUS AND FUTURE PROSPECTS OF THE USE OF BRM (BIOLOGICAL RESPONSE MODIFIERS) IN VIRAL INFECTIONS

TAKUSABURO EBINA AND NAKAO ISHIDA

Department of Bacteriology, Tohoku University School of Medicine, Sendai, Japan

We have tested many immunopotentiators of biological response modifiers (BRM) such as Streptococcus pyogenous preparation, OK-432 in our laboratory and have reported that a considerable number of these are interferon-γ inducers that can be used as anti-virals.

Here I would like to describe our reslts with an organic germanium compound, Ge-132 and glycyrrhizin preparation, SNMC.

I. Ge-132

Ge-132 is a carboxyethelgermanium sesquioxide having the structure shown in Fig. 1. It was syntesizied in 1967 by the Asai Germanium Research Institute.

Fig. 2a shows the time course of the interferon titer in mouse sera following oral asministration of 300 mg/kg of Ge-132. Fig. 2b shows the dose response effect of interferon induction after 24 hours.

As shown in Fig. 2, the antiviral activity appears 24 hours after oral administration and reaches a peak after 24 hours of 320 U/ml of interferon. Although the data is not shown in Figure, natural killer cell activity in the spleen cells is enhanced after 24 hours of adminstration and cytotoxic macrophages are also induced in the peritoneal cavity after 24 hours.

Next, we conducted an influenza virus infection experiment in mice to investigate the antiviral activity of Ge-132. We used the Kumamoto strain of the A2 influenza virus, and the pneumonia symptoms are shown by the lung consolidation scores.

After intranasal administraiton of the influenza virus in DDI mice, Ge-132 administered for 6 days in the doses shown in Fig. 3 produced these survival rates. As shown in Fig. 3, 100 mg/kg was the most effective dose for protection against influenza virus infection.

Fig. 4 shows the changes in lung consolidation score in the days after influenza virus infection. There is no progression in the Ge-132 group from the 5th day after administration.

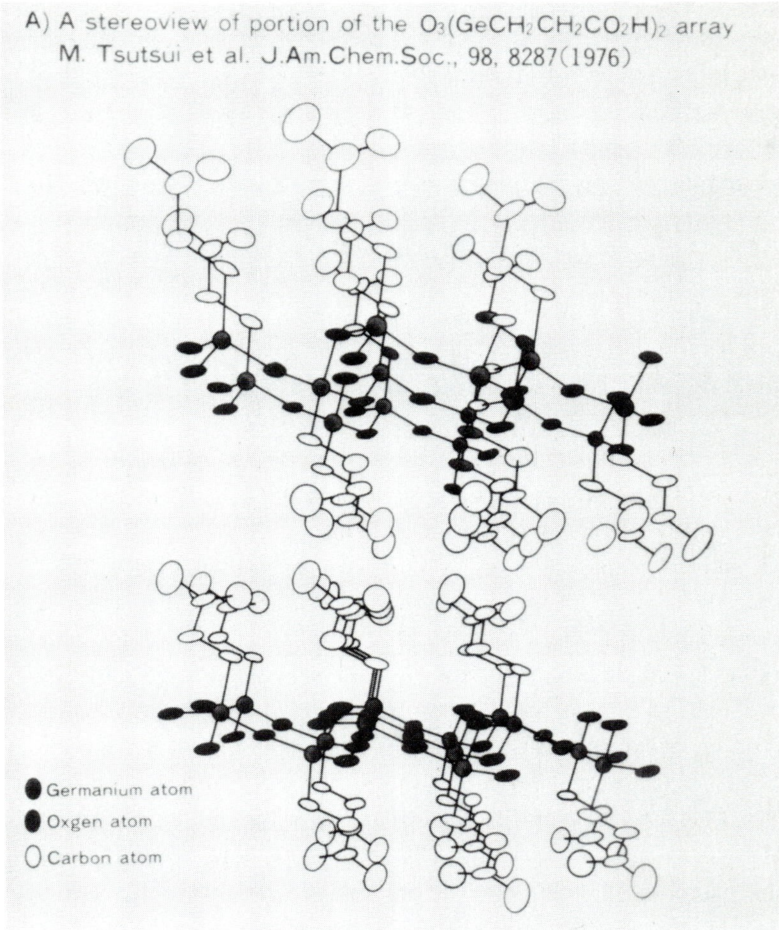

INTERFERON INDUCTION IN MICE BY ORAL ADMINISTRATION OF GE-132

Fig. 2.

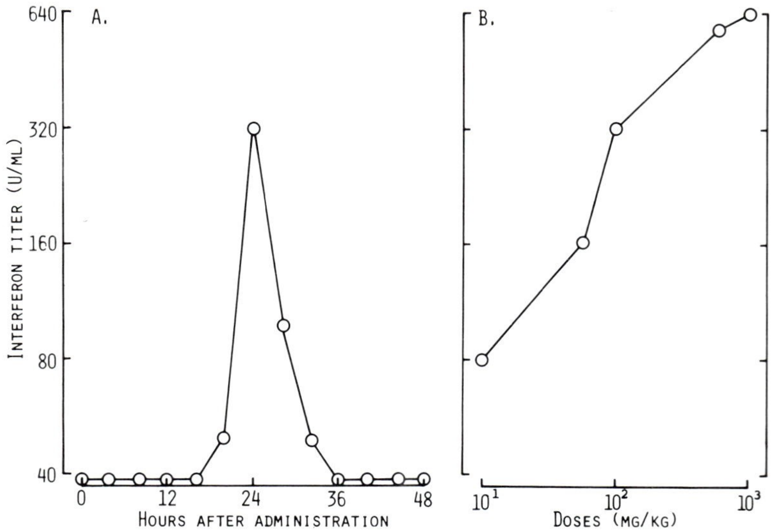

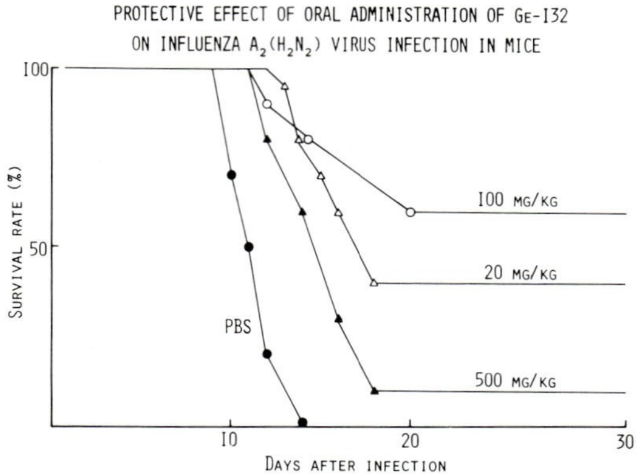

Fig.3.

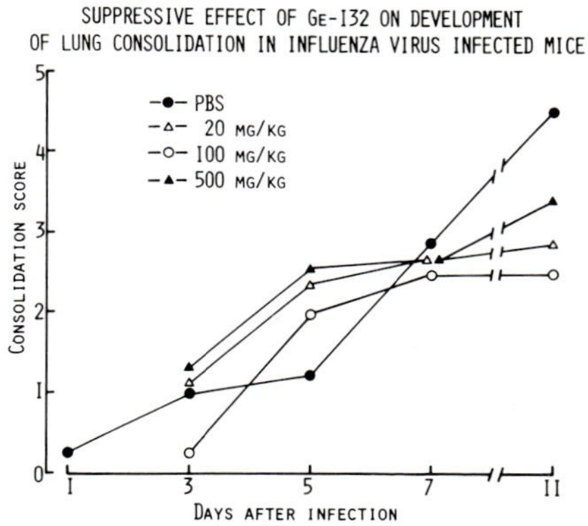

Fig. 4.

Fig. 5 shown inhibitory effect on virus growth in the lung after influenza virus infection. In the 100 mg/kg group, which was the most effective dose, virus growth is inhibited from the 5th day.

NK cell activity in the lung is clearly enhanced from the 3rd day after infection, and is further enhanced by administration of Ge-132. The infected cells in the lung are presumably killed by this enhanced NK cell activity.

II.SNMC

The glycyrrhizin preparation SNMC (stronger neo-minophagen C®) is shown in Fig. 6. It is composed of glycyrrhetinic acid and glucuronic acid and is extracted from licorice root.

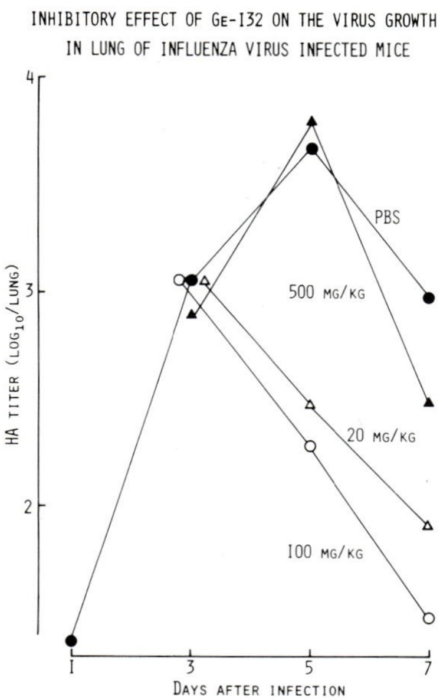

Fig. 5.

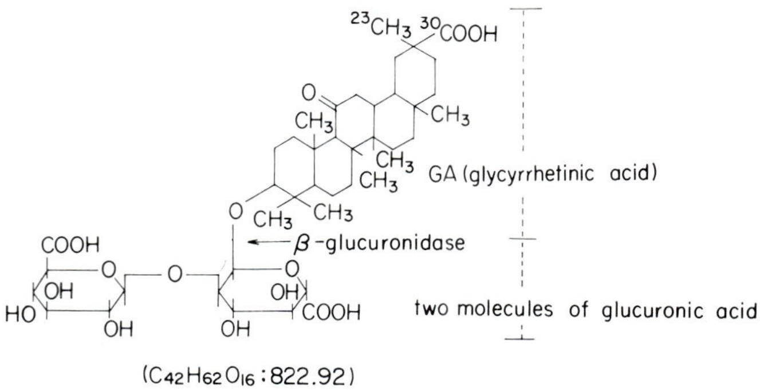

Fig. 6

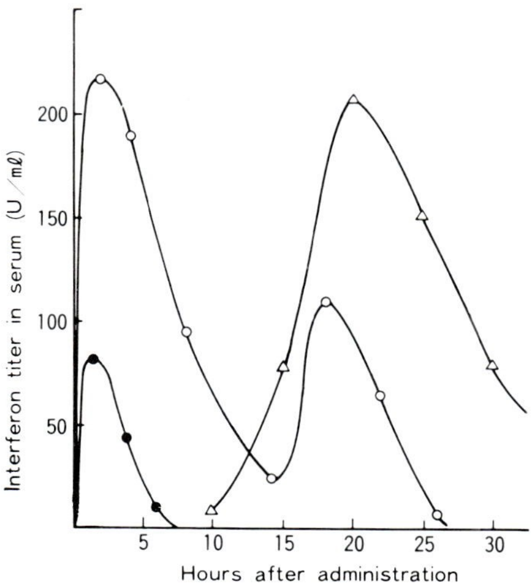

Fig. 7.

Using DDI mice, we examined its interferon inducing ability as shown in Fig. 7. The open circles indicate intravenous administration of glycyrrhizin and show 2 peaks. We believe that glychrretinic acid, which is indicated by the closed circles, also has interferon-inducing ability, and that glycyrrhizin is broken down and becomes glycyrrhetic acid after i.v. administration to cause a second interferon induction.

After 20 cancer patients were given intravenously 40 ml of SNMC containing 80 mg of glycyrrhizin, the relationship between interferon induction and enhancement of NK cell activity in the peripheral blood was examined. This result suggests that patients having general immunity showed both induction of interferon and enhancement of NK cell activity. However, patients lost general immunity showed no induction of interferon and no enhancement of NK cell activity.

Fig. 8 shows data obtained from Dr. Kiyoshi Fjisawa and his group at Jikei University, who conducted studies on the therapeutic effect of SNMC on patients with chronic hepatitis cases were given 40 ml each of SNMC every after day for several weeks by intravenous injection. Subsequently, they received the same dose 2 to 4 times a week for several months and finally once a week. The treatment was continued for an average of 2 years, and 8 months. The results of such intermittent administration are shown in Fig. 8. 7 out of 18 cases showed seroconversion from HBe Ag (+) to anti-HBe (+), 4 became HBe Ag-negative and in total 61% showed disappearance of the HBe antigen.

Changes in Serum HBeAntigen-Antibody System and the Long-Term Intermittent Abministration of SNMC on HBe-Antigen Positive Chronic Hepatitis

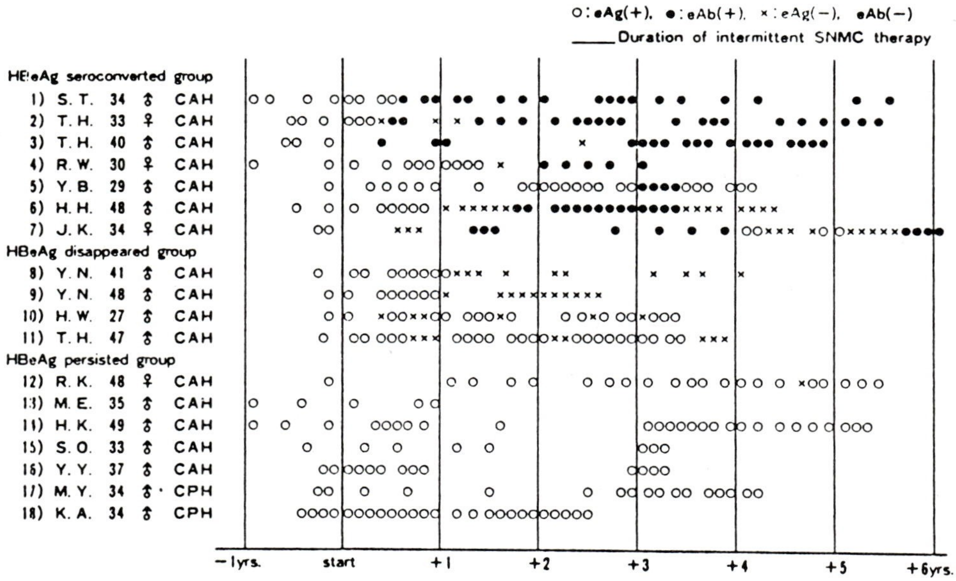

Fig. 8.

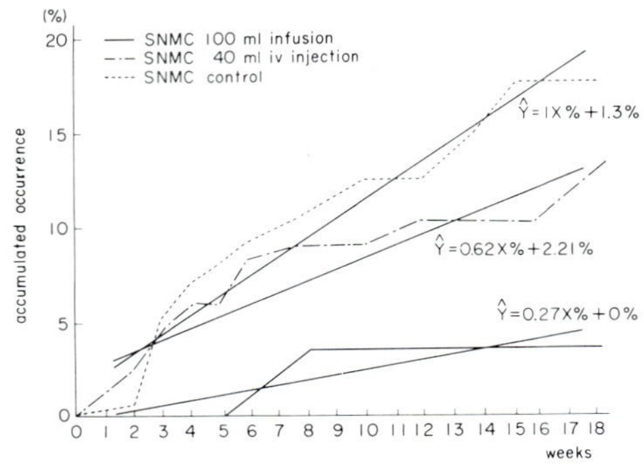

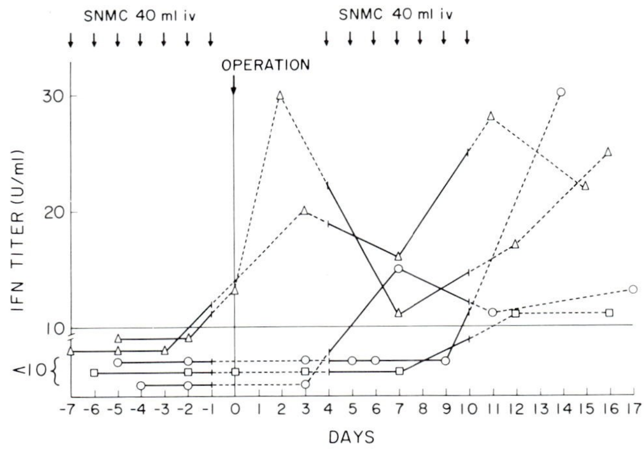

Fig. 9 shows the data concerning prevention of post-transfusion hepatitis that occurs after surgery. This is work from the lab of the late Prof. Kasai of Hokkaido University. The occurence of post transfusion hepatitis can be singificantly prevented by i.v. administration of 40 ml each for 2 weeks. However, when 91 transfusion cases were given 100 ml each of SNMC daily for 1 to 2 weeks by drip infusion, only 3 cases (3.6%) showed occurrence of hepatities, indicating that this glycyrrhizin preparation is effective for prevention post-transfusion hepatitis.

Our group conducted a study with a total of 20 surgical cases who were given 40 ml of SNMC by the i.v. route before and after surgery. Interferon was induced in all the patients as shown in Fig. 10. Furthermore, none have had hepatitis during the follow-up period of more than 2 years. These results suggest the involvement of interferon induction in the prevention of hepatitis by SNMC administration.

Herpes Viruses and Virus Chemotherapy, R. Kono, editor

CURRENT STATUS AND FUTURE PROSPECTS OF HERPES VIRUS VACCINES

FRANCIS L. BLACK
Dept of Epidemiology and Public Health, Yale University, New Haven, CT 06510 (USA)

Drugs have been used to prevent activation of latent herpes group virus when the risk is especially high, and vaccines can ameliorate persistent infections in animals. However, these are exceptions. Because drug administration must be sustained, it is unlikely to be suitable for prevention of herpesvirus disease in healthy persons, and because of the time needed for an immune response, vaccines will rarely be useful in treatment of active infection. Nearly everybody is now naturally infected with at least four of the five human herpesviruses and much of the disease with which we are concerned occurs in persons who possess naturally derived immunity. If herpesvirus vaccines must provide levels of immunity superior to those induced by natural infection, the prospects appear dim. However, in fact, most of us have adequate immunity most of the time. The vaccines must simply mimic the effective natural stimulation, while avoiding the pattern which, in nature, leads to inadequate protection.

The successful programs for vaccination against common childhood diseases have not been without problems, and these problems are relevant to avoidance of inappropriate herpesvirus vaccines. An inactivated measles virus vaccine can induce sensitivity without preventing virus replication and live measles vaccine, suppressed by maternal antibody, elicits a low titer that does not prevent infection but interferes with booster doses. Such pitfalls seem particularly hazardous when one deals with herpesviruses.

Drugs, replicating and non-replicating vaccines, each have distinct potential roles in controlling herpesvirus diseases. To identify the best solution in any particular situation, one must carefully identify the goal, the persons to be treated, and the natural course of the disease. Drugs will remain the agent of choice for control of some of these diseases, but a modified live virus vaccine or a vaccine composed of virus protein antigens hold promise in numerous specific situations. Primary infections with HSV1, CMV and EBV, when they occur in early childhood, are ordinarily sufficiently innocuous that there is little reason to try to meddle with the natural course of events. Primary infections with the other herpes group viruses might be prevented with vaccine. Though better prevented, HSV2 can give such a prolonged primary disease that drugs are useful in limiting it. Drugs will usually be chosen for treating serious localized infections such as keratis and encephalitis and, except in those instances when there is time to vaccinate before immunosuppression is effected, drugs will remain the most useful agent for controlling virus activation in persons with depressed immune responses. Drugs have proven extraordinarily effective in treatment of EBV associated tumors, but we might hope to supercede this with prevention by vaccination.

In those situations where vaccines may be useful, the preferred type of vaccine will depend on the goal which is sought. Safety tests of replicating vaccines pose serious problems because of the long delay between infection and appearance of some of the most serious sequelae. Hope is placed on the prospect that the genes responsible for latency and oncogenicity can be identified and removed so that we do not have to wait a lifetime to determine safety. It remains to be shown, however, if a virus which is incapable of latency can retain the ability to induce long term immunity. It may be preferable to leave latency in and remove only the capacity to reactivate. Because these vaccines must replicate to deliver sufficient antigen, they may be ineffective in boosting immunity in the partially immune recipient.

TABLE 1. POTENTIAL OF VACCINES IN CONTROL OF VARICELLA-ZOSTER DISEASES

GOAL #1. To prevent varicella in immunosuppressed children.
STRATEGY: Selectively immunize susceptible children.
AGENT: Attenuated live virus.
REQUIREMENTS: Minimal pathogenicity even when immune response is impaired.

GOAL #2. To prevent Varicella and Zoster in normal persons.
STRATEGY: Immunize young children.
AGENT: Attenuated virus without reactivation potential.
REQUIREMENTS: Long term protection; Long term innocuity.

GOAL #3. To reduce Zoster in immunosuppressed adults.
STRATEGY: Boost immunity levels in adults at special risk.
AGENT: Glycoproteins of infected cell surface.
REQUIREMENTS: Enhancement of cytolytic action toward infected cells. Effective even when immune system is impaired.

The other major direction being followed in vaccine development is to use only selected proteins to immunize. These antigens may be obtained by fractionating whole virus, synthesizing specific amino acid sequences, or transferring a key gene into a foster virus or bacterium for *in vitro* culture. The specific source does not affect general considerations of applicability. These vaccines avoid problems of reactivation and oncogenicity, but there are other difficulties. Adequate antigenic potency is difficult to attain without an undesirable adjuvant, wild virus will more easily mutate to resistance if antibody is generated against only one site, and, most important, narrowly defined antigens may not give a balanced immune response with destruction of actively infected cells, but few normal cells.

I will now consider the potential for vaccines against each of the five human *Herpesviridae*, starting with Varicella-Zoster because, thanks to Dr. Takahashi's group, most progress has been made here (Table 1). Three distinct goals can be identified. The first has been essentially achieved with a live virus vaccine developed by traditional methods of attenuation. Relative to the serious nature of this disease in immunosuppressed children, the fact that some of these children may later develop zoster is unimportant. Once the short term safety and efficacy of the vaccine was established, it could be used with assurance of benefit. The same is not true of Goal #2. Zoster is often a more troublesome disease than primary chickenpox. Takahashi reported no zoster in this group, but eight years is an inadequate follow-up. The Oka vaccine, or one like it, may also prove useful in boosting immunity in adults with cancer or undergoing transplant. For short term protection, such as this, in persons who have had prior experience with the virus, a subunit vaccine would be more logical, but it is unlikely to merit priority as long as the live virus vaccine promises to solve the more general problem, and drug therapy continues to improve in treatment of acute disease.

Turning to HSV1 (Table 2), such a small proportion of primary HSV1 infections are serious, their prevention is not urgent. Any vaccine would have to guard against the possibility that it might replace effective naturally derived immunity with an inadequate one, which would leave a greater number of persons subject to repeated attacks. A live virus engineered to remove troublesome genes holds the best prospect. By blocking access of superinfecting wild virus to the sites of latent persistence, such a vaccine might confer life-long protection. The situation is different for persons who are already afflicted by recurrent herpetic lesions. The prospect of reversing latency with a vaccine is not realistic and a live virus vaccine would not replicate well in a previously sensitized host. It is not clear what triggers reactivation. If it is determined by the nature of the latent state, drugs may offer the best prospect of control; but if it occurs

TABLE 2. POTENTIAL OF VACCINES IN CONTROL OF HSV_1 DISEASE

Goal #1. To prevent primary herpes virus infections.
STRATEGY 1: Immunize persons reaching adulthood without primary
2: Immunize everybody in infancy.
AGENT: Virus engineered to remove potential for reactivation, or selected balanced, highly immunogenic viral proteins.
REQUIREMENTS: Freedom from pathogenicity by reactivation
Longterm immunity to superinfecting virus.
Latency may be essential.
Absence of sensitization to superinfecting virus.

Goal #2. To prevent disease caused by established latency.
STRATEGY: Enhance cytolysis of infected non-neuronal cells.
AGENT: Viral glycoprotein presented in appropriate form, to affected persons, possibly in association with specific HLA antigens, and perhaps at regular intervals.
REQUIREMENTS: Immunogenicity even where natural infection failed to immunize, and even in the presence of pre-existing non-cytolytic immunity.
Absence of activity versus neurones.

---

whenever immunity wanes, stimulation of the deficient immune elements would rectify the situation and a vaccine containing selected virus proteins offers the best prospect. These proteins should probably be those which appear on the surface of virus infected cells and, to present them effectively, it may be necessary to incorporate them into lipid micelles, perhaps together with specifically appropriate histocompatibility antigens.

Prevention of primary infection by HSV2 is more important than HSV1, especially if we envision immunizing persons who reach puberty without immunity to either of the herpes simplex viruses (Table 3). Inasmuch as the cross immunity derived from HSV1 offers some protection against HSV2 it seems probable that some benefit might be achieved relatively easily. A genetically modified replicating vaccine may present fewer risks. For the treatment of established recurrent infections, the same premises hold as with HSV1: selected proteins would seem to offer a better prospect than live virus, but the possibility that drugs will remain the agent of choice cannot be discounted.

The only cytomegalovirus disease of great import is that in the newborn. Repeated CMV infections occur in women of childbearing age, but the primary infections are much more likely to affect the infant. We therefore have the

---

TABLE 3. POTENTIAL OF VACCINES IN CONTROL OF HSV_2 DISEASE

Goal #1. To prevent infection with wild HSV2.
STRATEGY: Provide solid durable immunity to all near puberty, perhaps by preempting sites of latency with non-reactivating virus.
AGENT: Live virus without potential for reactivation or oncogenicity, or selected viral proteins in balanced and highly immunogenic form.
REQUIREMENTS: Near absolute safety.
Solid and durable immunity.

Goal #2. To prevent reactivation of virus established in latency
STRATEGY: Enhance cytolysis of infected cells.
AGENT: Viral glycoprotein in appropriate form, perhaps at regular intervals, to affected persons.
REQUIREMENTS: Immunogenicity even where natural infection failed to immunize and even in presence of pre-existing non-cytolytic immunity.

TABLE 4. POTENTIAL OF VACCINES IN CONTROL OF CYTOMEGALOVIRUS DISEASE

Goal #1. To prevent primary CMV in pregnant women.	
STRATEGY:	Induce longterm immunity in girls approaching childbearing age.
AGENT:	Slightly modified live virus.
REQUIREMENTS:	Induction of solid long-term immunity.
	Safety if inadvertently given to woman already pregnant.
Goal #2. To prevent secondary infection in pregnant women	
STRATEGY:	Boost immunity in pregnant women.
AGENT:	Selected virus proteins in highly immunogenic form.
REQUIREMENTS:	Absolute freedom from transplacental infection.
	Induction of balanced immunity in immunologically inexperienced women.

prospect of eliminating most disease by immunizing women who have never been infected but the need to immunize many women repeatedly , if all infant disease is to be prevented (Table 4). If the first goal is sought, long term protection is important and a live virus vaccine offers the best prospect. Selection of an appropriate strain should be relatively easy. If, however, we seek to prevent secondary infections, we would have to immunize women who are already pregnant a subunit vaccine would be safer. Because women could be boosted each time they became pregnant, long term efficacy would not be important.

Epstein-Barr virus is associated with both infectious mononucleosis and tumors in special groups of persons. Immunization of persons who reach puberty without immunity to this virus would be highly relevant, but not easy to achieve safely (Table 5). Latency is so universally associated with the post infection period, its unlikely lasting immunity could be established without it. If a vaccine which establishes latency is chosen, it would have to be freed of oncogenic potential and it is not clear that the two properties are separable. As for a deliberate attempt to prevent EBV associated tumors by vaccination, that too would seem to be a cogent goal, but I would want to know more of the role of other associated factors such as malaria and HLA genes before embarking on such a project.

Clinical problems due to the Herpesvirididae usually arise because of ineffective natural immunological responses. Nevertheless, this does not destroy the potential of vaccination provided the vaccines are designed to accomplish specific goals in defined groups of people. It does make the field more complicated than vaccination against common childhood diseases, and no more than a start has been made as yet.

TABLE 5. POTENTIAL OF VACCINES IN CONTROL OF EBV DISEASES

GOAL #1. To prevent infectious mononucleosis.	
STRATEGY:	Immunize persons who reach puberty without natural immunity.
AGENT:	An attenuated or specifically modified live virus.
REQUIREMENTS:	Immunity must be durable.
	Free of oncogenicity.
	Administered prepubertal, attenuation could be minor.
GOAL #2. To prevent EBV associated tumors.	
STRATEGY:	Immunize at age or by route which circumvents associated causes.
AGENT:	Virus engineered to remove oncogenicity; possibly subunit vaccine.
REQUIREMENTS:	Better knowledge of associated causes in EBV oncogenicity.
	Probably immunization early in life.
	A subunit vaccine might protect by limiting subsequent natural infections.

Herpes Viruses and Virus Chemotherapy, R. Kono, editor

CURRENT STATUS AND FUTURE PROSPECTS OF ANTIVIRAL DRUG DEVELOPMENT

W.H. PRUSOFF, T.-S. LIN, S.A. SIEGEL, M. ZUCKER, W.F. BRUBAKER, JR. AND J.J. LEE

Department of Pharmacology, Yale University School of Medicine, New Haven, Connecticut, USA

There are many compounds that have potent antiviral activity in cell culture and in experimental animals, but only 5 have been approved by the FDA in the United States for use in man. These are shown on the first slide. In addition to these drugs, a number of other compounds are undergoing either clinical or pre-clinical evaluation. Unfortunately none of the compounds either in clinical use or on the horizon are without some adverse characteristics, and hence there is a need to develop antiviral drugs with improved properties.

The ideal approach is to identify potential targets for attack that are unique to the virus, and if successfully attacked would not produce any detrimental effect to the uninfected host tissues.

What are the prospects for future antiviral drug development? Is there a rational approach? Two major problems exist: first to identify virus specific targets, and second to develop a compound that selectively interacts with the target. Today we know of a number of viral specific targets. These have been found either from elucidation of the molecular basis for the activity of compounds that were serendipitously identified as being antiviral, or from studies of the molecular biology of viral replication. What are these targets? The virion per se when present in the blood stream, or during the phase of reversible adsorption to the cell prior to penetration is an important target for a vaccine.

Dr. Black has presented the current status and future prospects for vaccines. The hope, of course, is to develop potent and safe vaccines, whether from the virion, a subunit of the virus or a synthetic polypeptide.

In the absence of an effective vaccine for interaction with the target virus, we are dependent upon the development of antiviral drugs. Ideally the drug should exert its antiviral activity as a consequence of interaction with a target that is unique to the virus. The interaction could consist of a specific inhibitory event unique for the virus, or of a preferential activation of the drug in the virus infected cell.

What are some of the targets that one can consider as potential sites for antiviral drug development? What are some of the strategies that one might employ to take advantage of the availability of these targets? What are some of the approaches that one might take to develop antiviral agents for specific interaction with known target sites, as well as those target sites yet to be uncovered as a consequence of future acquired knowledge of the biochemistry of viral replication, the physiology of host cell-virus interrelationships, and the physical chemistry of drug-target interactions.

At this time we know very few targets that we have been able to take advantage of, and so it is not surprising that we have as of today very few clinically useful drugs.

The various targets for which antiviral agents have been demonstrated to exert an inhibitory effect, or are potential targets for future drug development are as follows:

(1) Adsorption of the virus to the cell surface.

(2) Transport of the virus across the cell wall.

(3) Uncoating of the virus.

(4) Transport of the viral genome into the cytoplasm or into the nucleus.

(5) Replication of the viral genome.

(6) Transcription.

(7) Methylation or polyadenylation of viral RNA.

(8) Protein synthesis and processing.

(9) Viral encoded enzymes.

(10) Assembly of macromolecules into a virion (maturation).

(11) Release of virion from the cell.

The difficult question is how to design an agent which uniquely interacts with the viral specific target. Today a great deal of effort is being expended not only to achieve this synthetic objective, but also on how to devise novel methods of drug delivery.

A POTENTIAL TARGET CONCERNS VIRAL ADSORPTION

With some viruses, such as the myxovirus (influenza) or the paramyxovirus (measles), a glycoprotein present on the surface of the virion must be cleaved by a host cell protease. This creates a new highly hydrophobic amino acid region, which is required for interaction of the virion with a receptor on the cell membrane. Dr. Choppin and his colleagues at Rockefeller University have found that oligopeptides with amino acid sequences similar to the N-terminal region of the cleaved viral glycoprotein compete with the virus for sites on the cell membrane. This results in the specific inhibition of the infection process. This is an example of how an antiviral agent can be designed based on basic knowledge of the structure and function of a viral protein.

Most of the new compounds under study have been prepared by the old fashion method of making specific structural modifications of known antiviral compounds, the synthesis of which is guided by classical structure-activity analysis. This has been very successful and no doubt will be continued, particularly since we now have the computer capability to visually examine a 3 dimensional (or stereo) graphic representation of a molecular shape.

Additional strategies for antiviral drug development include the design of suicide inhibitors, transition state analogs, or affinity compounds that must <u>first</u> be activated by a virus-encoded enzyme before proceeding to lethal synthesis.

The clinically useful antiherpetic drugs exert their activity as a consequence of interaction with a viral encoded enzyme or receptor. Can we determine which moieties on the substrate are critically involved in the viral enzyme-substrate interaction. This would be of value in the design of a more specific and potent antiviral agent. Nuclear magnetic resonance can be used to define the nature of the interaction. If the enzyme can be prepared in the crystalline state, it would be possible to combine cryoenzymology with X-ray diffraction to provide structural information with high resolution. The major problem has been to obtain the enzyme in a sufficient amount, and then to obtain crystals of an appropriate size for X-ray crystallography.

Recombinant DNA technology affords the potential for cloning the viral gene and thereby make adequate amounts of the desired enzyme or protein. A recent report by Littke and John (Science 255 203, 1984) described the formation of large protein single crystals suitable for X-ray analysis under conditions of microgravity. Crystals of β-galactosidase and lysozyme obtained in space were 27 and 1000 times larger than those produced under otherwise identical conditions, but subject to gravitation here on earth. If the viral enzymes behave similarly then we can expect great strides in the development of antiviral agents with increased specificity and potency.

Another approach for the design of an antiviral agent, that my laboratory is using may be termed Directed Serendipity, and is based on biochemical and pharmacological considerations. We have studied a number of antiviral nucleosides such as 5-iodo-2'-deoxyuridine (IdUrd), 5-iodo-5'-amino-2',5'-dideoxyuridine (5'AIdUrd), 5'-amino-5'-deoxythymidine (5'-AdThd) and 5(2-bromovinyl)-2'-deoxyuridine and have found a direct correlation between incorporation of the drug into the herpesvirus DNA and loss of infectivity.

We are interested in the physical and biological consequence of such uptake into the viral DNA in an attempt to elucidate the ultimate biochemical event that is responsible for the decreased formation of infectious virions.

To date we have found specific effects on the formation of herpesvirus RNA and proteins.

Whereas incorporation of [^{3}H]uridine into total RNA of HSV-1 infected Vero cells is not appreciably affected by IdUrd, 5'-AIdUrd or 5'-AdThd, the amount of viral poly A^+ RNA formed in the presence of these analogs were reduced markedly within 8 hours after infection. This effect continued throughout the infectious cycle (18 to 24 hours post infection).

The amount of viral poly A$^-$ RNA formed in the presence of IdUrd within 8 hours after infection, for example, was significantly greater than in the untreated controls, and at 18 to 24 hours post infection, the virus specific poly A$^-$ RNA was increased by as much as 400%. The molecular basis for the decrease in polyadenylated viral RNA is presently under investigation.

The effect of IdUrd on the formation of herpesvirus specific proteins was then investigated. There is no inhibition by IdUrd of the synthesis of immediate early (alpha) virus specific proteins, but the rates of synthesis of most early and late proteins (beta and gamma) are markedly decreased with the possible exception of the 2 beta polypeptides ICP #36 and 39 and the gamma protein ICP #35 which were not affected.

The objective of these experiments was to determine the critical event that is a consequence of incorporation of an antiviral nucleoside into the viral DNA. We hope to be able to uncover a novel virus-specific target, which would avoid the use of antiviral agents that may also be incorporated into the DNA of uninfected cells.

In conclusion, I feel that we have just scratched the surface in our attempts to develop antiviral agents. The future looks great, but we have a lot of hard work to do before we realize our potential.

ACKNOWLEDGEMENTS

The research performed in this laboratory was supported by United States Public Health Service Grant, CA-05262, from the National Cancer Institute.

CURRENT STATUS AND FUTURE PROSPECTS OF ANTIVIRAL DRUGS IN CLINICAL USE

GEORGE J. GALASSO, Ph.D.
National Institutes of Health, Bethesda, Maryland 20205 (U.S.A.)

Acquired immune deficiency syndrome (AIDS) is of major concern to the medical and the medical research community, not only for its threat to the target population but also because of its potential threat to the rest of the population, particularly recipients of blood products. AIDS has proven once more, if further proof were needed, that viral infectious diseases are perhaps the greatest public health problem. Although AIDS is an immune disorder, it is caused by a virus and, in addition, the greatest difficulty in dealing with these patients is their inability to cope with other infectious agents, including a variety of viruses. Nature is continually alerting us to the need for virus control measures which translates to the need for antiviral agents. Tremendous strides have been made in this area in the past 15 years but new innovative research is needed. We have now unequivocally proven that antiviral agents are clinically useful; this has come about through screening programs that have identified potential agents. We are now at the stage where targeted antiviral agents should be pursued. We have made a good start and need to maintain the momentum.

This meeting has served to focus the current status of antiviral agents - steady progress continues to be made. The eye still serves as an ideal organ for studies with antiviral agents; it is isolated and therefore amenable to studies with more toxic agents. Idoxuridine, vidarabine, and trifluro-thymidine continue to be effective against herpetic keratitis, although idoxuridine is now probably obsolete. Acyclovir and bromovinyldeoxyuridine also appear to be successful in treatment of this disease. Of particular interest, however, are the impressive studies with combination therapy. It has been demonstrated that interferon plus acyclovir, or interferon plus triflurothymidine are more efficacious than either drug alone.

An extremely effective and underrated antiviral agent against influenza A is amantadine. Amantadine has been available for many years, however, it was only made readily available in the U.S. against all influenza A infections in the late 70s. The reluctance to use amantadine was the reputed neurological side effects and its prophylactic nature. Studies have demonstrated that amantadine is no more harmful than many antihistamines readily available. It has also been demonstrated that amantadine is therapeutic as well as prophylactic against influenza A. This disease, which can be devastating in terms of mortality as well as morbidity, lends itself well to prophylactic treatment. As soon as influenza A is identified in a given area, the community can take the drug for approximately 4-6 weeks, the usual duration for an influenza outbreak in a given area. Treatment is especially important in at-risk groups such as those with chronic pulmonary problems, the aged, as well as certain essential personnel. More recent studies with the analog rimantadine have demonstrated that it is almost as effective as amantadine with no neurological side effects, making it the drug of choice. Additional studies are needed to evaluate their role against influenzal pneumonia.

Vidarabine was most successful in demonstrating that an antiviral agent could be used systemically to treat serious ongoing viral diseases (herpes encephalitis, neonatal herpes and herpes infections in immunosuppressed patients). The analog cyclaradine obviates the need for slow drip infusion since it is readily soluble and equally effective when given topically or orally. Acyclovir (ACV) has also proven useful against herpes viruses in treatment of immunosuppressed patients and in prevention of herpes infections in bone marrow transplant patients. It is also the first drug to be found efficacious in the treatment of initial genital herpes. Studies have shown that patients with serious and frequent recurrences could be put on a daily regimen which would prevent recurrences while on treatment. The prodrug deoxyacyclovir seems particularly suited as an oral drug. It is able to achieve the same plasma levels of the active compound as intravenous ACV. It even appears to be more effective than ACV when given topically. The daily administration of ACV or deoxyacyclovir raises several questions concerning the potential development of resistant virus strains and toxicity to the patient with prolonged treatment, however, to date there is no indication of either.

Several papers have been presented at this meeting indicating that ACV will prove beneficial in a variety of herpes infections, however, control of cytomegalovirus (CMV) infections will probably depend on its analog DHPG. Studies thus far indicate that CMV may be controlled by this drug. DHPG appears to have the same spectrum as ACV in addition to its effectiveness against CMV. Preliminary experiments indicate that a synergistic effect can be achieved when used with interferon. Two other drugs with clinical potential against herpes viruses are bromovinyldeoxyuridine (BVDU) which appears to be useful against HSV I and VZV and phosphonoformate (PFA) which is effective against HSV I and II and CMV. The fluoropyrimidines should not be overlooked as possible anti-herpes agents. Definitive clinical studies are needed to properly define their efficacy. However BVDU, PFA and the fluoropyrinudines all have toxic side effects such as myelosuppression which must be overcome. A possible solution for BVDU is the analog BVaraU which has antiviral properties similar to BVDU but appears less toxic. Ribavirin raises hopes for the control of a serious infection in newborns caused by respiratory syncytial virus. This drug appears to be useful when administered by aerosol not only against this disease but also against influenza A or B pneumonia. It is particularly exciting for its effectiveness against arena viruses. Lassa fever is a very serious disease in Africa with considerable mortality. This mortality could be reduced substantially, particularly if ribavirin is administered intravenously within the first six days of illness.

The greatest worldwide cause of morbidity is the common cold; the major causative agent involved is rhinovirus. Many attempts are currently underway in an effort to control this infection. Thus far there are no exciting leads however, this is not to say that there is no hope. The antirhinovirus chalcones and drugs such as enviroxime indicate that control is possible but the drug of choice still eludes us. Interferon has been used to prevent the common cold with some success but side effects which cause symptoms similar to those of the common cold dampen enthusiasm. A possible use may be in the family setting where close contacts can be put on prophylaxis for short periods of time. Interferon has been tested against a variety of infectious diseases. Thus far, although it has shown some efficacy against zoster, chronic hepatitis, CMV, adenovirus, and the common cold, it has not demonstrated sufficient beneficial effect to be accepted for general clinical use. However, interferon is finally beginning to demonstrate some of its early promise. The most exciting results with interferon are against warts. There have been a number of impressive studies where interferon appears to be efficacious against laryngeal papilloma and genital warts. What is needed now are studies in sufficient numbers of patients to give statistical significance. Both these clinical entities show spontaneous cures and care must be taken to assure that disappearance of the growth is due to the agent and not chance. The other area where interferon is proving to be of great value is in combination therapy. It has demonstrated synergy with drugs against herpetic keratitis and preliminary studies show potential with other drugs such as DHPG.

Depending on where one sits it could be said that antiviral research is progressing at a rapid rate with impressive results or at a very slow rate. Within the past 15 years, in addition to IDU and amantadine, we have seen the clinical acceptance of vidarabine, trifluorothymidine, ACV and the proven efficacy of rimantadine. The pessimist will complain that these drugs have been available for some years and nothing new has been approved by national authorities since. The optimist will point out the clinical potential of interferon by itself and as a synergistic agent, cyclaradine, deoxyacyclovir, BVaraU, DHPG, as well as BVDU, PFA, and the fluoropyrimidines, if the side effects can be controlled. This is remarkable in view of the nature of the problem. Inhibition of viral replication requires the agent to be effective intracellularly - the potential for toxicity is considerable.

As to the future, the prospects appear great. To continue to be successful there are six points that need to be stressed:

1. We need to learn as much as possible about the natural history of the disease. The severity of the disease and the stage that is appropriate for intervention needs to be clarified.
2. It is obvious that antivirals are most effective when applied early. This necessitates greater efforts in rapid viral diagnosis.
3. As indicated above, effective antivirals are available but more potent agents are needed. To date all the agents have been developed through serendipity; it is time to use a more targeted approach. The molecular virologist has taught us a great deal about the virus and we need to take advantage of this knowledge. There are several viral enzymes and proteins which can serve as targets. We need to get the molecular virologist, chemist and pharmacologist to combine their talents and produce more effective agents for the clinician to evaluate.
4. We must develop more effective delivery systems. We must take advantage of penetrating agents such as azone, DMSO and perhaps iontophoresis as well as the use of liposomes for prolonging the availability of the drug. It is also conceivable that antivirals could be combined with monoclonal antibodies to more effectively deliver the agent to the target organ or cell.
5. Combination of drugs will also prove very important. We are just beginning to investigate the various possibilities. We are learning about the synergistic effect of interferon with various drugs such as ACV, TFT and DHPG. It has been suggested that combination will also be useful in avoiding the development of resistance, particularly if the

drugs inhibit different stages of viral replication. This is also an excellent method of avoiding toxicity; subtoxic dosages of two drugs can be used which have an additive positive antiviral effect.

6. The importance of randomized double-blind, placebo-controlled studies cannot be overemphasized. It is only through such studies that the true efficacy of antiviral agents can be truly assessed.

In conclusion, I am optimistic about the future of antiviral agents for the control of viral diseases. The glass is indeed half full and it will continue to be filled over the next several years with newer and more exciting compounds.

Index of authors

Subject index

Prepared by A.C. Hekker, Bilthoven